To Stan,

My friend & colleague

Pete

ESSENTIAL HEPATOLOGY

THOMAS S. CHEN, M.D.

Department of Medicine and Department of Pathology,
New Jersey Medical School,
Veterans Administration Hospital, East Orange, NJ

PETER S. CHEN, M.D.

Department of Radiology,
Harvard Medical School and the
University of Massachusetts, School of Medicine,
St. Vincent's Hospital, Worcester, MA

BUTTERWORTH COMPANY
MASSACHUSETTS   TORONTO   LONDON

The Butterworth Group

United States

Butterworth (Publishers) Inc.
19 Cummings Park
Woburn, MA 01801

England

Butterworth & Co. (Publishers) Ltd.
Borough Green
Sevenoaks, Kent TN15 8PH

Australia

Butterworth Pty Ltd.
586 Pacific Highway
Chatswood, NSW 2067

Canada

Butterworth & Co. (Canada) Ltd.
2265 Midland Avenue
Scarborough, Ontario M1P 4S1

New Zealand

Butterworths of New Zealand Ltd.
26–28 Waring Taylor Street
Wellington 1

South Africa

Butterworth & Co. (South Africa)
(Pty) Ltd.
152–154 Gale Street, Durban

Printed in the United States of America.
Library of Congress Catalog Card Number: 76-44437   ISBN: 0–409–95005–X

Library of Congress Cataloging in Publication Data

Chen, Thomas S
  Essential hepatology.

  Includes bibliographical references and index.
  1. Liver—Diseases.   I. Chen, Peter S., joint author.   II. Title.
RC845.C46   616.3'62   76-44437
ISBN 0–409–95005–X

*For Margaret and Shirley and
our children*

We have written this book for medical students and physicians whose interests and needs lie in a concise and basic text on liver disorders. Others also may find it useful for review or as an introduction to the field of hepatology. Our coverage of the subject is broad and up to date. Recent developments such as bile salt metabolism, new biochemical and radiologic tests, immunologic perturbations, hepatotoxicity of ethanol, hepatitis virus A and B, and the treatment of chronic active hepatitis are discussed. We have adopted the standard nomenclature and diagnostic criteria for liver diseases that have been recently established by the International Association for the Study of the Liver and the World Health Organization (see H. Popper et al. in General References). We believe the standardization enhances the clarity of our text.

The book is organized into four units. Liver structure and function are discussed initially (Chapter 1). The presentation of each metabolic function is correlated with a summary of its clinical aberrations. The second unit, Chapters 2–4, details the biochemical, morphologic, radiologic, and immunologic methods of diagnosis. The manifestations of liver disease and its pathophysiology and clinical recognition are discussed in the third unit, Chapters 5–8. The final unit includes Chapters 9–18 and gives a comprehensive account of individual liver diseases.

Our association with the Division of Hepatology and Nutrition, New Jersey Medical School, over many years has provided us with a splendid opportunity to serve and to learn. We are grateful to past and present colleagues, and especially Dr. Carroll M. Leevy, Director of the Division, for encouragement and guidance. We are also indebted to Drs. F. George Zaki, Paul Jap, Lazar M. Schwartz, and Karl T. Benedict, Jr., for advice and support. We thank Juliette Rattner and Virginia Campan for their assistance on the draft. Finally, our publisher Thomas V. Kelley and his staff, Mike Scott and Catherine Engel, have been most cooperative and helpful.

CONTENTS

LIVER STRUCTURE AND FUNCTION

1

LIVER STRUCTURE

Gross Features[1,2]

The adult liver is the largest of internal organs, weighing 1500 g ± 100 g and accounting for 1/50 of the body weight (Fig. 1.1). The bulk of the hepatic mass occupies the right hypochondrium. The upper border reaches the level of the nipples; the lower edge is palpable below the right costal rib. The contour of the liver can be determined by percussion. In the right midclavicular line liver dullness extends 15 cm ± 2 cm; in the midsternal line, 4 cm ± 1 cm. Percussion of these margins provides a clinical, and fairly reliable, method of assessing liver size.

The liver is suspended from the parietes posteriorly by the coronary and triangular ligaments. Formerly, it was thought that these ligaments suspended the liver from the diaphragm, but careful anatomic dissection has shown this belief to be in error. The importance of this finding is that a more anterior displacement of the ligaments led to the creation of nonexistent subphrenic spaces. Clinically, there are two important perihepatic spaces in which an abscess may form. The subphrenic or suprahepatic space is represented by a potential space between the inferior surface of the diaphragm and the dome of the liver. The falciform ligament divides the compartment into two spaces, but functionally both sides communicate freely. The importance of distinguishing an abscess in the subphrenic space from one in the subhepatic space lies in the fact that the former abscess is more likely to perforate into the lung and may lead to a fatal outcome. The diaphragm offers much less resistance to perforation than does the liver. Furthermore, the surgical approach to the two differently located abscesses is not the same. Below the right lobe of the liver there is one right subhepatic space. When an intraabdominal abscess occurs, the right subhepatic space is the most frequently involved of upper abdominal spaces. This is because the right subhepatic space represents the watershed for the biliary tract, duodenum, and appendix.

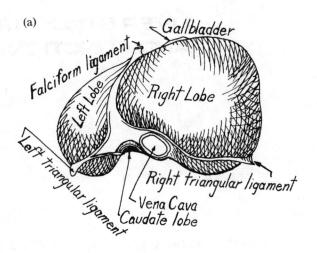

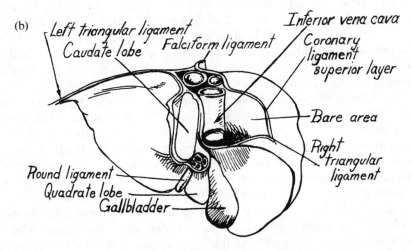

Fig. 1.1 (a) Superior and (b) posterior views of the liver.

Anatomically, the right and left lobes of the liver are divided by the falciform ligament on the smooth diaphragmatic surface. The division is unequal, so that the right lobe is about six times larger than the left lobe. The free margin of the falciform ligament contains the round ligament representing the fibrous obliteration of the umbilical vein. In adults the umbilical vein retains its patency, so that a catheter may be threaded through it to reach the portal vein. This anatomical pathway forms the basis of the umbilicoportal vein catheterization, which is one of the ways to study hepatic hemodynamics. The coronary ligament, a continuation of the right layer of the falciform ligament, is also on the diaphragmatic surface. The coronary ligament outlines one margin of the bare area of the liver which is devoid of peritoneum. At the extremes of the bare area, the coronary ligament continues on the right as the right triangular ligament, and the falciform ligament on the left as the left triangular ligament.

The visceral surface of the liver bears fissures for the round ligament and venous ligament (the obliterated remains of the ductus venosus) connecting the portal vein and the left hepatic vein and fossa markings for the gallbladder, inferior vena cava, and porta hepatis structures. These markings divide the visceral surface of the right lobe into two lobes. The more anterior quadratic lobe is bounded on the right by the gallbladder fossa, on the left by the round ligament, and posteriorly by the porta hepatis. The posterior caudate lobe is bounded by the inferior vena cava on the right, the venous ligament on the left, and the porta hepatis anteriorly. The caudate lobe drains directly into the vena cava. This lobe is not involved in hepatic vein obstruction, and it may undergo hypertrophy.

The anatomical divisions have little functional significance. They bear no relationship to the physiological bisection of the liver by its afferent vascular supply and biliary drainage. Perfusion and the cast corrosion studies indicate a nearly equal division of the right and left lobes by the portal vein, hepatic artery, and bile ducts. No functional anastomosis apparently exists between the terminal branches of the vascular and biliary systems of both lobes. Furthermore, a segmental division of the liver can be recognized that is comparable to the segments of the lung. The hepatic segments are based on the distribution of the major vascular and biliary branches. An understanding of the segmental anatomy has enabled surgeons to resect the liver with minimal bleeding and side effects. On a functional basis the liver can be bisected into right and left lobes by a line extending through the gallbladder fossa and vena cava. The left lobe is further divided into medial and lateral segments, and the right lobe into anterior and posterior segments. The falciform ligament marks the left segmental fissure, the juncture between the medial and lateral segments. The right segmental fissure separates the anterior and posterior segments of the right lobe. Other smaller segments are also present but these have little surgical significance.

The several anomalies of lobulation produce rare clinical disturbances. They are usually recognized at autopsy or as incidental findings at surgery; these anomalies are discussed below.

Riedel's lobe.   The tongue-like prolongation of the right lower lobe is probably caused by adhesions to the mesocolon. This lesion is common.

Accessory lobes. In this rare condition the mesenteric attachments of the small lobes may twist and infarct.

Atrophy of left lobe. The degenerative change is common in infants. It is thought that sudden withdrawal of oxygenated blood from the placenta and perfusion by poorly oxygenated portal venous blood at birth cause atrophy and fibrosis of the left lobe. Clinically, this is correlated with prolonged perinatal cyanosis.

Vascular Supply[1,2]

The liver receives one-fifth of the cardiac output, about 1500 ml blood/minute, by two vascular channels: the portal vein and hepatic artery. The portal vein, 5.5–8 cm long and 2 cm wide, is formed by the union of the splenic and superior mesenteric veins just behind the head of the pancreas. Although designated as a vein, the portal vein functions as an arterial nutrient vessel carrying blood from the intestines. The hepatic artery branches off the celiac axis, courses along the upper border of the pancreas, and turns at the porta hepatis where it divides into a right and left branch. It lies medial to the common bile duct and in front of the portal vein. Aberrant arterial branches and variations in origin are reported in 50% of cases.

The portal vein contrasts with the hepatic artery functionally, as shown below.

	Pressure	Blood flow	Oxygen supply
Portal vein	8–10 mm Hg	1200 ml/min (80%)	40 ml/min (75%)
Hepatic artery	120 mm Hg	300 ml/min (20%)	20 ml/min (25%)

These figures are obtained under standard fasting conditions. They vary considerably for other settings, for example, postprandial. Portal vein pressure is regulated by both inflow and outflow factors. Mesenteric and splenic arteriolar tone control inflow, whereas portal venular tone and hepatic sinusoidal pressure control outflow. Both hepatic arteriolar tone and hepatic venous pressure, in turn, determine sinusoidal pressure. Portal venous pressure and total hepatic flow are also subject to active contractions of the portal and hepatic veins. Small variations in portal venous pressure result in marked changes in total hepatic flow. In isolated liver preparations, an increase of perfusion pressure decreases the portal venous resistance and augments portal flow. This is in contrast with the autoregulation of the hepatic arterial system. Hepatic arterial flow is maintained at near constant rates when perfusion pressure varies within the physiological range. Splanchnic nerve stimulation causes an increase in both hepatic arterial and portal venous pressures and reduces blood flow in both systems. The effects of epinephrine and norepinephrine mimic in some respects those of splanchnic nerve stimulation. In humans, epinephrine increases total hepatic flow, although portal vein pressure is elevated. Norepinephrine causes a decrease in total liver flow.

Within the porta hepatis, the artery, vein, and bile duct bifurcate and penetrate the liver substance together, carrying a coat of connective tissue—an extension of Glisson's capsule. These structures are conducted in a cylindrical space (portal canal) surrounded by a limiting plate of hepatocytes. Each ramus of the portal vein is usually accompanied by a comparable subdivision of the hepatic artery and hepatic bile duct. The portal vein gives rise to conducting veins of decreasing caliber which drain into the inlet venules perforating the limiting plate or into the terminal venules representing the direct continuation of axial veins. Both venules discharge portal flow into sinusoids, which are arranged in a candelabra or monopodial pattern (Fig. 1.2). Sinusoidal blood empties into the central hepatic veins which enter perpendicularly into the sublobular veins, then continue into collecting and hepatic veins, and finally into the inferior vena cava. Although both the hepatic artery and hepatic duct follow the portal vein, the branching of both artery and duct is subject to variations and may deviate independently of the portal vein branches. In the liver, hepatic arteries supply the portal triad structures by minute branches which eventually drain into the inlet venules of the portal system and the parenchyma by long, straight arterial capillaries or arterioles, which enter into the sinusoids. Arterial flow is controlled by sphincters in branching arterioles and in arterioles entering sinusoids. Functionally, arterioles represent end-arteries, with no demonstrable intrahepatic communications between the right and left hepatic arteries.

Biliary Network

In contrast to the vascular flow, the biliary flow is directed away from liver cells. About 600–800 ml of bile is secreted daily into a system of ducts which increases in complexity and size. Bile excretion begins in the bile canaliculi represented by spaces between two or rarely three hepatocytes.[3] The cell membranes of these hepatocytes are folded into microvilli for increased secretion. Flow continues into the canals (ampulla) of Hering, constructed by one or two ductular cells sharing a canalicular lumen with hepatocytes. The basement membrane is scanty around these lining cells. The Hering canals drain into small and large bile ductules.

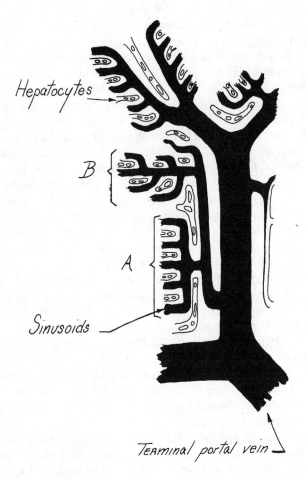

Fig. 1.2. Schematic representation of the liver sinusoidal pattern. A refers to the most common arrangement, the candelabra-type; B refers to the monopodial pattern of sinusoids. (After H. Elias and J. C. Sherrick.[2])

The small ductules are lined by three or less cells, and the large ductules by six or less cells on cross section. The basement membrane surrounds these tributaries, although they are not accompanied by neighboring arteries or veins. Bile ductules converge into interlobular ducts. The latter are differentiated by an epithelium of cuboidal cells and association with terminal portal veins in portal triads. Interlobular ducts empty into intrahepatic ducts, which have a mucosal wall of tall, folded epithelium and a coat of dense connective tissue with elastic fibers. Bile subsequently drains into the lobular ducts, common hepatic duct (3 cm long), and finally into the common bile duct (7.5 cm long by 0.6 cm in caliber).

The cystic duct draining the gallbladder joins the common hepatic duct at an angle. The two ducts form the triangle of Calot, in which the cystic, right hepatic, and other aberrant hepatic arteries are also found. Identification of Calot's triangle is important during hepatobiliary surgery.

Microstructure

Hepatic lobule and liver acinus. Two contrasting hypotheses account for the organization of liver cell parenchyma.[1,2] According to the classical concept of hepatic lobule, liver cells are arranged as two cell-thick cords enclosing a bile canaliculus and bathed by sinusoids. The network of liver cords radiates from the central hepatic vein, with portal tracts located at the periphery of the pyramidally shaped lobule. This concept of the hepatic structure is no longer tenable in view of the perfusion studies of A. M. Rappaport, and tridimensional reconstructions by H. Elias. The basic functional unit of the liner is the acinus, defined as an irregularly sized and shaped clump of cells clustered around an axis of terminal portal venule, hepatic arteriole, and bile ductule, which branch out together from a small portal field. The simple liver acinus lies between two or more central veins with which the vascular and biliary networks intertwine. It overlaps and fuses with an adjacent acinus. Larger acinar agglomerates are formed from these units. Both the acinus and lobule concepts of hepatic substructure are functional, not anatomical, units. The liver exists as a continuum without dissectable divisions, as do the renal nephrons. Liver cells are stacked as one-cell-thick plates or sheets which are tunneled by many lacunae forming the hepatic labyrinth (Fig. 1.3). The plates are continuous with one another. Sinusoids and bile ducts occupy the labyrinth system.

Zonal activity.[1] A zonal relationship exists between cells in the acinus and the blood flow (Fig. 1.4). The cellular rim closest to the portal space, zone I, receives fresh blood rich in nutrients and oxygen. It is metabolically most active and resistant to injury. The intermediate area, zone II, and the distant sector, zone III, are supplied by a poorer quality of blood with corresponding differences in metabolic activity and susceptibility to injury. The metabolic heterogeneity of the separate zones is expressed by the distribution of organelles in cells, enzyme activity and concentration, and cytogenic potential for regeneration (Table 1.1).

Liver histology. Conventional usage divides the hepatic fields seen on liver biopsy into centrolobular, periportal, and midzonal areas. The ratio of 2 or 3 portal triads to 1 central vein is rarely visualized. The uniformity

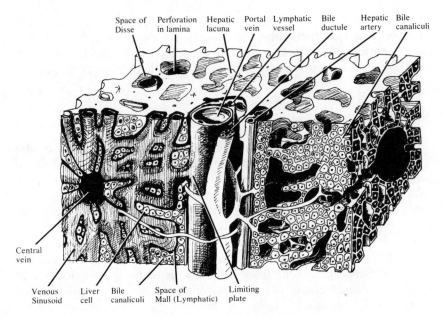

Fig. 1.3. Microstructure of the liver.

of hepatocytes, delicate central veins, and compact portal triads demarcated by a limiting plate of liver cells are features demonstrated in the normal liver biopsy (Fig. 1.5). Hepatocytes account for about 65% the total hepatic cell population; sinusoidal and ductular cells comprise the remaining 35%. It is estimated that each milliliter of mammalian liver contains 169×10^6 hepatocytes, and 90×10^6 other cells.[4]

Ultrastructure. The liver cell shares an ultrastructure similar to other tissue cells. Much of the fine structure and the major function of cell organelles are familiar knowledge (Figs. 1.6 and 7).[3] Appreciation of the ultrastructural alterations in liver disease adds little to diagnostic accuracy but does provide insights into the pathologic process.

Liver Cell Proliferation

A striking feature of liver cells is the capacity to proliferate during physiological and pathological states. Proliferation during physiological conditions includes initial growth prior to maturity and renewal growth after attainment of maturity. Cell proliferation during pathological states refers to reparative growth or regeneration, pathological hyperplasia, and neoplasia.[5]

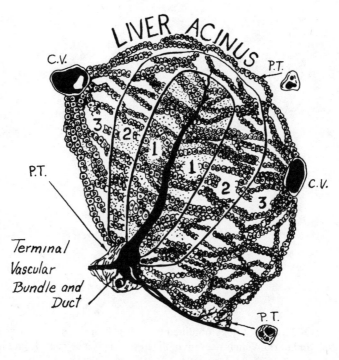

Fig. 1.4. Functional acinus of the liver, with zonal arrangement of cells. Zones 1, 2, 3 mark areas which are supplied by blood of decreasing quality in terms of oxygen and nutrient content. P.T. = portal tract; C.V. = central veins. (After Dr. A. M. Rappaport.[1])

Table 1.1. Cell heterogenity in the hepatic acinus.[1]

Zone I	Zone III
Mitochondria: Numerous, larger	Few, rounded
Bile canaliculi: Wide	Narrow
Canaliculi and sinusoids: Higher ATPase activity	Higher 5'-nucleotidase activity
Glycogen deposition: Usually occurs here first	Lipid deposition: Frequently seen here first
Enzymes: Glucose-6-phosphatase, succinc dehydrogenase, and others in Kreb's cycle more active	Glucose-6-P-dehydrogenase, lactic dehydrogenase more active
Cytogenesis: DNA synthesis after partial hepatectomy	Later event

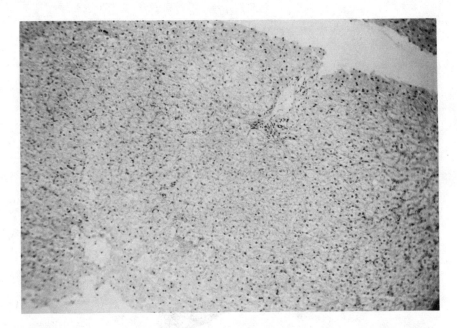

Fig. 1.5. Normal liver histology obtained by needle biopsy. A small triad containing bile duct and portal vein is present in the upper right quadrant. H and E, X100.

Initial growth. Physiological proliferation prior to maturity involves a limited number of cells, estimated at 10% of the total hepatic cell population.[5] At any given time only 4% of the population are actually synthesizing DNA.

Renewal growth. Renewal growth after maturity seems virtually absent in mammalian livers. In the adult organ approximately 1 mitosis per 10,000–20,000 hepatocytes is enough to maintain the renewal process. Judging by ^{3}H thymidine uptake, less than 1% of liver cells are engaged in DNA synthesis. The proportion of labeled Kupffer cells and mesenchymal cells is higher than labeled hepatocytes. In rats the level of liver cell turnover is so low that the life span of these cells is similar to the remaining life span of the animal.

Reparative growth. This may be defined as growth which occurs in response to liver injury: compensatory hyperplasia after partial hepatectomy or hyperplasia in the liver damaged by other agents.

Partial hepatectomy. The sequence of events following partial hepatectomy in the rat (68% of the liver mass removed) is particularly

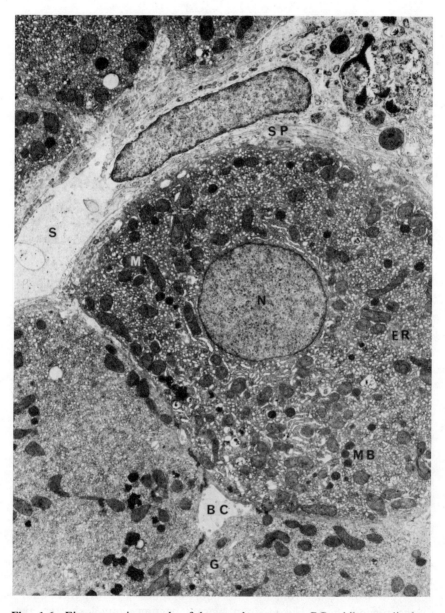

Fig. 1.6. Electron micrograph of human hepatocyte. BC = bile canaliculus; ER = endoplasmic reticulum; G = Golgi complex; M = mitochondria; MB = microbody; N = nucleus; S = sinusoid; SP = space of Disse. X10,000. Courtesy of Dr. F. G. Zaki (Squibb Institute of Medical Research).

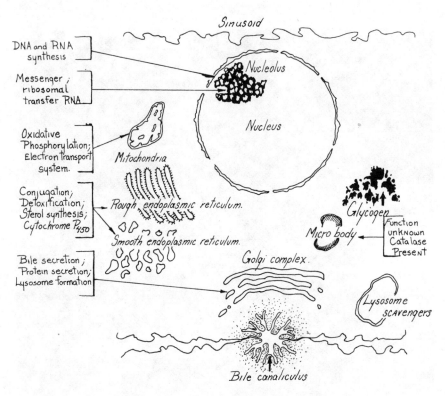

Fig. 1.7. Functions of liver cell organelles.

well documented. Histologically, fat appears within 2–3 hours in remaining cells.[6] Glycogen stores disappear and are depleted by 10 hours. Cells, as well as nuclei and nucleoli, enlarge by 6–12 hours and double by 24 hours. Biochemically, there is an increase in RNA synthesis by six hours and protein synthesis by 12 hours. After a lag of about half a day, DNA synthesis becomes activated, first in cells of the lobule periphery and later spreading to the center. Peak DNA synthesis (about 30% of hepatocytes are labeled by ^{3}H thymidine) occurs after 20–24 hours and declines slowly. Cell mitosis (up to a peak level of 3.5% of hepatocytes with nuclear division) follows the same pattern by a delay of 6–8 hours. The cell cycle is shortened from about 21 hours in renewal growth to 16 hours during regeneration. The G_1 (gap) period becomes much shorter; the other periods of the cycle, S (synthesis) and G_2 + M (mitosis), remain relatively constant. Binucleate cells which account for 20–30% of normal adult rat hepatocytes (60–70% are tetraploid) fall to 10%, and polyploidy is increased. Nonparenchymal cells which are diploid and form 30–40% of the total liver cell count lag by 24 hours behind hepatocytes in initiating DNA synthesis and mitosis. Nonparenchymal cell division occurs randomly throughout the lobule. Both the size and numbers of lobules increase to the extent that, by the end of the first week, the original liver weight is approached. Closely coupled with hepatocellular division is the production of alpha-fetoprotein. DNA synthesis following partial hepatectomy varies in timing and magnitude with (1) the age of the animal, the older the animal the slower the rise in hepatic DNA synthesis; (2) nutrition, starvation depresses the hepatic response; (3) hormonal status, absence of pituitary or adrenal hormones decreases hepatic regeneration; and (4) the amount of liver removed.

Control systems.[7]   The regulatory mechanism which activates hepatic regeneration is the subject of lively interest and controversy. Many stimuli are proposed and include: hemodynamic factors, especially the upsurge in portal blood flow carrying hepatotrophic substances (insulin and glucagon); functional demand due to overloading by metabolic products; changes in blood hormone levels, e.g., corticosteroids; modulation by blood-borne stimulator(s); and loss of blood-borne inhibitor(s). Cross-circulation and exchange transfusion experiments suggest the existence of stimulating humoral agent(s). Several factors are identified: fetal calf serum factors (FF_1 and FF_2) and regenerating liver serum factor (RF) with an MW of 17,000 daltons, heat stability at 100°C, and resistance to neuraminidase digestion. The proliferative stimulus, such as RF, may act by several speculated mechanisms. First, RF may cause a change in the permeability of the cell membrane. This leads to loss of cytoplasmic inhibitors, permitting synthesis of cytoplasmic messengers and activation of the nucleus. A second model may involve the chalones, specific inhibitors of mitosis. RF blocks chalone function at the cell membrane or metabolically decreases synthesis or enhances degradation of the inhibitor. In any case, reversal of chalone activity leads to mitosis.

Hepatic regeneration in humans.   After a hepatectomy, the human liver rebuilds itself at a rate as rapid as 100 g/day, and by 1–2 months full restoration of the liver takes place.[8] Recent scanning evidence shows that the rate of regeneration exceeds the previous estimates of 50 g/day and attainment of full size by 4–6 months. Regeneration commences soon after surgery and is well advanced within 10 days of an operation. Up to 80% of the liver may be removed with little permanent impairment of hepatic function. Prothrombin time, fibrinogen, and cholesterol are reduced temporarily, but blood ammonia concentration remains unchanged. Transient jaundice may appear, with serum bilirubin returning to normal by the third week. Serum alkaline phosphatases and BSP retention may increase and subside within the first postoperative week. The serum albumin level falls within 24 hours of hepatic resection, but normal value is attained by the fifth to sixth postoperative week. Hypoglycemia may persist for two weeks following a lobectomy, although clinical signs of this metabolic problem are not often apparent. Postlobectomy replacement with glucose and albumin is advisable to correct hypoglycemia and hypoalbuminemia.[9] Prevention of these two common biochemical consequences improves the chances of survival. In contrast to the normal liver, the cirrhotic liver does not regenerate or regain function after partial hepatectomy.

A normal liver biopsy incubated with tritiated thymidine shows 4–5 labeled nuclei per 10,000 liver cells, with hepatocytes constituting 10–20% of the labeled population.[10] Mesenchymal and ductular cells make up the remainder. Liver damage or necrosis, as seen in viral hepatitis, alcoholic hepatitis, and active cirrhosis, is associated with a ten to fifty-fold increase in DNA synthesis. Labeled hepatocytes increase to 50% of the total cell uptake. About 10% of the patients with active liver disease have absent or deficient hepatic DNA synthesis. The explanation is uncertain but may include circulating inhibitors of DNA synthesis found in various chronic liver diseases.

METABOLIC FUNCTIONS

Amino Acid Metabolism

The liver is the major site of amino acid metabolism, forming precursors for a variety of nitrogenous compounds (Fig. 1.8).[11] Both the carbon and nitrogen atoms of the amino acid molecule undergo degradation. The carbon atom is ultimately oxidized to CO_2 by entering into the acetyl-CoA pool or into the citric acid cycle. The fate of the nitrogen atom is somewhat more complex. Under normal conditions the average diet and tissue breakdown provide about 17 g of nitrogen per day which must be ex-

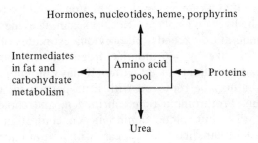

Fig. 1.8. Metabolism of amino acids.

creted. The basic step is removal of the alpha-amino group (containing the nitrogen atom) from amino acids. Several hepatic reactions are involved: (1) Transamination. This step is catalyzed by aminotransferases or transaminases and involves a transfer of a pair of alpha-amino groups by interconversion between pairs of alpha-amino acids and alpha-keto acids. Two major enzymes play a role: aspartate aminotransferase (AsAT) and L-alanine aminotransferase (AlAT). (2) Oxidative deamination. This process produces a keto acid and ammonia. (3) Trapping of ammonia. Both reactions (1) and (2) liberate free ammonia, which is rapidly cleared from the circulaton and converted principally to urea or to glutamate and glutamine. Glutamate entraps ammonia by the glutamate dehydrogenase reaction, and glutamine formation removes ammonia in a process involving the enzyme glutamine synthetase. (4) Urea synthesis. The formation of urea entails a series of reactions known as the ornithine (Krebs-Henseleit) cycle. $[NH_4]^+$, $[HCO_3]^-$, and L-aspartate enter into the cycle to generate urea, fumarate, and water (Fig. 1.9). Urea constitutes the major pathway of nitrogen excretion (80–90% of all excreted nitrogen) in humans. Most of the urea is eliminated through the urine; about 5% is passed through the stool.

Abnormalities in liver disease. Since the liver contains all the enzymes involved in urea synthesis, a fall in serum BUN may occur in massive hepatic necrosis. Altered patterns of plasma and urine amino acids are common in liver disease, but their determinations are rarely utilized for diagnosis (Table 1.2). This is in part due to lack of specificity and a simple method of determination. Study of amino acid metabolism in hepatic coma has provided new insights into the pathogenesis of this disorder (see Chapter 8).

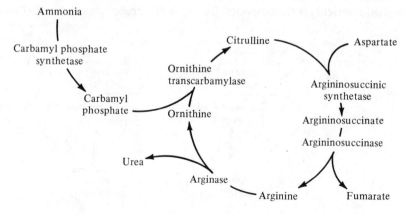

Fig. 1.9. Urea (Krebs-Henseleit) cycle.

Table 1.2. Altered plasma and urine amino acid patterns in liver disease.

Disease	Amino acids	Mechanism
Acute, severe, viral hepatitis; massive hepatic necrosis	Cystine, leucine, tyrosine	Liver cell necrosis; overflow into urine
Cirrhosis	Tyrosine, methionine, phenylalanine	Unknown
	Valine, leucine, isoleucine	Hyperinsulinemia
Hepatic coma	Lactic acid, pyruvic acid, ketoglutaric acid	Impaired carbohydrate metabolism

Bile Salt Metabolism

The bile salt pool in humans is 3 g (Fig. 1.10). This amount recycles through the enterohepatic circulation 10 times each day, so that 30 g of bile salts perfuse the liver and small intestine. Synthesis and fecal loss are balanced at 0.5 g/day. The pool size and rates of formation are variable and affected by diet, hormones, and the enterohepatic cycle. Bile salts represent the major catabolic and excretory pathway for cholesterol. The metabolic steps take place in the liver (Fig. 1.11).[12] The first step, 7-α-hydroxylation of cholesterol, is the site for feedback inhibition of cholesterol by bile salts. Following a shift of double bond (Δ5 to Δ4) and oxidation of the 3-α-hydroxyl group, the molecule undergoes either 12-α-hydroxylation to become ultimately cholic acid or bypasses this step to form eventually chenodeoxycholic acid (CDCA). The hydroxylases and dehydrogenases required for these reactions are all localized on the endoplasmic reticulum (microsomal fraction) of hepatocytes. The next two

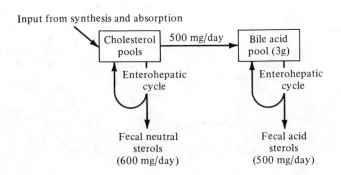

Fig. 1.10. Bile acid turnover.

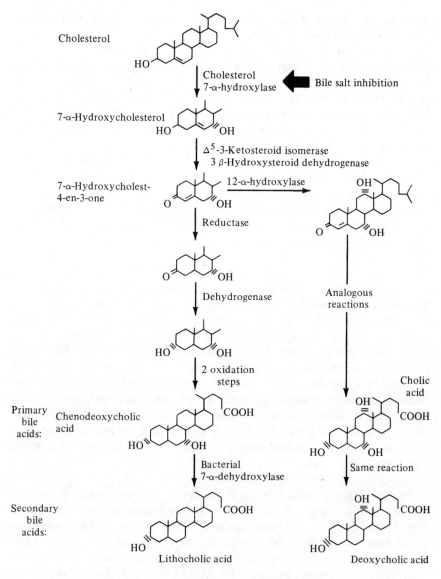

Fig. 1.11. Synthesis of bile salts.

steps, saturation of the 5-β-double bond and reduction of the 3-keto group, are mediated by soluble enzymes.

This completes the hydroxylation of the steroid ring nuclei. Oxidation then occurs at C26 carbon of the side chain in two steps, yielding cholic acid and CDCA (trihydroxy and dihydroxy bile acids). The oxidative enzymes are found in the mitochondrial fraction of liver homogenate. Since cholic acid and CDCA are produced directly from cholesterol, they are referred to as primary bile acids. The third major bile acid, deoxycholic acid, is derived from 7-α-dehydroxylation of cholic acid by intestinal bacteria. Bile acids are conjugated in the liver with glycine or taurine to form bile salts. Unconjugated bile acids do not exist in normal bile. Bile salts are reabsorbed in the small intestine; a small amount escapes to the colon where bacterial enzymes remove the 3,7,12-hydroxyl groups and the amino acid conjugates to form secondary bile acids. Besides deoxycholic acid, the other major secondary bile acid, lithocholic acid, is also derived by a 7-α-dehydroxylation step from CDCA. Secondary bile salts also undergo an enterohepatic cycle and conjugation with amino acids. Normal bile contains both primary and secondary bile salts, in a concentration ratio of 10:10:5:1 for cholate, chenodeoxycholate, deoxycholate, and lithocholate, respectively.

Function.   The presence of both hydroxyl and carboxyl groups on the bile salt molecule confers upon it an amphipathic property. This refers to the ability of the molecule to orient itself at an oil-water interphase. Such molecules above a critical concentration and temperature form aggregates called micelles. Bile salt micelles can solubilize less soluble lipids such as cholesterol and lecithin. Mixed micelles in bile contain bile salts-cholesterol-lecithin in molar ratios of 6:2:1. The amount of cholesterol solubilized depends on the relative concentrations of bile salts and lecithin. Bile with a composition outside the micellar zone of solubility is lithogenic, and associated with a high incidence of cholesterol gallstones. In addition to this major function of solubilizing cholesterol, bile salts have an important role in the emulsification and absorption of fat in the small intestine.

Bile Secretion.   Bile formation begins at the microvilli of the bile canaliculi. Bile composition is determined by both canalicular and ductal functions (Fig. 1.12). The canalicular function has two components, one dependent upon and the other independent of bile salt secretion. At this level of bile flow at least three active transport systems are identified: bile salts secretion, organic anions (such as BSP and dehydrocholate) secretion, and sodium excretion. The latter accounts for the bile-salt independent fraction of canalicular flow, the quantitative aspects of which are unknown in humans. In other mammalian livers the bile salt independent fraction constitutes as much as 75% of basal bile flow. Both bile salts and sodium exert in addition an osmotic driving force for bile flow. Water and other small solutes are secreted by diffusion. Beyond the canaliculi, at the small ductules, bile composition is further modified by net isosmotic

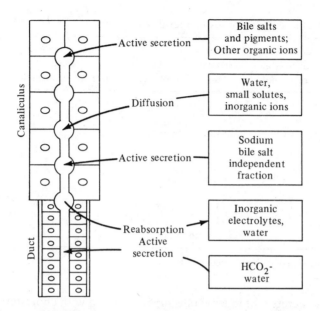

Fig. 1.12. Formation of bile at the canaliculus and duct.

reabsorption or secretion of inorganic electrolytes and water. Multiple factors, including secretin, gastrin, glucagon, and vagal stimulation, influence ductular bile secretion. The osmolality of bile mirrors the plasma osmolality, approximately 300 mOsm/l. The total volume of bile produced daily averages 15 ml/kg body weight.

Bile salt alterations. Abnormal bile secretion and metabolism are observed in cholestasis (Chapter 5) and in other liver diseases (Table 1.3).[13,14,15,16] Altered rates of synthesis are described particularly for alcoholic cirrhosis and during the formation of gallstones. In alcoholic cirrhosis, reduction of biliary deoxycholate due to lack of cholic acid substrate and deficient intestinal conversion of cholic acid to deoxycholic acid, decreased biliary output of cholic acid ascribed to deficient 12-α-hydroxylase and impairment in snythesis from cholesterol precursor, relative normal secretion of CDCA, and lower rates of biliary phospholipid and cholesterol secretion are present.

Lithogenic bile. An estimated 10% of the white American population and 80% of young American Indian women harbor gallstones.[17] Gallstones occur three times more frequently in women than in men. Eighty-five percent of gallstones are composed mainly of cholesterol, the remainder of bilirubinate pigment stones. Patients with cholesterol

Table 1.3. Bile salt alterations in liver disease.[13,14,15,16]

	Conjugation (glycine/taurine ratio)	Trihydroxy/dihydroxy ratio	Cholate		Chenodeoxycholate		Serum monohydroxy bile salts
			Pool	Production	Pool	Production	
Normal	3.4:1	1.0					Absent
Biliary obstruction	<1.0	>1.0	Incr*	Incr			Present
Primary biliary cirrhosis	<1.0	>1.0					High
Alcoholic cirrhosis	<3.0	<1.0	Decr†	Decr	?	Incr	Absent
Viral hepatitis		>1.0 then ↓ to 1.0	Decr	Decr		Incr	

*Incr = increased; † Decr = decreased.

gallstones secrete a lithogenic bile supersaturated with cholesterol. In the supersaturated state, the bile-acid-phospholipid to cholesterol fraction exceeds the normal molar ratio of 10:1. Lithogenic bile results from (1) decrease of bile-acid pool size and (2) increase of hepatic synthesis and secretion of cholesterol (Fig. 1.13).[18] Bile acid synthesis may be reduced by an intrinsic hepatic defect or by an abnormal recirculation of bile acid. Extrahepatic factors also may play a role. Diets high in calories and rich in protein and the obese condition increase the cholesterol content of bile. Highly refined and cholesterol-lowering diets contract the bile acid pool.[19] Altered gallbladder contractibility reduces the bile-acid pool size

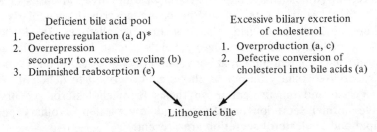

Deficient bile acid pool
1. Defective regulation (a, d)*
2. Overrepression secondary to excessive cycling (b)
3. Diminished reabsorption (e)

Excessive biliary excretion of cholesterol
1. Overproduction (a, c)
2. Defective conversion of cholesterol into bile acids (a)

Lithogenic bile

*Observed in a = American Indian women
b = Caucasian patients
c = Obese patients
d = Oral contraceptive therapy
e = Postileoctomy state

Fig. 1.13. Causes of lithogenic bile.

by increasing the frequency of bile acid recirculation. Whether a cholecystectomy corrects the defect is not clear. The role of the gallbladder in producing lithogenic bile is not completely understood. Treatment with oral CDCA improves cholesterol solubility in bile by depressing cholesterol secretion into bile, thereby dissolving radiolucent gallstones.[20] Radiopaque stones are not affected.

Sixty to seventy percent of patients with radiolucent gallstones and functioning gallbladders respond to CDCA therapy.[21] Small gallstones (< 5 mm in diameter) are dissolved either completely or partially within 12 months of treatment, larger stones within a period of two years. Failure of gallstones to decrease in size within this interval should raise questions about the type of gallstones present. Once CDCA is withdrawn, the bile reverts to the pretreatment status and supersaturation with cholesterol. Recurrence of gallstones is reported in 10% of the patients within a year. This suggests that lifelong treatment may be required in some cases. Side effects are dose-related.[22] Diarrhea, due to the effect of the primary bile acid in the colonic mucosa, is the most common undesirable effect. It does not occur if the CDCA dose is less than 500 mg/day. About 25% of the patients on doses of 750–1000 mg/day show mild serum aminotransferase elevation (twice the normal level.)

Liver biopsies generally show normal histology, although fatty change, portal triaditis, periportal inflammation, and mild fibrosis have been observed.[23] The long-term toxicity of CDCA has not been fully evaluated since its usage is still in its infancy. The drug is not available for the general public in the United States. Lithocholic acid, a secondary bile acid derived from CDCA, is a known potent hepatotoxin but little lithocholic acid is absorbed during CDCA therapy. At the moment, there is no indication that therapy is hazardous. Increasing doses of CDCA increase not only cholesterol solubility in bile but side effects as well. As an alternative to CDCA, the secondary bile acid, ursodeoxycholic acid (UDCA), the 7-β epimer of CDCA, may be used.[24] The effectiveness and safety of UDCA compared to CDCA are under current evaluation. During CDCA therapy, UDCA concentration increases in the bile. On the other hand, the biliary CDCA level does not change with UDCA therapy. It is not clear if UDCA alone, CDCA alone, or both combined dissolves gallstones. Another therapeutic agent, beta-glycerophosphate, has been suggested for dissolution of cholesterol gallstones.[25] This precursor of phospholipid crosses the intestinal mucosa intact and increases the hepatic synthesis of biliary phospholipids. Although cholesterol concentration remains unchanged, hepatic bile becomes less lithogenic. The efficacy of beta-glycerophosphate in dissolving gallstones remains to be tested on a large scale.

Bilirubin Metabolism[26]

The formation of bilirubin has been studied with radioactive glycine, a precursor of the prosthetic group heme of the molecule hemoglobin. Twenty percent of the isotopic label appears in fecal stercobilin within a week, referred to as the early-labeled peak of pigment formation. Eighty percent of the excreted label occurs in 120 days after administration of the glycine. This major peak represents the bilirubin derived from senescent erythrocytes. Degradation of the heme group of hemoglobin accounts for 80% of the 250–300-mg daily production of bilirubin. Intact erythrocytes are catabolized in the reticuloendothelial system, whereas circulating free or haptoglobin-bound hemoglobin and other transport hemoproteins such as methemalbumin and hemopexin are degraded in hepatic parenchymal cells. The early-labeled peak of bilirubin formation originates from the destruction of maturing erythrocytes, so-called ineffective erythropoiesis, and turnover of tissue hemoproteins. Degradation of hepatic cytochrome P-450 is the major source of nonhemoglobin heme.

Intracellularly, the cyclic tetrapyrrole, heme, is converted to the open, linear tetrapyrrole, biliverdin. Cleavage of the ferroprotoporphyrin ring of heme requires the enzyme, microsomal heme oxygenase, with NADPH and O_2 as cofactors (Fig. 1.14). Heme oxygenase increases in response to stimuli other than heme, such as starvation, glucagon, epinephrine, cyclic AMP, and endotoxin. Activity of the enzyme also varies with another microsomal heme enzyme, cytochrome P-450. Biliverdin is subsequently reduced to bilirubin, catalyzed by the cytosol enzyme, biliverdin reductase, with NADPH as cofactor.

Following its appearance in the plasma, 95% of the unconjugated bilirubin becomes tightly bound to albumin at a molar ratio of 1. This allows for a maximum possible serum level of 60–80 mg/dl of unconjugated bilirubin in the normal adult. Other metabolites such as free fatty acids may compete with bilirubin for binding to albumin. The albumin-unconjugated bilirubin complex, after reaching the hepatic sinsusoids, rapidly disassociates at the liver cell membrane. The carrier mechanism responsible for the hepatic uptake of bilirubin across the membrane has not been identified. Within the cell cytoplasm bilirubin is bound by two recently discovered cytosol proteins, Y and Z. Y, also known as ligandin, and Z are low-molecular weight, soluble proteins which bind a variety of other organic anions. Y is more abundant than Z in the liver, comprising about 5% of the cytosol protein. Y plays the more important role in the binding of bilirubin. The acceptor proteins are subject to induction by the drug phenobarbital. Y protein is identical to the B-type isoenzyme of glutathione transferase, indicating an enzyme function. Bilirubin is subsequently conjugated in hepatic microsomes to form predominantly

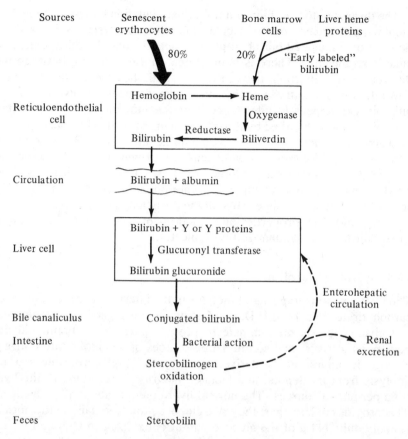

Fig. 1.14. Metabolism of bilirubin.

bilirubin diglucuronide. This process converts a water-insoluble unconjugated pigment to a water-soluble conjugated derivative. Conjugation is catalyzed by glucuronyl transferase located on the smooth endoplasmic reticulum:

Bilirubin + Uridine diphosphate glucuronic acid (UDPGA) →
Bilirubin diglucuronide + Uridine diphosphate (UDP)

Bilirubin monoglucuronide and other conjugates with carbohydrate moieties are also formed in small amounts. Their role in biliary excretion is unknown. Transport of the conjugated bilirubin from the cytosol into the bile canaliculus involves the Golgi apparatus and possibly lysosomes. The transport process can be saturated, may be inhibited by cholecystographic agents, and appears to require energy. Bile salt micelles also play an important role by creating a concentration gradient which favors the movement of pigment into bile.

The disappearance of bilirubin from the circulation has been studied by employing a tracer dose of labeled bilirubin. Analysis discloses three pools of unconjugated bilirubin: plasma, hepatic, and the third, extravascular, extrahepatic. There is bidirectional flux of bilirubin between the different pools. Bilirubin derived from hepatic heme may directly enter into bile without entry into the other compartments. Only conjugated bilirubin can appear in bile. Once excreted into the feces, conjugated bilirubin is not reabsorbed by the intestinal mucosa. It is instead degraded by bacterial action in the small and large intestines. By a series of reduction steps colorless urobilinogens are formed. Further oxidation of the urobilinogens yields the colored urobilins. Urobilinogen is reabsorbed by the small intestine to enter the enterohepatic circulation. A small amount is excreted into bile. Most of the urobilinogen appears in the urine (< 4 mg/day). The properties and reactions of conjugated and unconjugated bilirubin are summarized in Table 1.4.

Carbohydrate Metabolism

The liver performs important functions in the intermediary metabolism of carbohydrate (Fig. 1.15).[11] During fasting, gluconeogenesis, ketogenesis, and glycogenolysis predominate to provide glucose for brain, kidney, hemopoietic tissue, and so on. Three sources of metabolite are utilized: glycogenic amino acids derived from muscle, glycerol released by lipolysis from fat depots, and lactate or pyruvate returning to the liver from peripheral sources. The normal liver contains about 80 g glycogen. This provides in large part the 180 g glucose produced daily in the normal fasting adult; 144 g of the glucose output is oxidized to CO_2 and water, and 36 g returns to the liver as lactate or pyruvate. After a meal, glycogenesis is increased at the expense of gluconeogenesis and ketogenesis. The amino acid influx from the intestine is deaminated for

Table 1.4. Comparison between conjugated and unconjugated bilirubin.[11]

Properties or reactions	Bilirubin	
	Conjugated	Unconjugated
Water solubility	+	0
Lipid solubility	0	+
Lipid membrane permeability	0	+
Albumin binding	±	+++
Renal excretion	+	0
Van den Bergh reaction	Direct	Indirect

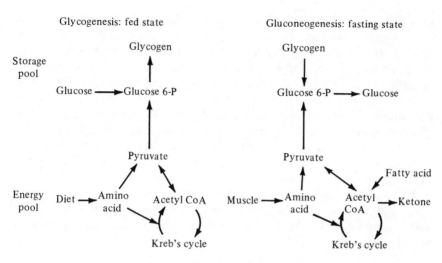

Fig. 1.15. Carbohydrate metabolism in the liver.

entry into the citric acid cycle. Ketone production ceases and circulating fatty acids fall. These processes together result in glycogen storage.

Viral Hepatitis. Although hypoglycemia is usually considered rare in liver disease, low fasting blood glucose is not uncommon in viral hepatitis. Both glycogen synthesis and gluconeogenesis are impaired in viral hepatitis.[27] Glucose response to glucagon is reduced to one-third of that in normal subjects. Reduction of amino acid concentrations does not occur after glucagon administration, as in the control group. Insulin secretion is not affected. Gross impairment in carbohydrate metabolism also occurs in fulminant hepatitis, in which hypoglycemia is a common finding.

Cirrhosis. Approximately 80% of the patients with alcoholic cirrhosis show glucose intolerance. This state has been attributed variously to hepatocellular damage, hypokalemia, hyperinsulinemia, insulin resistance, pancreatitis, hemosiderosis, diabetogenic drugs, elevated serum growth hormone, and glucagon concentrations.[28,29] An abnormal oral glucose tolerance test occurs four times more frequently than the intravenous glucose tolerance test, indicating that the cirrhotic process is partly responsible for impaired glucose metabolism. A correlation exists between the high incidence of glucose intolerance and portacaval shunting. Since glucagon and insulin are degraded by the liver, impaired hepatic cell function and the spontaneous or surgically induced portacaval shunting of cirrhosis may account for the hyperglucagonemia and hyperinsulinemia. The secretion of both hormones is also influenced by altered plasma amino acid concentrations found in this condition, eg, elevation of tyrosine, methionine, and phenylalanine, and reduction of the branched-chain amino acids valine, leucine, and isoleucine. Providing potassium supplement to cirrhotics who have had a total body loss of potassium in spite of normokalemia reverses the diabetic response to glucose. Potassium supplementation also corrects the reduced insulin and growth hormone outputs associated with potassium depletion.[30] The increased growth hormone is ascribed to the stimulatory effect of the hyperestrogenism occurring in cirrhotics. The clinical manifestations of diabetes mellitus are usually absent in cirrhotics with abnormal carbohydrate metabolism. This group does share common biochemical features with maturity onset diabetics, and the disease has been termed hepatogenous diabetes.

Hepatic coma.   Rises in pyruvic acid and alpha-ketoglutaric acid are correlated with the neurologic deterioration in this condition (see Chapter 8).

Cholesterol Metabolism

Cholesterol synthesis takes place primarily in the liver, and to a lesser degree in the intestine, adrenal cortex, skin, and testis. Endogenous synthesis accounts for the greater part of the total cholesterol pool (1 g/day), whereas the average diet provides about 0.3 g/day. All 27 carbon atoms of the cholesterol molecule are derived from acetate units. The first step in the synthesis is the formation of mevalonate, a 6-carbon compound, from acetyl-CoA.[11] The reaction is catalyzed by the enzyme beta-hydroxy-beta-methylglutaryl (HMG) CoA reductase. By a series of steps mevalonate is converted to isoprenoid, then to squalene and lanosterol, and finally to cholesterol. Adrenal cortical hormones, estrogen, and bile acids are end products derived from the cholesterol molecule. Cholesterol is eliminated by two pathways: formation of bile salts, and fecal excretion as neutral sterols. Regulation of synthesis in the liver is exerted by a negative feedback mechanism whereby cholesterol inhibits the enzyme HMG CoA reductase at an early step of cholesterol metabolism. Cholesterol is esterified with fatty acids in the liver, intestine, and plasma. The enzyme lecithin cholesterol acyltransferase (LCAT), produced in the liver, catalyzes the esterification reaction. LCAT transfers the fatty acid from the beta position of lecithin to the 3-β-OH group of free cholesterol, producing both cholesterol ester and lysolecithin. Cholesterol is transported predominantly as low-density (beta) lipoproteins (LDL). Serum cholesterol varies 150 mg–250 mg/dl, depending on age, diet, and race. Esterified cholesterol constitutes 50–70% of the total serum concentration.

Alterations in liver disease. The two important changes are:

1. In cholestasis, total serum cholesterol usually becomes elevated. The rise is predominantly in the nonesterified cholesterol fraction.[31] Very high levels of cholesterol > 600 mg/dl are associated with chronic extrahepatic biliary obstruction or primary biliary cirrhosis. Low serum cholesterol ester indicates severe parenchymal damage. The ratio of free to esterified cholesterol may rise in acute and chronic hepatocellular injury, indicating diminished esterification and LCAT activity.[32] The decrease of LCAT activity in chronic liver disease without marked jaundice is in contrast to the normal activity in chronic extrahepatic cholestasis.

2. Decreased LCAT enzyme, due to chronic hepatic dysfunction, especially in alcoholic cirrhosis, results in lipoproteins inordinately rich in free cholesterol.[33] The erythrocyte cell membrane bathed by these lipoproteins acquires more surface area and a scalloped contour. These spur cells have an increase of membrane "microviscosity" which undergoes splenic conditioning. In the spleen there is loss of surface area and finally transformation to mature spur cells. The membrane rigidity of spur cells, similar to that observed in hereditary spherocytosis, leads to hemolysis.

Lipid Metabolism

Lipids account for 5% of the normal liver weight, consisting chiefly of triglycerides but also including phospholipids, fatty acids, cholesterol, and cholesterol ester.[11] The liver rapidly extracts free fatty acids from plasma derived from fat depots and diet (Fig. 1.16). Some unsaturated fatty acids are synthesized within the liver from acetate. Breakdown of the long-chained fatty acids proceeds in the liver in a step-by-step sequence of 2-carbon cleavage. The eventual product consists of molecules of acetyl-CoA and acetoacetyl-CoA. Acetyl-CoA represents a central intermediary which enters into a number of different metabolic processes. It may be oxidized to CO_2 and water via the citric acid cycle. Or it may enter the major synthetic pathway of forming triglycerides: acetyl-CoA → phosphatidic acid → diglyceride → triglyceride. The same diglyceride may enter into the precursor pool producing phospholipid. Acetyl-CoA may also be diverted into the production of cholesterol. Most of the triglycerides formed are exported extracellularly by combining with specific apoproteins to yield very-low-density pre-beta-lipoprotein (VLDL), low-

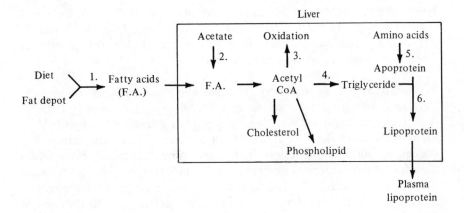

Fig. 1.16. Lipid metabolism in the liver. The numbers represent the possible sites of interference which may produce fatty livers (see text and Table 1.5). (Adapted from Alpers and Isselbacher, Gen Ref No 14, p 820.)

density beta-lipoprotein (LDL), and high-density alpha-lipoprotein (HDL). Trigylceride secretion by the liver depends on intact protein synthesis.

Fatty livers. In fatty livers the chief lipids which accumulate are the triglycerides. The lipid content of the liver increases from the normal 5% of liver weight to 10–40% (see also Chapter 14). Fatty livers may be classified functionally, depending on the site of interference with lipid metabolism (Table 1.5).

Serum lipids in infectious hepatitis. Serum total cholesterol (particularly cholesterol ester), triglycerides, and total phospholipids increase with the onset of jaundice in acute type A viral hepatitis.[34] The elevated levels persist throughout the active phase, regardless of the change in other liver function tests, and return to normal in about one month after the onset of symptoms. The finding that the concentrations of lipids increase while bilirubin and alkaline phosphatases recede to normal range suggests that intrahepatic biliary obstruction does not play a major role in the elevation. Overproduction is a likely factor for the increase. The triglyceride fatty acids show a gradual decline in relative linoleic acid concentration. This can be attributed to faulty absorption of fat or to increased utilization of carbohydrates during recovery. Another possible explanation for the rise in serum lipids is a deficiency of lecithin-cholesterol acyltransferase occurring in acute viral hepatitis.

Table 1.5.   Causes of fatty liver.

  I. Increased mobilization of fatty acids from fat depots or diet
    1. High-fat diet
    2. Early stage of starvation
    3. Uncontrolled diabetes mellitus
    4. Alcohol
  II. Increased hepatic synthesis of fatty acids
    1. High-carbohydrate diet
    2. Obesity
    3. Diabetes mellitus
    4. Alcohol
 III. Decreased hepatic oxidation of fatty acids
    1. Alcohol
 IV. Increased hepatic esterification of fatty acids
    1. Alcohol
  V. Decreased hepatic apoprotein synthesis
    1. CCl_4
    2. Phosphorous
    3. Tetracycline
    4. Ethionine (This specific antagonist replaces methionine in 5-adenosyl methionine, trapping available adenine. ATP synthesis is prevented, and both messenger RNA and protein synthesis decline.)
    5. Puromycin
 VI. Decreased formation of hepatic lipoprotein
    1. Essential fatty acid deficiency
    2. Choline deficiency (This is not encountered in humans, except perhaps in kwashiorkor or severe chronic starvation. It serves, however, a useful and time-honored method of inducing fatty liver and cirrhosis in animals. Diets low in methionine or choline may be used. As choline can be synthesized using the labile methyl group donated by methionine, choline deficiency is basically a shortage of methyl groups. Other methyl-rich compounds, such as betaine, can substitute for choline as lipotropic agents in preventing this type of fatty liver.)

Lipoproteins in liver disease. Hepatocellular liver disease is associated with decreased serum concentrations of HDL and VLDL, while in cholestasis all fractions of lipoproteins are raised (Table 1.6).[31] The decrease in HDL is primarily due to the impaired lipid-binding capacity of apolipoprotein A (apoA), the major protein in HDL. This results in a high protein to lipid ratio and an HDL disassociated into two polypeptides. The low VLDL has a composition that, although resembling normal VLDL, lacks apoA. The damaged liver synthesizes an altered apoA which does not properly bind neutral lipids. The decrease of both HDL and VLDL is

Table 1.6.   Serum lipoprotein patterns in liver disease.[31]

	Lipoproteins		
	Low density (beta)	Very low density (pre-beta)	High density (alpha)
Acute viral hepatitis	↑↑	↓↓	↓↓
Alcoholic cirrhosis	↑	↓↓	↓
Primary biliary cirrhosis	↑↑	N	N
Cholestasis	↑↑	↑↑	↑↑

↑ or ↑↑ = mild or marked increase;   ↓ or ↓↓ = mild or marked decrease; N = normal level.

accounted for on this basis. These changes occur independently of the production of the abnormal lipoprotein, LP-X, in cholestasis.

Alterations in cholestasis.   For a full treatment of the topic see Chapter 5.

Serum free (nonesterified) fatty acids.   Elevations are encountered in acute and chronic liver diseases of diverse origins. They are due to an increased mobilization from peripheral fat stores and to impairment of carbohydrate metabolism.

Protein Metabolism

The human liver synthesizes albumin, alpha- and beta-globulins, blood-coagulation factors (fibrinogen, prothrombin, factors VII, IX, and X), haptoglobin, glycoprotein, transferrin, and certain enzymes (pseudo-cholinesterase and ceruloplasmin).

Albumin.[35]   At any given time one-third of the hepatocytes is engaged in albumin synthesis by the rough, endoplasmic reticulum with bound polysome RNA units. Albumin is made at the rate of 120–200 mg/kg body weight per day, with a degradation rate expressed as 6–10% plasma albumin pool per day. The intravascular mass is 35–45% of the total pool. The total exchange mass is in the order of 4–5 g/kg body weight. All this provides for a serum concentration of 3.5–4.5 g/dl. The half-life of albumin is 17–20 days. For this reason acute liver injury does not affect the serum levels initially. Complete cessation of albumin production for a week is required to produce a 25% decrease of serum values. Advanced chronic liver disease, regardless of etiology, is attended by a fall in serum albumin concentration. Although it is not a good index of the liver's ability to synthesize albumin, the level of hypoalbuminemia serves as a useful guide to therapy in active cirrhosis. Adequate nutrition, corticosteroids, and thyroid and growth hormones stimulate hepatic synthesis of albumin. Malnutrition, analbuminemia, cirrhosis, general stress including infection and heat, carcinoma, and hypothyroidism all decrease albumin production. Although cirrhosis is characterized by depressed serum albumin levels, albumin synthesis is variably affected and the exchangeable albumin pool is decreased only in one-half of the patients. Once the alcoholic effect is discontinued and adequate nutrition provided, the cirrhotic liver rapidly regains its capacity for albumin production. This suggests that the albumin-synthesizing ability of the liver may be restored to normal in alcoholic cirrhosis.

Globulins. In normal human serum five distinct moving boundaries are identified on paper electrophoresis. They are designated in order of increasing mobility as albumin, alpha$_1$- and alpha$_2$-globulins, beta-globulin, and gamma-globulin (Fig. 1.17). Variations of globulin level in liver disease are summarized in Table 1.7. The half-life of the globulins are much shorter than albumin, except for IgG. Their rapid turnover rates

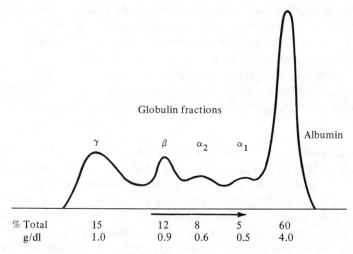

Fig. 1.17. Serum protein electrophoretic pattern.

Table 1.7. Globulin levels in liver disease.

	Globulins			
	Alpha$_1$	Alpha$_2$	Beta	Gamma
Viral hepatitis	N	↑	↑	↑
Fulminant hepatic failure	N	↓↓	↓↓	N
Extrahepatic cholestasis	↓	↑↑	↑↑	N
Cirrhosis	↑	↑	↑	↑↑

↑ or ↑↑ = mild or marked increase; ↓ or ↓↓ = mild or marked decrease; N = normal level.

account for early fluctuations in liver disease. The pattern of changes is not diagnostic for any single disease. Other serum proteins show variations which are of little practical significance. In general, prealbumin and retinol-binding protein (RBP) are decreased in most types of liver disease, except for fatty liver and chronic persistent hepatitis.[36] Alpha-lipoprotein is also lowered in most liver disorders, except for cholestasis and primary biliary cirrhosis. Levels of prealbumin, RBP, alpha-lipoprotein, albumin, and certain clotting factors are highly intercorrelated for the different hepatic diseases. Decreased protein synthesis in the liver probably accounts for the low concentrations. Alpha$_1$-antitrypsin is increased, while haptoglobin and total iron-binding capacity are depressed in acute and chronic hepatic disorders. Ceruloplasmin is increased especially in primary biliary cirrhosis and liver tumors. Alpha$_2$-macroglobulin appears elevated in all types of cirrhosis. Ceruloplasmin, haptoglobin, total iron-binding capacity, and alpha-antitrypsin to a certain extent behave like acute-phase reactants. Cholestasis is associated with high concentrations of ceruloplasmin, C3 complement, alpha-lipoprotein, and certain clotting factors.

Coagulation factors. The liver generates prothrombin (factor II) and factors V, VII, IX, and X. All except factor V are vitamin-K-dependent in their metabolism. In severe cirrhosis and fulminant hepatitis these factors are depressed. A lack of response to vitamin K given parenterally within 24–48 hours indicates parenchymal damage. The half-lives of coagulation proteins are relatively short, ranging from six days for prothrombin to 20 minutes for factor VII. For this reason replacement therapy with these factors is not a practical procedure in liver disease.

Table 1.8. Coagulation abnormalities in liver disease.*

1. Viral hepatitis, toxic hepatitis, infiltrative disease:
   a. Variable ↓ of factors I, II, V, VII, IX, X, XI
   b. Thrombocytopenia
   c. ↑ Fibrinolysis
2. Cirrhosis, Wilson's disease, hemochromatosis:
   a. Same as 1a, plus ↓ in factor XIII
   b. Thrombocytopenia and thrombocytopathy
   c. ↑ Fibrinolysis and ↓ antithrombin II, III
   d. Dysfibrinogenemia
3. Cholestasis, biliary cirrhosis
   a. ↓ Factors II, VII, IX, X
   b. Normal or ↑ factors I, V
   c. ↑ Antithrombin III (biliary cirrhosis only)
4. Primary or secondary liver cancer
   a. ↑ Factors I, V, VIII
   b. ↓ Factors II, VII, IX, X, XIII
   c. ↑ Fibrinolysis
   d. Thrombocytopenia and thrombocytopathy
   e. ↓ Antithrombin II, III
   f. Abnormal fibrinogen production (hepatoma)

* From H. R. Roberts and A. I. Cederbaum, *Gastroenterology* 63: 297–320, Williams and Wilkins Co, 1972.

Coagulation defects in liver disease. Variations in coagulation proteins accompany many types of liver disease (see Table 1.8).[37]

Cholestasis. Cholestasis due to biliary obstruction or primary biliary cirrhosis is associated with decreased plasma fibrinolysis (plasminogen activator activity), decreased urokinase inhibitors, and increased fibrinogen.[38] Plasma fibrinolysis and fibrinogen correlate with the degree of cholestasis and vary inversely with serum triglyceride level in primary biliary cirrhosis. Fibrin/fibrinogen degradation products are normal in PBC but increased in bile duct obstruction. Antiplasmin activity is raised in extrahepatic cholestasis, but not in PBC. The serum inhibitors of fibrinolysis, urokinase, and antiplasmin do not correlate with liver function tests or serum triglyceride concentration. Cholestasis impairs fibrinolysis by increasing serum lipids. This may predispose patients undergoing surgery for biliary obstruction to develop venous thrombosis.

Fulminant hepatic failure. This liver disorder is discussed in Chapter 8.

REFERENCES

1. Rappaport AM: Anatomic considerations, in Gen Ref No. 14, pp 1–50.
2. Elias H, Sherrick JC: Gross anatomy of the liver, pp 265–277, and Microscopic anatomy of the liver, pp 5–135, in Gen Ref No. 4.
3. Shaffner F, Popper H: Electron microscopy of the liver, in Gen Ref No. 14, pp 51–86.
4. Weibel ER, et al: Correlated morphometric and biochemical studies on the liver cell: 1: Morphometric model, stereologic methods, and normal morphometric data for rat liver. *J Cell Biol* 42:68–91, 1969.
5. Steiner JW, Perez ZM, Taichman LB: Cell population dynamics in the liver: A review of quantitative morphological techniques applied to the study of physiological and pathological growth. *Exp Molec Path* 5:146–181, 1966.
6. Bucher NLR, Malt RA: Morphological and biological aspects, in Gen Ref No. 2, pp 23–54.
7. Morley CGD: Humoral regulation of liver regeneration and tissue growth. *Persp Biol Med* 17:411–428, 1974.
8. Blumgart HL, Vajrabukka T: Injuries to the liver: Analysis of 20 cases. *Brit Med J* 1:158–164, 1972.
9. Mays ET: Physiologic consequences of hepatic lobectomy in man. *South Med J* 68:399–406, 1975.
10. Leevy CM: Liver regeneration in man. Springfield, Il, Charles C Thomas, 1974, pp 31–78.
11. Whitby LG: The metabolic functions of the liver, in Passmore R, Robson JS (eds.), A companion to medical studies. *Blackwell Sci Publ*, Oxford, 1968, pp 31.1–31.18.
12. Hardison WGM: Bile salts and the liver, in Gen Ref No. 9, pp 83–95.
13. Vlahcevic ZR, et al: Bile acid metabolism in cirrhosis: II: Cholic and chenodeoxycholic acid metabolism. *Gastroenterology* 62:1174–1181, 1972.
14. Murphy GM, Ross A, Billing BH: Serum bile acids in primary biliary cirrhosis. *Gut* 13:201–206, 1972.
15. Palmer RH: Bile acids, liver injury and liver disease. *Arch Intern Med* 130:606–617, 1972.
16. Einarsson K, Hellstrom K, Schersten T: The formation of bile acids in patients with portal liver cirrhosis. *Scand J Gastroent* 10:299–304, 1975.
17. Editorial: Medical treatment of gallstones. *Lancet* 1:360–361, 1972.
18. Grundy SM: Cholesterol-bile acid interactions in gallstone pathogenesis. *Hosp Pract* 8:57–65, 1973.
19. Editorial: Diet and gallstones. *Lancet* 1:471, 1973.
20. Thistle JL, Hofmann AF: Efficacy and specificity of chenodeoxycholic acid therapy for dissolving gallstones. *New Eng J Med* 289:655–659, 1973.
21. Iser JH, et al: Chenodeoxycholic acid treatment of gallstones: A follow-up report and analysis of factors influencing response to therapy. *New Eng J Med* 293:378–383, 1975.

22. Mok HYI, Bell GD, Dowling RH: Effect of different doses of chenodeoxy-cholic acid on bile-lipid composition and on frequency of side-effects in patients with gallstones. *Lancet* 2:253–257, 1974.

23. Bell GD, et al: Liver structure and function in cholelithiasis: Effect of chenodeoxycholic acid. *Gut* 15:165–172, 1974.

24. Carey MC: Cheno and urso: What the goose and the bear have in common. *New Eng J Med* 293:1255–1257, 1975.

25. Linscheer WG, Raheja KL: Effect of glycerophosphate on lithogenic bile: A new approach to treatment of cholelithiasis. *Lancet* 2:551–553, 1974.

26. Bissell DM: Formation and elimination of bilirubin. *Gastroenterology* 69:519–538, 1975.

27. Felig P, et al: Glucose homeostasis in viral hepatitis. *New Eng J Med* 283:1436–1440, 1970.

28. Conn HO, Schreiber W, Elkington SG: Cirrhosis and diabetes: II: Association of impaired glucose tolerance with portal-systemic shunting in Laennec's cirrhosis. *Amer J Dig Dis* 16:227–239, 1971.

29. Marco J, et al: Elevated plasma glucagon levels in cirrhosis of the liver. *New Eng J Med* 289:1107–1111, 1973.

30. Podolsky S, et al: Potassium depletion in hepatic cirrhosis: A reversible cause of impaired growth-hormone and insulin response to stimulation. *New Eng J Med* 288:644–648, 1973.

31. Seidel D: Plasma lipids and lipoproteins in patients with liver disease. *Scand J Gastroent* 7:105–108, 1972.

32. Kepkay DL, Poon R, Simon JB: Lecithin-cholesterol acyltransferase and serum cholesterol esterification in obstructive jaundice. *J Lab Clin Med* 81:172–181, 1973.

33. Cooper RA, Kimball DB, Durocher JR: Role of the spleen in membrane conditioning and hemolysis of spur cells in liver disease. *New Eng J Med* 290:1279–1284, 1974.

34. Tamir I, et al: Behavior of serum lipids in children with hepatitis A. *Clin Chem Acta* 56:113–120, 1974.

35. Rothschild MA, Oratz M, Schreiber SS: Albumin metabolism, in Gen Ref No. 9, pp 19–29.

36. Skrede S, et al: Serum proteins in diseases of the liver. *Scand J Clin Lab Invest* 35:399–406, 1975.

37. Roberts HR, Cederbaum AI: The liver and blood coagulation: Physiology and pathology. *Gastroenterology* 63:297–320, 1972.

38. Jedrychowski A, et al: Fibrinolysis in cholestatic jaundice. *Brit Med J* 1:640–642, 1973.

LABORATORY TESTS AND MORPHOLOGIC EVALUATION

2

LIVER FUNCTION TESTS

Hepatic disease is evaluated in the laboratory by a group of procedures known as liver function tests or profiles (Table 2.1). Discriminant analysis demonstrates that the individual test alone has limited diagnostic effectiveness.[1] The frequency of correct diagnoses of hepatitis, fatty liver, and chronic liver disease is about 80% when six measurements (aminotransferase, alkaline phosphatases, gamma globulin, prothrombin time, bilirubin, and albumin) are made. Correct allocation to the disease groups of hepatitis, fatty liver, chronic liver disease, duct obstruction, and tumor is approximately 60% when tests of aminotransferase, alkaline phosphatases, prothrombin time, and bilirubin are used. In general, the above battery of hepatic tests makes it possible to discriminate between hepatitis and fatty liver and between hepatitis and duct obstruction. Other diagnostic procedures are most needed in the diagnosis of chronic liver disease and liver tumors.

LABORATORY TESTS

Blood Ammonia

Determination of blood ammonia confirms the presence of existing or impending hepatic coma. Two basic methods are available: enzymatic or diffusion techniques. The enzymatic method is based on the reaction:

$$\text{Alpha ketoglutarate} + NH_4^+ + NADH \xrightarrow[\text{dehydrogenase}]{\text{Glutamine}} \text{glutamic acid} + H_2O + NAD^+$$

Quantitation is obtained by measuring the decrease of optical density as NADH is converted to NAD. The older diffusion method releases ammonia in the blood by the addition of potassium carbonate, after which the free ammonia is reabsorbed by acid. The amount of ammonia is

Table 2.1. Types of liver function tests.

Function	Tests
Hepatocellular necrosis	Aminotransferases
Cholestasis	Alkaline phosphatases 5'-Nucleotidase Gamma-glutamyl transpetidase
Organic anion metabolism	Bilirubin Bile salts BSP Indocyanine green
Metabolic function	Ammonia
Synthetic capacity	Albumin Prothrombin time
Immunologic reactivity	Gamma globulin Immunoglobulins Autoantibodies
Disease markers	HAAg HB$_s$Ag Alpha-1-fetoprotein

determined by titration (Conway method), nesslerization, or the Berthelot reaction. The precaution for all procedures is that fresh blood must be drawn and the test must be done immediately since ammonia accumulates on standing.

The normal level for whole blood and plasma ammonia is less than 1 μg/ml. About 10% of the cases of hepatic coma do not show elevated ammonia concentrations. Increased levels of ammonia are encountered in patients with ureterosigmoidostomy, or with inborn errors of the urea cycle.

Serum Bile Acids

In general, three methods of detection are used:[2] (1) Gas-liquid chromatography. This technique requires extraction of conjugated bile acids from serum, hydrolysis into free nonconjugated forms, and preparation of volatile derivatives. For quantitation, an internal standard is added to the serum prior to determination. (2) Radioimmunoassay. A method of estimating cholic acid and its conjugates in plasma has been described.[3] The technique is rapid, sensitive, and specific. (3) Enzymatic method. 3-α-Hydroxysteroid dehydrogenase in the presence of NAD oxidizes the 3-α-hydroxy group of bile acids to a keto derivative. The NADH generated is measured spectrophotometrically. Bile acids with ester sulfate or glucuronide at the C3 position are not quantitated.

The clinical applicability of these procedures is still under study. With the introduction of simple and sensitive methods, determination of serum bile salts will undoubtedly be extensively employed and become a standard test of hepatic function. Measurement of individual bile acids also provides diagnostic information. Severe parenchymal diseases such as cirrhosis and viral hepatitis show a predominance of chenodeoxycholic acid (CDCA) in serum. In extrahepatic and intrahepatic cholestasis, cholic acid is predominant in serum. The ratio of cholic acid to CDCA characteristically exceeds unity. During the newborn period the main serum bile acid is cholic acid. Infants with extrahepatic biliary atresia show a predominant rise of CDCA, prognostically a poor sign associated with early demise. Those infants with serum cholic acid higher than CDCA generally do better. Their jaundice may spontaneously remit, although other signs of cholestasis may persist and hepatic complications may appear during early adolescence.

In practice, bile acid metabolism is tested in two functional ways. First, serum bile acids may be determined during the fasting stage or after a test meal.[4] The two-hour postprandial bile acid determination appears to be a sensitive test of hepatic dysfunction. In a study of 26 patients with liver disease, only three showed abnormal fasting bile acid levels, whereas all 26 exceeded the two-hour postprandial value of 1.5 μg/ml.[5] Second, bile acid may be used as a clearance test. Small doses of cholylglycine (glycocholate) injected into normal subjects are rapidly cleared by the liver. Cholylglycine disappearance may be estimated by radioimmunoassay.[6] The sensitivity of cholylglycine clearance exceeded that of the standard BSP retention test when both were used to evaluate patients treated for chronic active hepatitis.[3,6]

Normal serum levels vary with the method of determination. Using gas-liquid chromatography, the normal fasting bile acid concentration in serum is 2–4 nanomoles/ml; whereas for the enzymatic method, the normal value is 4–8 nanomoles/ml.

Serum Bilirubin

Serum total bilirubin does not exceed 1 mg/dl in healthy persons. The conjugated bilirubin fraction ranges up to 0.3 mg/dl, and the unconjugated fraction up to 0.7 mg/dl. The basis of determination continues to be the van den Bergh reaction, which utilizes the different solubility of the two bilirubin fractions (see Table 1.4). In aqueous solution conjugated, direct-reacting bilirubin is diazotized with sulfanilic acid, and the chromogen developed is read at one minute. In dilute methanol, the diazo reaction measures total (both conjugated and unconjugated) bilirubin. In the Malloy-Evelyn method this is read at 30 minutes. Total bilirubin minus the conjugated fraction represents the unconjugated, indirect-reacting bilirubin. The technique suffers from several drawbacks: poor reproducibility due partly to the dilution of serum, instability of pure bilirubin standard, and interference from hemolyzed blood. In clinical practice direct-reacting and indirect-reacting pigments are regarded as equivalent to conjugated and unconjugated bilirubin, respectively. They are in fact not identical. The direct-reacting fraction is measurable even though normal serum contains only trace amounts of true conjugated bilirubin. Pure crystalline unconjugated bilirubin shows 10% direct-reacting pigment on conventional assay. Other variants of the Malloy-Evelyn technique utilize accelerators other than methanol to speed up the diazo reaction. In this way unconjugated bilirubin which normally reacts slowly may be estimated more rapidly. A popular modification is the Jendrassik method which uses caffeine as an accelerator. An advantage of this modification is its reproducibility. Fasting increases bilirubin values, particularly in Gilbert's disease. High bilirubin levels can interfere with the determination of albumin and cholesterol when all three are performed on the Autoanalyzer. False reductions of serum albumin and cholesterol are obtained.

Urine Bilirubin

Unconjugated bilirubin, being tightly bound to albumin, does not clear the renal glomerulus. Conjugated bilirubin above the serum threshold of 0.4 mg/dl appears in urine. Renal excretion of the conjugated bile pigment is affected by the level of serum bile salts. In extrahepatic biliary obstruction, the increased concentration of bile salts enhances the excretion of conjugated bilirubin. Hence, serum bilirubin usually does not exceed 40 mg/dl in obstructive jaundice. In hemolytic states the elevated unconjugated bilirubin and normal bile salts concentration do not produce any significant bilirubinuria. Qualitative detection of urine bilirubin is usually carried out with Ictotest, a tablet containing p-nitrobenzenediazonium, p-toluenesulfonate, and sulfosalicylate acid. The test is specific and utilizes the diazo reaction to detect bilirubin. For a quantitative procedure the Harrison test can be employed: The principle is based on concentration of bilirubin with barium sulfate, and oxidation to chromogenic biliverdin with Fouchet's reagent (trichloroacetic acid and ferric chloride).

Urine Urobilinogen and Urobilin

Urobilinogen is colorless; when in excess, the colored urobilin imparts an orange color to urine. For semiquantitative determination the Watson-Schwarz procedure may be employed. The test is based on Ehrlich's aldehyde reaction with p-dimethylaminobenzaldehyde. The urobilinogen-aldehyde complex provides a strong chromogen after intensification with sodium acetate. The normal urine urobilinogen value is less than 2 Ehrlich units (roughly equivalent to 2 mg urobilinogen) per two hours. Urobilin fluoresces green with alcoholic zinc acetate solution. This forms the basis of the Schlesinger test for urobilin.

Fecal Urobilinogen and Urobilin

The principles of determination are those outlined for the urinary counterparts. The brown color of feces usually indicates an adequate presence of urobilin. With gray, clay-colored stools, urobilin and urobilinogen may be present, decreased, or absent. The qualitative screening test for bile pigment should be done first to ascertain if bile derivatives are present.

Clearance Tests

Clearance tests measure the liver's capacity to eliminate organic anions. Commonly employed test materials are dyes such as sulfobromophthalein and indocyanine green and endogenous anions such as bile salts. Clearance of the test substance depends on several discrete steps: transport of the substance to the liver cell (blood flow); uptake by the hepatocyte; intracellular binding by Y and Z proteins; metabolic alteration or conjugation, although this is not an obligatory step with some substances; and biliary excretion. The sensitivity of clearance tests as monitors of liver function increases when the doses of the various substances approach the maximum uptake capacity (V_{max}). At high doses some substances are toxic and their usefulness becomes limited. In general, clearance tests are among the most sensitive indicators of liver dysfunction that we have at present.

Sulfobromophthalein (BSP) Test[7]

After its intravenous administration, sulfobromophthalein (sodium phenoltetrabromphthalein, BSP) appears bound to albumin and alpha$_1$-

lipoprotein. The dye is rapidly cleared from the blood by the liver at the rate of 10–16% of the residual concentration in blood per minute and is slowly excreted into bile. The liver, however, removes only 70–80% of the injected dose, the remainder being removed by extrahepatic mechanisms: 2% appears in the urine, and in liver damage up to 10% is excreted by the kidney. Hepatic uptake of BSP is carrier-mediated, utilizing the same organic anion transport mechanism as bilirubin, indocyanine green and rose bengal. Competitive saturation may occur with these compounds. In liver cells BSP is conjugated primarily with glutathione, catalyzed by soluble cytoplasmic enzymes. Some BSP remains unconjugated and is freely excreted into bile. Transport across the canalicular membrane is also carrier-mediated and competes with other organic anions for saturation.

The standard BSP test is based on a dose of 5 mg/kg body weight and estimation of the dye retained at 45 minutes after injection. Normal value is less than 5% BSP retention at 45 minutes. Determination of BSP rests on the development of a purple color in an alkaline solution. This is measured spectrophotometrically and compared to a standard curve.

Infusion of BSP at two rates and periodic determinations of plasma values may provide estimates of the hepatic storage of BSP (relative storage capacity, S) and active secretion of BSP (transport maximum, Tm). Determination of Tm and S is useful in estimating the excretory defect in cholestasis. In primary biliary cirrhosis the Tm is markedly decreased but S remains normal. In Dubin-Johnson syndrome, S is normal but Tm value is reduced. In cirrhosis both Tm and S are decreased.

Although it is one of the most sensitive of hepatic tests, an abnormal serum BSP level does not indicate the type of liver dysfunction. In the jaundiced patient a BSP determination is useless and redundant since evidence for liver disease already exists. BSP values are increased by anemia, shock, fever, certain drugs, and advanced age. The standard test presumes that the same plasma volume to the total body weight, 50 ml/kg body weight, holds in all subjects. This is not true in the obese patient who has a plasma volume less than the ideal 50 ml/kg body weight. Rare allergic manifestations and death have been reported after BSP administration.

Indocyanine Green Dye

This tricarbocyanine dye possesses several advantages over BSP as an excretory test. There is no extrahepatic mechanism of removal. Indocyanine green dye (ICG) is not conjugated in hepatocytes and practically all the dye is recovered in bile. Furthermore, toxic reactions have not been reported, except for rare hypersensitivity to the iodine present in the molecule.[8] Its disadvantages are expense and the relatively more cumbersome assay compared to BSP. ICG is injected intravenously at a dose of 0.5 or 5 mg/kg body weight and the disappearance from the circulation followed by ear densitometry or by serial blood samplings and spectrophotometric determinations. The normal percentage disappearance rate (PDR) is $28.2 \pm 2.7\%$ per minute for the 0.5 mg/kg dose. If the result is normal, the larger dose of 5.0 mg/kg body weight may be given. This dose approaches the maximum uptake capacity in the normal adult liver. The normal PDR for the 5 mg/kg dose is $23.4 \pm 2.3\%$ per minute.

Serum Protein

Serum protein tests measure total serum protein, albumin, and globulins. Total serum protein is usually determined by the biuret method, which utilizes the color formed between copper and the peptide bond of protein. Normal values vary 6–8 g/dl. Variations in liver disease occur in a narrow range and are not diagnostic. Serum albumin is measured by the dye-binding method or by electrophoresis. The former procedure is subject to interference by high bilirubin levels, resulting in false reduction. Serum albumin concentration in normal adults ranges 4–6 g/dl. Globulin level is usually not measured by specific methods but derived by subtracting the albumin value from the total protein concentration (normally 1–2 g/dl). Albumin to globulin (A/G) ratio has no physiological significance and the term is best avoided.

A reduction in serum albumin level and an inverse rise in serum globulin is a common change in chronic liver disease, particularly cirrhosis. Hypoalbuminemia itself reflects loss of hepatocellular mass. Serial determinations of serum albumin provide a useful indicator of prognosis and therapeutic response. Hyperglobulinemia suggests chronic inflammation and a continuing process of cell destruction. It serves as an index of activity in diseases such as chronic active hepatitis and active cirrhosis.

Fractionation of alpha-, beta-, and gamma-globulin is accomplished by electrophoresis or salting-out procedures. Alpha$_1$-globulin tends to parallel serum albumin and declines in severe hepatocellular disease. A rise is common in neoplasms. Alpha$_2$-globulin and beta-globulin are low in fulminant hepatitis but high in cholestasis, reflecting the increased lipoprotein content of these two globulin fractions.

Serum Flocculation Tests

The empirical procedures such as cephalin-cholesterol flocculation, thymol turbidity, and zinc sulfate turbidity have been largely abandoned. They add little that is not revealed by other hepatic tests. Positive flocculation depends on the elevation of globulin and the decrease of the inhibiting power of albumin. Both fractions are better served by direct measurement.

Immunoglobulin

Of the five known immunoglobulins, only three (IgG, IgA, and IgM) are routinely determined. The assay is performed on immunodiffusion gel plates with antibodies directed against respective immunoglobulins. Normal serum levels are IgG 800–1500 mg/dl, IgA 90–325 mg/dl, IgM 45–150 mg/dl (see Chapter 4 for immunoglobulin changes in liver disease).

Plasma Prothrombin

This clotting factor requires vitamin K for its synthesis. A marked decrease in prothrombin levels, to about 10% of normal, must occur before bleeding tendencies appear. For this reason, spontaneous bleeding due to prothrombin deficiency is rare in obstructive jaundice or hepatitis. Furthermore, a deficiency of prothrombin usually involves other clotting factors. The one-stage (Quick's) assay allows oxalated plasma to react with excess thromboplastin (prepared from rabbit brain) and calcium. The clotting time is determined and expressed in seconds or as percentage of normal activity. Normal control varies but is generally in the range of 11.5–12.5 seconds. This procedure measures not only prothrombin concentration but also factors V, VII, and X and fibrinogen in plasma. Depression of fibrinogen to less than 100 mg/dl or any one of the other required factors to less than 20–40% of normal levels results in prolongation of the prothrombin time. The prothrombin test is not a sensitive indicator of liver disease. It is, however, valuable in that it provides an early clue in acute viral hepatitis to the development of fulminant hepatic necrosis. Depressed prothrombin time often precedes other manifestations of liver failure in this disease. Additionally, the prothrombin test permits an assessment of coagulation homeostasis before any surgical or diagnostic procedure, such as liver biopsy, is attempted. It helps to screen out patients who might bleed excessively.

Serum Enzymes

Alkaline phosphatases.[9]   Alkaline phosphatases hydrolyze the monoesters of orthophosphorate acid at an alkaline pH (8.6–10.3). They are present in many human tissues, primarily in bone, liver, intestine, placenta, leukocytes, and kidney. In normal individuals, serum phosphatases perform no known physiological function. Serum alkaline phosphatases are derived from three sources: liver, bone, and intestine. During the third trimester of pregnancy an additional fourth source contributes toward the serum level, the placenta. Electrophoretic pattern reveals two major isoenzyme bands representing alkaline phosphatases derived from bone and liver (the major band). The third component, intestinal alkaline phosphatase, is found in serum of 20–60% of normal persons who have blood type O or A, secrete ABH red cell antigens, and are positive for Lewis antigen.

The liver does not excrete serum alkaline phosphatases into the bile, as it does bilirubin. The enzymes are catabolized like other serum proteins, and their turnover is independent of the patency of the bile ducts. Unlike the aminotransferases, they are not simply leaked from injured hepatocytes. Biliary obstruction, in unknown ways, activates the hepatic synthesis of alkaline phosphatases which then regurgitate into the general circulation. The increased serum levels in liver disease represent the appearance of newly synthesized hepatic enzymes.

In normal adults serum alkaline phosphatases range 1.5–4.0 Bodansky units, or 3–15 King-Armstrong units, or 20–85 International units (IU). Growing children and women in late pregnancy have higher levels. High values are found in bone diseases associated with increased osteoblastic activity or in biliary obstruction. Values greater than 15 Bodansky units in patients with liver disease suggest cholestasis; in infiltrative lesions of the liver, such as granuloma and tumor metastases, slightly lower values are encountered; increases in the 6–12 Bodansky unit range indicate other liver disease such as cirrhosis or viral hepatitis (Table 2.2). Liver-derived enzyme is identified from other isoenzymes by electrophoresis on starch gel or by its heat stability (15 minutes at 56°C) or by urea resistance (18 minutes in 3 M urea). Bone alkaline phosphatases lack either heat or urea stability. Serum alkaline phosphatases form the single most useful enzyme indicator of cholestasis.

Aminotransferases. Aminotransferases (transaminases) are enzymes which catalyze the interconversion between a pair of amino acids and a pair of keto acids. The two enzymes most commonly measured are aspartate aminotransferase (AsAT), formerly GOT, and L-alanine aminotransferase (AlAT), previously known as GPT. AsAT occurs in all tissues, especially the heart, skeletal muscle, brain, liver, and kidney, in descending order of concentration. AlAT is present primarily in the liver, and to a lesser extent in kidney and skeletal muscle. High serum values of AsAT are found mainly in myocardial infarction or acute hepatocellular necrosis. Presumably necrotic or damaged cells with altered membrane permeability release the enzyme into the general circulation. AlAT is somewhat more specific for acute liver injury due to its greater hepatic

Table 2.2. Serum enzyme changes in liver disease.

	Aminotransferases	Alkaline phosphatases	5'-Nucleotidase
Acute viral hepatitis	>500 IU/l rise during preicteric and icteric phases; returns to normal within 6 weeks after onset of jaundice	6–12 BU* during cholestatic phase; 5%[†] > 15 BU	
Chronic active hepatitis	< 500 IU/l during active stage	< 12 BU in 30%	
Cirrhosis	< 200 IU/l in 50%[†]	< 12 BU in 40%	
Extrahepatic cholestasis	< 100 IU/l early; may return to normal in 1–2 weeks	80% > 15 BU, frequently > 25 BU	> 18 BU
Granulomatous infiltration	20% < 100 IU/l	50% < 12 BU	
Metastatic tumors	50% < 100 IU/l	90% < 12 BU	

* BU = Bodansky units; [†] % = percent of total cases.

concentration. The kinetic test for AsAT is based on two coupled reactions:

$$\text{Asparate + Alpha-ketoglutarate} \xrightarrow{\text{AsAT}} \text{oxaloacetate + glutamate}$$

$$\text{Oxaloacetate + NADH} \xrightarrow[\text{dehydrogenase}]{\text{Malic}} \text{malate + NAD}$$

NADH is quantitated as its optical density decreases in its conversion to NAD. Normal serum level of AsAT is 15–20 IU/l and for AlAT 3–25 IU/l. In acute viral hepatitis and fulminant hepatitis, the aminotransferases reach 1000–2000 IU/l. Other hepatic disorders such as cirrhosis, cholestasis, and tumor involvement without necrosis usually do not show serum levels exceeding 250 IU/l (Table 2.2). The ratio of AsAT to AlAT (GOT/GPT) is less than one in 90% of the patients with acute viral hepatitis or infectious mononucleosis, but exceeds one in 95% of cases of cirrhosis. Patients with alcoholic liver disease and deficiency of vitamin B_6 (pyridoxine), a coenzyme required for transamination reactions, may have a reduction of serum AlAT despite acute hepatic damage. Although the height and duration of serum changes generally correlate with the severity of liver disease, precise parallels cannot be drawn in all instances. Serial estimations are invaluable in following the course of illness.

5'-Nucleotidase. This enzyme, found primarily in hepatic microvilli, hydrolyzes the phosphate ester bond of the nucleotide attached to the 5 position of pentose. In one commonly employed method the substrate is adenosine 5'-monophosphate (AMP). Either adenosine or phosphorus which splits off after incubation may then be quantitated. Alkaline phosphatase interferes with the reaction since it also hydrolyzes AMP. Hence, in parallel assays an inhibitor must be used which suppresses the activity of one of two enzymes. In bone disorders serum values are normal (0.3–3.2 Bodansky units, or less than 15 IU).

The enzyme is mainly useful in distinguishing bone diseases from cholestatic syndromes. 5'-Nucleotidase is probably more sensitive and definitely more specific than alkaline phosphatases in the diagnosis of cholestasis.[10]

Other enzymes. Ornithine carbamoyltransferase (an indicator of mitochondrial injury), lactic-dehydrogenase fraction 5, phosphofructose aldolase, and sorbitol dehydrogenase are used as indicators of hepatocellular damage.[10] Leucine aminopeptidase (LAP) appears elevated in cholestasis. Since LAP is not present in bone, it is considered more specific than alkaline phosphatases. All of the aforementioned enzymes are not widely employed and add little to diagnostic accuracy.

Serum gamma-glutamyl transpeptidase (GGTP). This enzyme catalyzes the gamma glutamyl group from aromatic amines to receptor amino acid or peptide. It is concentrated mainly in the kidney, with only a tenth as much in the liver and less in the pancreas and gut. Although serum levels are increased in several renal diseases and various cardiac disorders, the enzyme serves as a sensitive indicator of liver cell dysfunction.[11] Hepatic GGTP is located mainly in the microsomes and undergoes nonspecific induction.[12] Elevated levels often occur in chronic alcoholics when other tests are normal. Serum GGTP activity does not parallel the increase in aminotransferase. In acute viral hepatitis, marked elevation of aminotransferase is accompanied by a modest GGPT increase which peaks after clinical recovery.[13] Very high levels of GGPT are found in cholestasis, where its usefulness parallels alkaline phosphatases. GGPT suffers from two handicaps: lack of specificity for liver disease and false elevations produced by drug induction.

Serum Cholesterol

Many procedures are available for the determination of serum cholesterol but the basic reactions are identical. Cholesterol reacts with strong acids to produce chromogenic products, chiefly cholestadiene sulfonic acids, which appear green in the Liebermann-Burchard reaction or red in the Salkowski reaction. Esters are determined as free cholesterol after a saponification step. Serum total cholesterol ranges 150–250 mg/dl, 50–70% of which comprises the esterified fraction. Diet and age may alter this concentration. Increased values are found in cholestatic syndromes, and decreased levels in severe hepatocellular necrosis.

Alpha-fetoprotein[14,15,16]

Alpha-fetoprotein (AFP) (MW 70,000 daltons; ½ life 3–5 days) is a normal fetal protein synthesized by embryonal liver and yolk sac cells. During normal gestation AFP reaches a peak concentration of 2–4 mg/ml in the first trimester and drops rapidly to less than 50 μg/ml in the newborn umbilical cord blood. AFP continues to be produced in normal adults at 1–17 ng/ml levels. AFP can be detected by: the immunodiffusion (Ouchterlony) method with a sensitivity of about 3000 ng/ml; the counter-current immunoelectrophoretic technique, with a sensitivity of 200 ng/ml; or the radioimmunoassay method, with a sensitivity about 0.3 ng/ml. AFP is increased in hepatectomy, liver trauma, acute and chronic liver diseases (Table 2.3), hepatoma, hepatoblastoma (but not cholangiocarcinoma), testicular embryonal carcinoma (one-third are AFP-positive), occasional carcinomas of the stomach or pancreas with or without hepatic metastases, pregnancy, ataxia telangiectasia, Indian infantile cirrhosis, and congenital tyrosinemia. AFP is also occasionally demonstrated in patients with other types of entodermally derived tumors and germinal cell cancer of the testis and ovary. Except for primary hepatic tumors, the raised AFP concentrations in these conditions usually do not exceed 500 ng/ml, well below the sensitivity of immunodiffusion techniques.

Among its diagnostic functions, AFP serves as a most useful biochemical marker for the development and growth of hepatoma. Up to 95% of patients with this primary liver carcinoma are AFP-positive. Quantitative levels of AFP in hepatomas vary widely and bear little clinical or prognostic significance. Large, poorly differentiated hepatomas often are associated with higher AFP levels than small, well-differentiated tumors. Serial measurement with the radioimmunoassay method provides a prognostic guide during treatment. A decline in AFP concentration occurs with response to surgery or chemotherapy. The older literature reports a lower incidence of AFP-positive hepatocellular carcinoma in Caucasians (50% of cases) compared to 95% positivity in Asians and Africans with the

Table 2.3. Alpha-fetoprotein in liver disease.[14,15,16]

Disease	% of AFP positive cases	AFP range ng/ml	Comments
Acute viral hepatitis	30*	250	
Acute fulminant hepatitis	30–80	?	Absence (no regeneration) prognostically unfavorable
Chronic HB$_s$Ag carrier	10	50	
Chronic persistent hepatitis	10	250	
Chronic active hepatitis	30	25–4000	Transient elevation; unrelated to HB$_s$Ag status
Alcoholic cirrhosis	10	50	
Hepatoma	95	150–5.5 $\times 10^6$	Persistently high levels
Extrahepatic cholestasis; primary biliary cirrhosis	0	0	

* Response often parallels aminotransferases level.

same tumor. This difference in the frequency of positive cases reflects the sensitivity of the technique employed and the level of AFP accepted as significant and diagnostic. A true discrepancy probably does not exist.[17] The increase of AFP in nonmalignant disease is usually transient, an important differential feature in the diagnosis of hepatoma. AFP may be used to screen conditions such as cirrhosis, hemochromatosis, Budd-Chiari syndrome, alpha-1-antitrypsin deficiency, and porphyria cutanea tarda known to be associated with a high risk of hepatoma development.

Alpha$_2$-H Globulin

Alpha$_2$-H globulin, a glycoferroprotein, originates in the fetal liver. Like alpha-fetoprotein, serum levels decline soon after birth, and only trace quantities are found in the bloodstream of healthy adults. Alpha$_2$-H behaves as an acute phase protein. It is elevated in many pathological conditions, especially when malignant disease is present. Serial observations of alpha$_2$-H titers in patients with cancer show a rise 1–2 months prior to clinical evidence of local recurrence or hepatic metastases.[18] In patients with hepatoma, an alpha$_2$-H increase precedes the elevation of alpha-fetoprotein as an early signal of relapse after treatment. The physiological role of alpha$_2$-H is unknown. Both alpha-fetoprotein and alpha$_2$-H glycoprotein have immunosuppressive activity, as demonstrated by the inhibitory action on PHA-induced lymphocyte transformation. The high levels of both fetoproteins may serve to protect the fetus as a privileged immunologic site in the maternal womb. Elevated titers may also facilitate the dissemination of tumors.

Carcinoembryonic Antigens (CEA)

These serum glycoproteins, representing shared antigens between neoplastic and embryonic tissue, are increased in malignancies of the gastrointestinal tract, pancreas, and bronchus, and in alcoholic liver disease and chronic renal failure. CEA can be quantitated by a commercially available radioimmunoassay method. CEA positivity is high in alcoholic cirrhosis and alcoholic hepatitis.[19] It is present in low titers in nonalcoholic liver disease. CEA levels exceed 2.5 μg/ml in 45% of patients with alcoholic liver disease, compared to 70–90% of cases of colonic or pancreatic carcinoma. Tumors of the colon and pancreas show much higher CEA concentrations than are found in liver disease. The raised CEA activity may represent a "derepressive dedifferentiation" of endodermal-derived cancer cells, or CEA may be produced continuously in minute amounts and become increased as a result of membrane changes. The liver may act as the site of synthesis and degradation of CEA.

Serologic Markers of Viral Hepatitis Type A and B

Viral hepatitis type A antigen, HAAg, is detected by radioimmunoassay. The antibody, HAAb, can be measured by several serologic methods: complement fixation, hemagglutination immune adherence, and radioimmunoassay. The viral antigen is prepared from the liver of a marmoset monkey infected with type A virus material. The procedure is relatively complex and cumbersome. Simple and refined techniques are being developed. Patients with acute type A hepatitis also excrete 27 nm viral particles in their stools. Immune electron microscopy may be employed to visualize the particles. In type B hepatitis, all three circulating viral particles carry the surface antigenic determinant, HB$_s$Ag (previously known as Australian antigen or hepatitis-associated antigen). The immunologic methods which detect HB$_s$Ag and its corresponding antibody, HB$_s$Ab, vary in sensitivity, specificity, speed of performance, reproducibility, and expense (Table 2.4). In order of descending sensitivity, radioimmunoassay, hemagglutination inhibition, complement fixation, counterelectrophoresis, and agar gel diffusion are all commonly employed techniques.[20] The large viral agent, the so-called Dane particle, may be identified by electron microscopy of the concentrated serum. The core of the Dane particle elicits an antibody HB$_c$Ab response during infection. HB$_c$Ab is measured by complement fixation and radioimmunoassay.

HBsAg in liver disease. For a full discussion of HB$_s$Ag in liver disease see Chapter 11.

MORPHOLOGIC EVALUATION

Liver Biopsy

Morphological evaluation of hepatic dysfunction is usually obtained by means of a percutaneous needle biopsy of the liver. The procedure is useful for determining the nature of the disease and monitoring its course. Liver biopsy is a safe and accepted technique, though not without the small risks of morbidity and rare fatality. It should be done only by a trained physician on selected patients for definite indications. Precautions should include:

1. Exclusion of those with a tendency to bleed or bruise spontaneously. A careful history, platelet count, and one-stage prothrombin time test should be obtained as minimum precautionary measures.
2. Exclusion of those with an allergic reaction to the anesthetic agent.
3. Postbiopsy care should include monitoring blood pressure and pulse, prescribed bed rest for 24 hours, and pressure hemostasis achieved by lying on the side of the puncture wound for two hours.
4. The services of a blood bank and surgical team available on short notice.

Indications for liver biopsies are:

1. Jaundice of nonhematological origin: The depth and duration of jaundice are not contradictions in themselves. The need for a diagnosis overrides any risks, particularly in order to differentiate intrahepatic from extrahepatic cholestasis.
2. Hepatomegaly: Fatty liver, cirrhosis, and tumor are among the more frequent causes of liver enlargement. Determination of liver size by

Table 2.4. Comparison of tests for detecting HB_sAg and HB_sAb.[20]

Technique	Sensitivity for detecting		Specificity	Time required	Comment
	HB_sAg	HB_sAb			
Agar gel diffusion	1	1	Excellent	> 24 hr	Standard test for antigen subtypes
Counterelectrophoresis	5–10	<1	Good	hours	
Complement fixation	20–100	1	Good	24 hr	Anticomplementary activity common
Passive hemagglutination	–	1,000–10,000	Good	hours	
Passive hemagglutination inhibition	100–200	–	Good	hours	Reproducibility may be difficult
Reverse passive hemagglutination	100–500	–	Poor	hours	
Radioimmunoassay: Solid phase	100–1000	?	?	24 hr	False positives due to presence of antiguinea-pig serum protein
Double antibody	100–1000	1,000–10,000	?	> 72 hr	

From A. M. Prince, in F. F. Becker (ed.), *The Liver: Normal and Abnormal Functions*, pt B, p 579, 1975; used with permission of author and Marcel Dekker, Inc.

physical examination correlates poorly with scintiphotographic estimations. False positive and negative errors occur in about 30% of cases.[21]
3. Abnormal liver function tests of uncertain etiology: These are often due to infiltrative disease such as granuloma, metastatic carcinoma, and lymphoma, or drug-induced liver injury.
4. Hepatic malignancies: The documentation of tumor involvement of the liver affects the course of treatment.
5. Granulomatous disease: Extension to the liver is often an early and definite clue to the presence of the disease, as in sarcoidosis.
6. Fever of unknown origin: The liver biopsy frequently clarifies this difficult diagnostic problem.
7. Assessment of therapy: This is advisable in corticosteroids for chronic active hepatitis, venesection for hemochromatosis, and anabolic steroids for fatty liver.
8. Delineation of the course of disease: This aids treatment and prognosis, as in the progression of acute viral hepatitis into chronic active hepatitis.

Contraindications include the following:

1. An uncooperative, depressed, or hyporeactive patient.
2. Evidence of a possible hemorrhagic tendency, such as an abnormal prothrombin test, low platelet count, and profuse superficial bleeding at the intended site of biopsy.
3. Disease near or at the proposed pathway of biopsy, including subphrenic abscess, empyema, and hydatid cyst of the liver.
4. Marked ascites, which hinders procurement of an adequate tissue specimen. Hemorrhage is likely due to the lack of tamponade effect.
5. Severe anemia.

Reactions, Complications, and Fatality Rate

Common reactions consist of referred pain to the shoulder, pain at the site of entry, and epigastric discomfort. The symptoms are caused by the perihepatitis or pleuritis that follows every biopsy. Rare complications commonly appearing within 12 hours of the procedure are: (1) Hemorrhage into the peritoneum or pleural cavity: The misadventure results from laceration of the portal and hepatic vessels or intercostal artery. (2) Hemobilia: Colicky pain, gastrointestinal hemorrhage, and fluctuating jaundice are characteristic symptoms[22] (see also Chapter 18). (3) Bile peritonitis: This is more apt to occur in severe chronic obstructive jaundice and chronic cholangitis when large ducts are punctured. (4) Acute transient hypotension: Blood loss is not involved and the hypotension presumably is neurogenic in origin. (5) Penetration of kidney, gallbladder, stomach, colon, and pancreas: Fortunately, septic or bleeding complications are rare. (6) Bacteremia: This is reported to occur in 3% of liver biopsies.[23] The offending organism often belongs to the gram-negative group. Not dangerous in itself, bacteremia could account for the fever, hypotension, and confusion once attributed to sterile bile peritonitis or hemorrhage. (7) Intrahepatic hematoma: This has a recorded incidence of 7%.[24] It is detectable by hepatic scintiscan and is accompanied by a slight rise in serum alkaline phosphatases and elevation of aminotransferases. The hematocrit often drops by 3% or more, indicating that at least 500 ml blood is trapped in the hepatic hematoma. Despite such losses, patients appear surprisingly well.

Fatality rates vary from 0.17% in 20,000 biopsies with the Vim-Silverman needle to 0.15% in 80,000 biopsies with the Menghini needle.[25,26] The risk of death from a liver biopsy is estimated as 1 in 6000 biopsies for the Menghini technique, and 1 in 1000 biopsies for the Vim-Silverman needle.[26] The Menghini technique is somewhat safer due to the smaller-bore size of the needle (1.2 mm bore width). The advantage of using the Vim-Silverman needle is that a larger specimen is obtained, which is useful for the diagnosis of extrahepatic cholestasis and primary biliary cirrhosis. More portal triads can be observed in a larger piece of liver. The chief cause of death in doing a liver biopsy is massive intraperitoneal hemorrhage.

Diagnostic Efficiency of Liver Biopsy

There are three factors involved: the experience of the interpreter, adequacy of the biopsy specimen, and nature of the disease process. In one series, observer error among three pathologists is reported as 48% for needle biopsies and 73% for wedge biopsies in the diagnosis of cirrhosis.[27] In another study, sampling error (the representative nature of the tissue acquired) for cirrhosis is large, about 67%, whereas it is minimal for acute viral hepatitis.[28] Observer error (reliability of a single interpreter) is on the order of 25% for cirrhosis, and 10% for acute viral hepatitis. This suggests that cirrhosis is a relatively more difficult lesion to recognize than acute viral hepatitis. In metastatic carcinoma and hepatic granuloma, approximately 70–80% of the cases yield positive findings by biopsy. A simple random liver biopsy detects tumor in 50% of the cases.[29] A second biopsy increases the positive yield by 10%. Cytologic examination of fluid aspirate adds another 10% to the positive cases. This is as compared to 80% positivity by a scan-guided liver biopsy and 70% by biopsy performed during a peritoneoscopy. The high percentage of positive cases is impressive considering that a biopsy specimen samples only

1:100,000 of the original mass (15 mg average biopsy weight from a 1500-g liver). Differentiation between certain liver diseases by needle biopsy may be difficult. This is particularly true in distinguishing extrahepatic from intrahepatic cholestasis. Liver biopsy is probably accurate in about 60% of these cases.

Peritoneoscopy

This procedure, usually done in conjunction with a liver biopsy, is practiced with enthusiasm in some areas of the world, but not in the United States. Reluctance stems partly from unfamiliarity with the technique and partly from the feeling that diagnosis can be established by other less invasive means. The time requirement and risks are higher than percutaneous liver biopsy. Cirrhosis, metastatic carcinoma, hemangioma, and tuberculosis are among the lesions readily recognized with confidence. Diagnostic accuracy is poor in the detection of hepatoma, and in discriminating between intrahepatic and extrahepatic jaundice.

Abnormal Morphology

Hepatic reactions to injury are limited in their range of morphological expression. The changes include increase of fat, degenerative changes, necrosis, inflammation, duct proliferation, fibrosis, pigment accumulation, and neoplasia (Table 2.5).[30] These alterations are not often specific for a disease process. For example, the appearance of fat in the liver does not by itself denote the etiologic cause. Likewise, the pattern of spotty necrosis and lymphocytic triaditis, although most commonly seen in viral hepatitis, occurs in other viral diseases. Widespread hepatocellular necrosis and chronic inflammation may indicate chronic active hepatitis without differentiating the various forms of chronic active liver disease. In cirrhosis the fibrosis and regenerative nodules do not signify the antecedent cause. In one form of pigment accumulation, cholestasis, the histological difference between extrahepatic and intrahepatic causes is not easily separated. It should be emphasized that the proper interpretation of liver histology must include a consideration of both clinical and laboratory data. Diagnosis on tissue reaction alone, without the aid of ancillary information, is either incomplete or erroneous.

Disease Markers in Liver Tissue

Alpha-1-fetoprotein (AFP). Immunofluorescence shows AFP in hepatocytes from patients with alcoholic hepatitis and hepatocellular carcinoma. AFP may be detected in the liver without its being present in the serum.

Table 2.5. Glossary of morphologic alterations in liver disease.[30]

Terms	Synonym	Change	Distribution	Disease
Bile infarcts, lakes		Extracellular accumulations of bile	Periportal	Extrahepatic cholestasis
Bodies:				
Acidophilic	Councilman bodies Acidophilic necrosis	Densely eosinophilic, round body with or without pyknotic nuclei (necrotic hepatocytes)	Extracellular intrasinusoidal	Viral hepatitis
Mallory	Alcoholic hyalin	Irregular, densely amphophilic or eosinophilic, usually intracellular inclusion.	Centrolobular, periportal	Alcoholic hepatitis, other liver diseases
Lymphoid aggregates	Lymphoid follicles	Round collection of mononuclear inflammatory cells	Portal	Primary biliary cirrhosis, chronic active hepatitis, drug abuse associated hepatitis
Necrosis:				
Acidophilic	Acidophilic bodies	Similar to above, except may not be extracellular		
Bridging		Collapse between portal to portal or central vein with condensation of stroma		Subacute hepatitis with bridging
Piecemeal		Destruction of portal limiting plates by lymphocytes, plasma cells, histiocytes		Chronic active hepatitis, active cirrhosis, absent or minimal in chronic persistent hepatitis
Sclerosing hyaline		Leukocytes, fibrosis, degenerated liver cells, Mallory bodies	Centrolobular	Early stage of alcoholic hepatitis

Table 2.5. Glossary of morphologic alterations in liver disease.[30] (*cont.*)

Terms	Synonym	Change	Distribution	Disease
Necrosis (*cont.*)				
Spotty		Foci of necrotic or damaged hepatocytes with mononuclear inflammation	Centrolobular, panlobular	Acute viral hepatitis
Pseudoglandular transformation		Formation of liver cells around false lumen mimicking acinar structure	Variable	Regenerative phase of fulminant hepatic necrosis, galactosemia
Regenerative nodule	Cirrhotic nodule	Disturbed lobular structure, with nodulation of liver cells, abnormal vascular relationships, different rates and directions of cell growth	Diffuse	Cirrhosis
Reverse lobulation		Portal triads become center of lobules with fibrosis linking central veins	Diffuse	Cardiac cirrhosis
Rosette		Nest of swollen hepatocytes outlined by compressed reticulum and inflammatory elements	Periportal	Chronic active hepatitis
Vacuolization:				
Nuclear		Glycogen in liver cell nucleus	Focal or diffuse	Diabetes mellitus, obesity, Wilson's disease, normal infants
Cytoplasmic		Fat or glycogen in liver cell	Focal or diffuse	Fatty liver, glycogen storage disease
Von Meyerberg complex	Microhamartoma	Dilated bile ducts in fibrous tissue	Portal	Normal liver, polycystic liver

Table 2.5.   Glossary of morphologic alterations in liver disease.[30] (*cont.*)

Terms	Synonym	Change	Distribution	Disease
Degeneration:				
Balloon		Swollen, distend-ed hepatocyte with clear cyto-plasm	Focal or diffuse	Acute viral hepatitis, alcoholic hepatitis
Feathery		Liver cell damaged by bile, with swollen, thin stranded cytoplasm	Periportal	Associated with bile infarcts
			Focal	Viral hepa-titis
Granuloma		Focalized in-filtrate of in-flammatory cells and modified cells (epitheloid cells, giant cells) with or without necrosis	Diffuse or focal	Sarcoidosis, tuberculosis
Pigment:				
Hemosiderin		Dark-brown color	Diffuse or focal in hepatocytes or Kupffer cells	Hemosiderosis, hemochromatosis
Lipofuscin		Yellow-brown color, AFB positive	Centrolobular	Normal, Gilbert's disease
Bile		Variable color, PAS positive	Centrolobular initially	Cholestasis
Dubin-Johnson pigment		Dark-brown or black color, often PAS and AFB positive	Centrolobular	Dubin-Johnson disease
Malaria pigment		Dark brown, iron negative	Diffuse in RE cells	Malaria
Schistosomal pigment		Dark brown, iron negative	Diffuse or focal in RE cells	Schistosomiasis

Alpha-1-antitrypsin deficiency.   Intracytoplasmic pink globules are seen in periportal hepatocytes in hematoxylin- and eosin-stained sections. The material represents accumulated antitrypsin and gives a positive PAS reaction after pretreatment with diastase. Immunofluorescence and biochemical extraction provide further identification. The tissue deposits of antitrypsin do not correlate with the severity of hepatic dysfunction or symptoms.

HB$_s$Ag and HB$_c$Ag. Under light microscopy, HB$_s$Ag may be observed in ground-glass hepatocytes which are easily identified by staining with Gomori aldehyde fuchsin or a modified orcein method.[31,32] The cytoplasm of these cells contains tubular and spherical viral particles in the cisterna of proliferated endoplasmic reticulum, confirmed by both electron microscopic and fluoresceinated antiserum techniques. Ground-glass hepatocytes are common in HB$_s$Ag carriers and are seen in serologically positive cases of chronic hepatitis and cirrhosis. In general, an inverse relationship exists between the amount of hepatic antigen and the severity of liver disease. Chronic carriers show abundant HB$_s$Ag particles, whereas the smallest numbers are found in fulminant viral hepatitis. The particles are not observed in the damaged areas but in the better-preserved parts of the liver. On immunofluorescence and electron microscopy, HB$_c$Ag is found in liver cell nuclei, and rarely in cytoplasm. The predominance of HB$_c$Ag suggests a persistent infection or a carrier state.

REFERENCES

1. Winkle P, et al: Diagnostic value of routine liver tests. *Clin Chem* 21:71–75, 1975.
2. Javitt NB, et al: Serum bile acids, in Gen Ref No. 10, pp 156–158.
3. Korman MG, Hoffman AF, Summerskill WHJ: Assessment of activity in chronic active liver disease: Serum bile acids compared with conventional tests and histology. *New Eng J Med* 290:1399–1402, 1974.
4. Barnes S, et al: Diagnostic value of serum bile acid estimations in liver disease. *J Clin Path* 28:506–509, 1975.
5. Kaplowitz N, Kok E, Javitt NB: Post prandial serum bile acid for detection of hepatobiliary disease. *JAMA* 225:292–293, 1973.
6. LaRusso NF, et al: Validity and sensitivity of an intravenous bile acid tolerance test in patients with liver disease. *New Eng J Med* 292:1209–1214, 1975.
7. Combes B, Schenker S: Laboratory tests, in Gen Ref No. 14, pp 212–217.
8. Tygstrup N, Senoir JR, Paumgartner G: Indocyanine green (ICG) elimination test, in Gen Ref No. 10, p 145.
9. Kaplan MM: Alkaline phosphatases. *New Eng J Med* 286:200–202, 1972.
10. Hutterer F: Recent progress in clinical enzymology for the diagnosis of liver diseases, in Gen Ref No. 12, p 145.
11. Whitfield JB, et al: Serum γ-glutamyl transpeptidase activity in liver disease. *Gut* 13:702–708, 1972.
12. Whitfield, JB, et al: Changes in plasma γ-glutamyl transpeptidase activity associated with alterations in drug metabolism in man. *Brit Med J* 1:316–318, 1973.

13. Cuschieri A, Baker PR: Gamma-glutamyl transpeptidase in hepatobiliary disease—value as an enzymatic liver function test. *Brit J Exp Path* 55:110–115, 1974.
14. Silver HKB, et al: Radioimmunoassay for human alpha₁-fetoprotein. *Proc Nat Acad Sci USA* 70:526–530, 1973.
15. Kew M: Alpha-fetoprotein in primary liver cancer and other diseases. *Gut* 15:814–821, 1974.
16. Silver HKB, et al: Alpha₁-fetoprotein in chronic liver disease. *New Eng J Med* 291:506–508, 1974.
17. Kohn J, Weaver PC: Serum-alpha₁-fetoprotein in hepatocellular carcinoma. *Lancet* 2:334–337, 1974.
18. Buffe D, Rimbant C: Immunosuppressive effect of a human hepatic glycoferroprotein, α 2H globulin: A study on the transformation of normal human lymphocytes. *Immunology* 29:175–184, 1975.
19. Moore T, et al: Carcinoembryonic antigen(s) in liver disease: I: Clinical and morphological studies. *Gastroenterology* 63:88–94, 1972.
20. Prince AM: The hepatitis B antigen, in Gen Ref No. 1, pt B, p 579.
21. Halpern S, et al: Correlation of liver and spleen size: Determinations by nuclear medicine studies and physical examination. *Arch Intern Med* 134:123–124, 1974.
22. Levinson, JD, et al: Hemobilia secondary to percutaneous liver biopsy. *Arch Intern Med* 130:396–400, 1972.
23. McCloskey RV, Gold M, Weser E: Bacteremia after liver biopsy. *Arch Intern Med* 132:213–215, 1973.
24. Raines, DR, Van Heertun RL, Johnson LF: Intrahepatic hematoma: A complication of percutaneous liver biopsy. *Gastroenterology* 67:284–289, 1974.
25. Menghini G: One-second needle biopsy of the liver: Problems of its clinical application. *New Eng J Med* 283:582–585, 1970.
26. Conn HO: Intrahepatic hematoma after liver biopsy. *Gastroenterology* 67:375–381, 1974.
27. Garceau AJ, and the Boston Inter-Hospital Liver Group: The natural history of cirrhosis: II: The influence of alcohol and prior hepatitis on pathology and prognosis. *New Eng J Med* 271:1173–1179, 1964.
28. Soloway, RD, et al: Observer error and sampling variability treated in evaluation of hepatitis and cirrhosis by liver biopsy. *Amer J Dig Dis* 16:1082–1086, 1971.
29. Conn HO: Percutaneous versus peritoneoscopic liver biopsy. *Gastroenterology* 63:1074–1075, 1972.
30. Scheuer, PJ: Glossary, in Gen Ref No. 13, pp 160–163.
31. Gerber MA, Paronetto F: Hepatitis B antigen in human tissues, in Gen Ref No. 12, pp 54–63.
32. Shikata T, et al: Staining methods of Australia antigen in paraffin section: Detection of cytoplasmic inclusion bodies. *Jap J Exp Med* 44:25–36, 1974.

RADIOLOGIC EVALUATION

3

The liver can be viewed as a vascular-biliary tree scaffold supporting the parenchymal tissues. Radiologic evaluation can be directed to the morphologic and functional aspects of the various components of the liver. In general, the various techniques are complementary in nature.

Plain Film

This is the simplest but least sensitive and specific method of evaluating liver disease. Enlargement of the liver, gallbladder, and spleen may be detected. Because the liver edge perceived by the radiologist may be the posterior edge and the liver edge palpated by the clinician is the anterior edge, there can be a discrepancy between the two methods.[1] Increased overall density of the liver may be seen in hemosiderosis and hemochromatosis. Discrete calcifications within the liver may indicate infectious processes such as tuberculosis, echinococcosis, granulomatous disease of childhood, or metastatic lesions from mucinous tumors of the gastrointestinal tract. Calcifications at the porta hepatis have been described in portal vein thrombosis in the newborn and infant. Of course, 15% of gallbladder stones are calcified and may be detected on plain film. Even common duct stones may be recognized.[2]

Upper Gastrointestinal Series

An enlarged liver may indent and displace the stomach and duodenum toward the left. A dilated common duct can produce a characteristic indentation of the postbulbar duodenum and indicate an extrahepatic cause of obstructive jaundice. Inflammatory and neoplastic diseases of the pancreas may widen or indent the duodenal C-loop, particularly pancreatic head lesions. Although not the most accurate method of detecting esophageal varices, the upper gastrointestinal (UGI) series is certainly the simplest.

Hypotonic Duodenography

This procedure permits detailed evaluation of the duodenum, particularly the C-loop in which the pancreatic head nestles. It may be obtained as an adjunct to a UGI series if the examination is unsatisfactory or equivocal in its examination of the duodenum or as a primary examination in the evaluation of obstructive jaundice. Duodenal atony has been obtained traditionally with intramuscular anticholinergics, but because of contraindications such as glaucoma, prostatic hypertrophy, severe cardiac disease, and frequent side effects, intramuscular glucagon has been advocated recently.[3] Use of this drug has resulted in good duodenal atony with virtually no side effects. Glucagon, in the doses employed, does not cause hyperglycemia in diabetics.

Enlargement of the duodenal papilla may indicate edema secondary to inflammatory disease such as impacted common duct stones, pancreatitis, or acute duodenal ulcers. Ampullary malignancy may also cause an enlarged duodenal papilla. Enlargement of the head of the pancreas is detected readily by the hypotonic study, although it is often difficult to differentiate between a benign and malignant process. In addition, there is sometimes concurrent inflammatory changes surrounding a pancreatic malignancy.[4]

Oral Cholecystography

An opacified gallbladder is about 95% accurate in the detection of stones. A nonopacified gallbladder after two consecutive doses of contrast material is similarly accurate in indicating intrinsic gallbladder disease after satisfying the conditions for a normal study. The normal study is predicated on the following:[5] (1) Ingestion of contrast material. (2) Satisfactory absorption, that is, the contrast material has passed beyond the stomach (no pyloric obstruction) and has not passed too rapidly out of the GI tract because of diarrhea. Both intake and absorption of contrast material can be evaluated readily by inspection of preliminary plain film of the abdomen. (3) Normal liver function. Oral cholecystography performed during an episode of acute pancreatitis may result in nonopacification due to transient liver malfunction without biliary disease. In this case, the study should not be performed until the BSP is normal.[6]

Multiple-dose oral cholecystographic studies should probably be avoided in patients with poor hepatic or renal function, since renal failure has been reported in such patients, especially after Orabilex administration.[7] This agent is no longer used. Iopanoic acid (Telepaque) is the most commonly used contrast agent, although the recently introduced iocetamic acid (Cholebrine) appears to have fewer side effects and a higher percentage of satisfactory opacification after a single dose.[8]

Intravenous Cholangiography[9]

Iodipamide methylglucamine (Cholografin methylglucamine) is injected intravenously with resulting opacification of the common duct and gallbladder, and excretion of the contrast material into the duodenum. Since approximately 10% of the contrast material is excreted by the kidney, there is usually a faint kidney opacification. Indications for the study are (1) nonopacification of the gallbladder on oral cholecystography and the detection of cholelithiasis and choledocholithiasis; (2) recurrent symptoms after gallbladder removal (postcholecystectomy syndrome); and (3) differentiation of acute cholecystitis and acute pancreatitis.

If the total serum bilirubin is 4 mg/dl or above or the BSP retention is above 40%, the chances of visualization of the biliary system are extremely low and the examination should be postponed. Reactions such as nausea, vomiting, urticaria, and hypotension are fairly frequent (approximately 10%), although severe fatal reactions are very rare. Elevated AsAT levels are reported postinfusion, the frequency being related to the dosage. Aside from a history of previous major allergic reactions, contraindications are relative and include poor hepatic and renal function and the precarious state of a patient who might not tolerate prolonged hypotension.

Tomography of the gallbladder and common duct should be employed almost routinely as a part of the examination in the detection of calculous disease, since this greatly increases the sensitivity of the procedure.

Percutaneous Transhepatic Cholangiography[10]

A catheter sheath needle is placed percutaneously into the liver substance in order to cannulate a bile duct with subsequent injection of contrast material. This is a direct method of visualizing the entire biliary system and is not dependent on hepatic function. It is best used in patients with obstructive jaundice in whom the intravenous study would be unsuccessful. The site and often the cause of obstruction (calculus, neoplasm, or stricture) may be demonstrated. If after several attempts no duct is cannulated, then it is probable that the intrahepatic biliary tree is not dilated. If the ducts are dilated, the rate of successful examination exceeds 90%.

Complications include intraperitoneal and intrahepatic bleeding, bile peritonitis, and septicemia. There is a mortality rate of 5%. It is general policy to follow the examination with surgery unless a normal duct system is demonstrated. The catheter is left in place to provide bile drainage until surgery. A transjugular catheter with a needle-tip approach has been developed to circumvent the problem of bleeding and bile leakage since the liver capsule is not punctured in this method. It is, however, more difficult to perform, and there has not been a significant decrease in complications.[11]

Recently a new thin needle from Japan, the "Chiba needle," has been employed in the performance of percutaneous transhepatic cholangiography. The success rate is 80% or higher in entering the biliary duct, especially in the presence of dilated ducts.[12] Unlike the traditional catheter sheath needle, surgery is not required in most cases after the procedure. Complications include bile leakage and septicemia. The thin needle may also be employed to visualize the portal venous system. Use of the thin needle is gaining popularity in the United States because of the ease and relative safety of the technique.

Peroral Endoscopic Cholangiography and Pancreatography

The development of the flexible fiberoptic, side-viewing duodenoscope and its extensive clinical application in Japan have resulted in the use of this new technique for evaluating the biliary and pancreatic ductal systems. The rate of success in cannulating the desired duct exceeds 90% in experienced hands; however, the technique is difficult and requires considerable expertise.

Ideally, the endoscopic examination should precede both the percutaneous cholangiogram and angiography in the evaluation of jaundice. The few complications include pancreatitis, cholangitis, and obscure febrile reactions. Acute pancreatitis is a contraindication to the study.

Radiologic interpretation of biliary tract disease is quite reliable; however, evaluation of pancreatic disease, particularly the differentiation between benign inflammatory and malignant disease, is less certain. Recently proposed criteria for this differentiation require more general confirmation as to its reliability.[13,14,15]

Angiography

The vascular compartments of the liver may be individually studied by selective angiography.

Celiac and superior mesenteric arteriography. In this method, the hepatic arterial and portal venous systems will be visualized, but not the hepatic venous system (Figs. 3.1–4). Subselective injections of the hepatic, splenic, left gastric, and pancreatic feeding arteries with magnification techniques may be performed to increase diagnostic information. If necessary, portal venous visualization can be enhanced by the infusion of vasodilators such as tolazoline hydrochloride (Priscoline) or papaverine prior to the injection of contrast material.

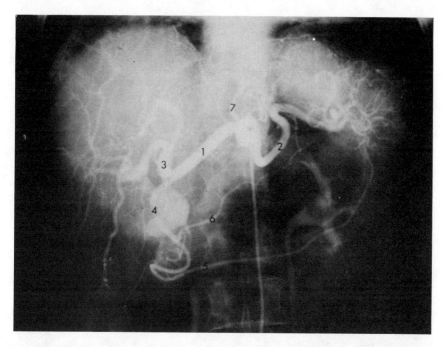

Fig. 3.1. Normal celiac arteriogram: (1) common hepatic artery, (2) splenic artery, (3) hepatic proper artery, (4) gastroduodenal artery, (5) gastroepiploic artery, (6) transverse pancreatic artery, and (7) left gastric artery.

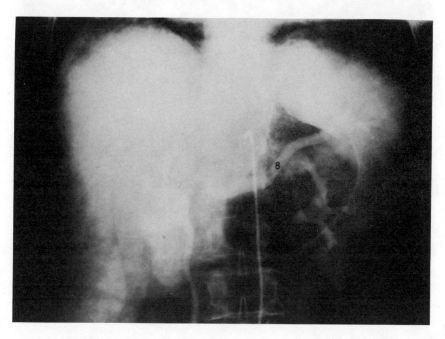

Fig. 3.2. Venous phase of celiac arteriogram: (8) splenic vein.

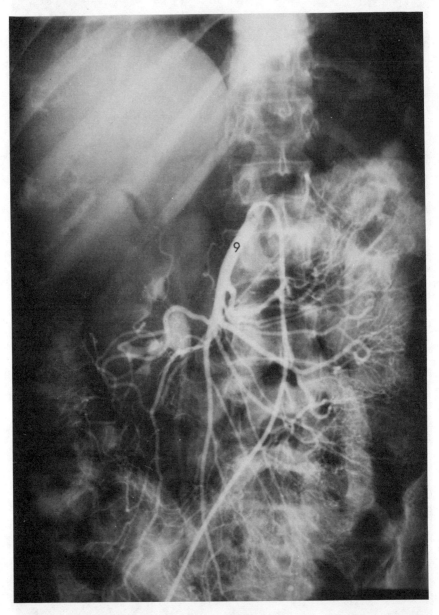

Fig. 3.3. Superior mesenteric arteriogram (post Priscoline): (9) superior mesenteric artery.

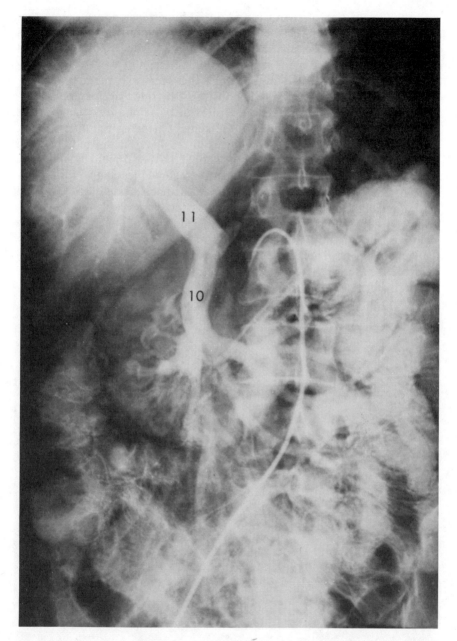

Fig. 3.4. Venous phase: (10) superior mesenteric vein, (11) portal vein. Note excellent opacification post Priscoline infusion.

In the evaluation of cirrhosis and portal hypertension, arterial portography[16] is of value in: (1) Detection of portal hypertension and varices (Fig. 3.5). The observation of hepatofugal flow (away from the liver) and visualization of esophageal varices would be diagnostic of portal hypertension. Selective injection of the left gastric artery may permit opacification of esophageal varices not demonstrated by other angiographic techniques (Fig. 3.6).[17] (2) Detection of sites of bleeding other than varices and therapy for such bleeding. In the acutely bleeding cirrhotic patient, other sites of bleeding are frequent, as in erosive gastritis and duodenal ulcer. Complementary gastroscopy should be performed in making a diagnostic evaluation. Therapy of gastrointestinal bleeding with the infusion of vasopressors, such as vasopressin, and occasionally embolization of autologous clots or other hemostatic material is well established.[18] (3) Detection of associated hepatomas. (4) Evaluation of portal vein patency and postoperative shunt patency (Fig. 3.7).

Tumors of the liver are fed by the hepatic arterial circulation. Well-vascularized tumors such as most hepatomas (Fig. 3.8), adenomas, metastatic hypernephromas (Fig. 3.9), choriocarcinomas, carcinoid tumors,

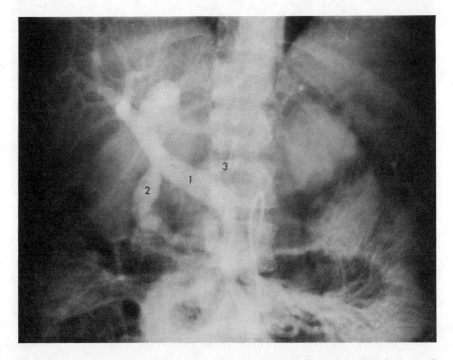

Fig. 3.5. Venous phase of superior mesenteric artery injection showing portal hypertension. Portal vein (1). Hepatofugal flow is seen with visualization of umbilical (2) and coronary (3) veins.

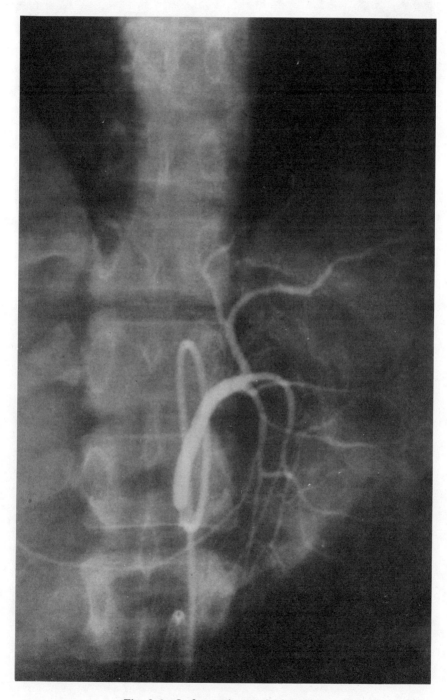

Fig. 3.6a. Left gastric arterial injection.

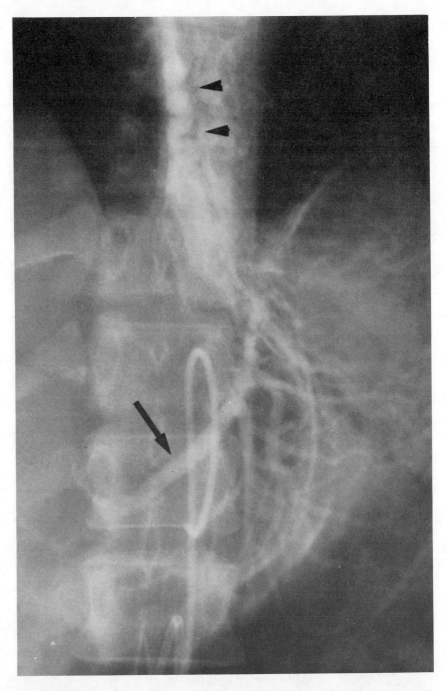

Fig. 3.6b. Venous phase shows esophageal varices (arrowheads). Note coronary vein (arrow) filling the normal drainage pathway.

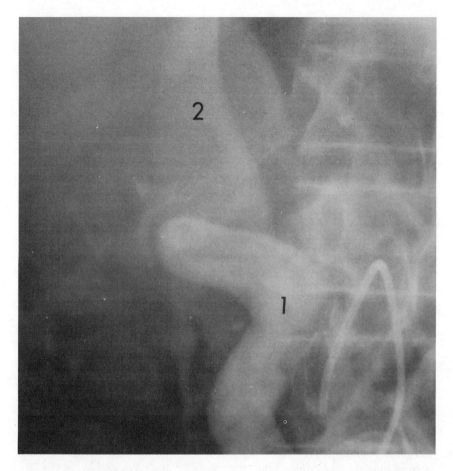

Fig. 3.7. Venous phase of superior mesenteric artery injection. Opacified portal vein (1) and inferior vena cava (2) indicates patent porto-caval anastomosis.

and islet cell tumors of the pancreas are easily detected angiographically. Avascular or poorly vascularized tumors in the liver are more difficult to detect since reliance is then placed on secondary signs such as displacement or dislocation of vessels and defects in the sinusoidal phase. Examples of such include cholangiocarcinomas, metastatic carcinomas from the breast or lung, and adenocarcinomas of the gastrointestinal tract and pancreas. Hepatic arteriography may be employed to determine the site and extent of a malignant lesion and to evaluate its resectability.[19] Abscesses and cysts of the liver are usually avascular masses. Traumatic and vascular lesions (eg, aneurysms) are most accurately assessed by angiography.

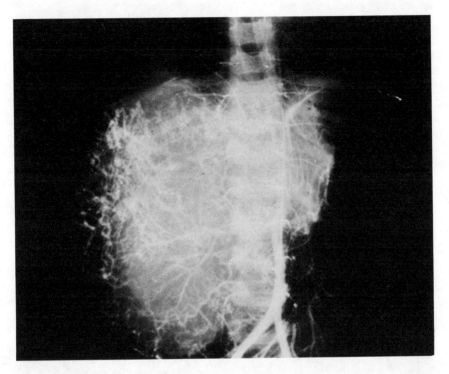

Fig. 3.8. Aortogram shows hepatoma in 4-year-old male: large liver with diffuse vascular tumor.

Hepatic venography and manometry.[16,20] Using the Seldinger method, a catheter is placed into the inferior vena cava and subsequently into a hepatic vein branch where both contrast and pressure studies may be obtained. The wedged hepatic venogram flow patterns are valuable in the evaluation of cirrhosis, as well as other causes of portal hypertension such as portal vein obstruction and hepatic vein thrombosis. The wedged hepatic vein pressure is a measure of sinusoidal pressure and indirectly reflects portal vein pressure in postsinusoidal obstruction. The catheter may also be used to record free hepatic vein, caval, and right atrial pressures, and to differentiate between suprahepatic sinusoidal hypertension (eg, congestive heart failure, constrictive pericarditis) and sinusoidal hypertension due to the intrahepatic postsinusoidal obstruction of cirrhosis.

Splenoportography.[20] Direct puncture of the spleen is performed to obtain direct visualization of the splenic and portal venous systems and to measure splenic pulp pressure. This method is used primarily in the

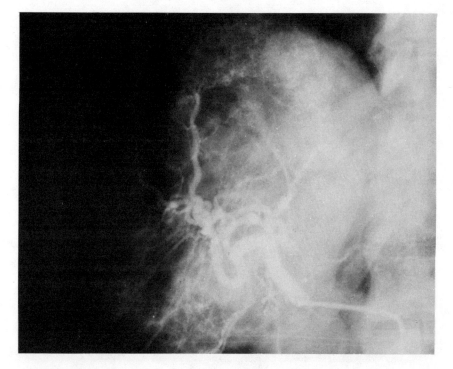

Fig. 3.9. Hepatic arteriogram: moderately vascular metastasis to liver.

evaluation of portal vein morphology and portal flow patterns in portal hypertension. Because of the possibility of splenic laceration and bleeding, this examination has been largely superseded by indirect portography following selective arterial injections. Generally, direct splenoportography is done prior to surgery or in the operating room.

Umbilical portography.[20] A catheter is placed into the left, main portal or splenic vein via an umbilical vein cutdown. Contrast opacification of the splenic and portal venous system is excellent and portal vein pressure can be measured directly. The technique has not been extensively employed because the cutdown required is usually done in the operating room, with some risk of entering the peritoneal cavity. In addition, the umbilical vein may not be entered successfully and once entered, may thrombose after the procedure, so that the procedure can be performed only once.

Transhepatic portography. Using a similar approach as in percutaneous transhepatic cholangiography, a catheter is placed into the portal vein and various branches may be selected and subsequently obliterated with

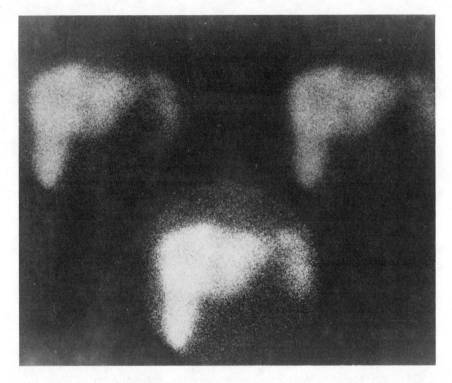

Fig. 3.10. Technetium sulfur colloid hepatic scan: enlarged liver with multiple focal defects due to colonic metastases.

injection of sclerosing agents followed with thrombin. This has been successfully employed to stop acute variceal bleeding,[21] but experience is limited.

Radioisotopic Scanning

Isotopic study of the liver is used mainly to determine gross hepatic morphology and patency of the biliary tree.[22] The localization of isotopes in the liver is based on uptake of the tracer by the reticuloendothelial cells in the liver (eg, [198]gold colloid, [99m]technetium (Tc) sulfur colloid, [67]gallium (Ga) citrate) or by the hepatocyte (^{131}I rose bengal, [67]gallium citrate, [75]selenomethionine). There are virtually no complications or contraindications and radiation dosage is minimal. Repeated follow-up studies may be obtained.

The liver size, shape, position, and integrity can be evaluated by scanning, and the most commonly used agent is ^{99m}Tc sulfur colloid. Any space-occupying lesion of the liver presents usually as a filling defect and occasionally appears as a "hot spot" on the scan, depending on the agent used. The limit of resolution is approximately 2–3 cm. The focal abnormality detected on scanning is nonspecific and may represent primary or metastatic malignancy, cyst, abscess, hematoma, and even regenerating nodules in cirrhosis (Fig. 3.10). The finding of a small liver with increased splenic and bone-marrow uptake of labeled colloid is consistent with cirrhosis and hepatocellular dysfunction (Fig. 3.11). Errors in the interpretation of scans are relatively high, approaching 20% overall, with a particularly high false negative rate.[23] A positive finding is generally more significant and would localize the site for liver biopsy.

More recently, ^{67}Ga citrate has been found to be of great value in the study of liver disease.[24] The exact mechanism of ^{67}Ga citrate uptake is unclear; however, the agent is taken up by tumor, inflammatory, reticuloendothelial, and normal liver cells. In conjunction with alpha-l-fetoprotein assay, ^{67}Ga citrate scanning of the liver is extremely accurate in the detection of primary hepatomas arising in cirrhotic livers. Detection

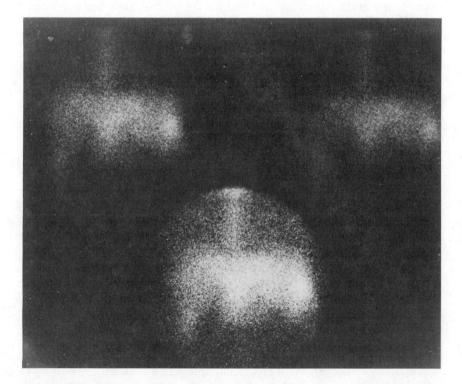

Fig. 3.11. Technetium sulfur colloid hepatic scan: small right lobe of liver with focal defects, enlarged left lobe, enlarged spleen and marrow uptake characteristic of cirrhosis. a = abscess; k = kidney.

of these hepatomas with conventional isotopic agent scanning may be difficult. ^{67}Ga citrate scanning is less useful in the detection of metastatic disease and bile duct carcinomas, but is valuable in the detection of intrahepatic and perihepatic inflammatory disease. It is of use in the staging of lymphomas, including detection of splenic and other extrahepatic sites of involvement.[25] In the liver, a ^{99m}Tc sulfur colloid scan should also be obtained, since an area of decreased uptake on the colloid scan, which appears normal on the ^{67}Ga citrate scan, would indicate an abnormal area of lymphoma.

^{131}I rose bengal is removed rapidly from the bloodstream by the hepatocyte and excreted together with bile into the gastrointestinal tract. The gallbladder is often visualized. Biliary tract patency is thus readily evaluated. Serial scans may be required to differentiate small bowel activity from renal excretion which may occur as an alternate pathway with severe liver disease or biliary obstruction. External blood clearance rate determination may be necessary to discriminate between hepatocellular disease and extrahepatic obstruction in cases where there is no excretion into the intestines. The test thus is most useful when it indicates biliary tree patency.[26]

Ultrasonics

Conventional ultrasound scanning of the liver has been of value in the evaluation of the liver size, shape, and volume. Diagnosis of focal lesions of the liver by ultrasonic investigation alone is difficult. When used in conjunction with other diagnostic methods such as the isotope scan, ultrasound is of value in differentiating a cystic from a solid lesion (Fig. 3.12). The limit of resolution of the conventional ultrasound scan is approximately 2 cm. Focal fluid collections around the liver such as hematomas or abscesses may be detected. Ascites can be detected with ease and reliability. Ultrasonic guidance of a biopsy of either a small liver or a focal hepatic lesion can be of value.[27] Ultrasound can be of value in differentiating obstructive from nonobstructive jaundice by the detection of dilated gallbladder, common duct, and also pancreatic masses.

With the development of gray-scale scanning which permits recording of intermediate levels of information lost in the conventional scan, the limit of resolution of focal lesions approaches several millimeters. The role of ultrasonic investigation of liver disease is expanding rapidly.[28]

Computed Tomography of the Liver

Computed tomography is a new technique adding computer analysis of x-ray transmission through body structures. The procedure has revolutionized evaluation of the skull, an area where its uses have been well

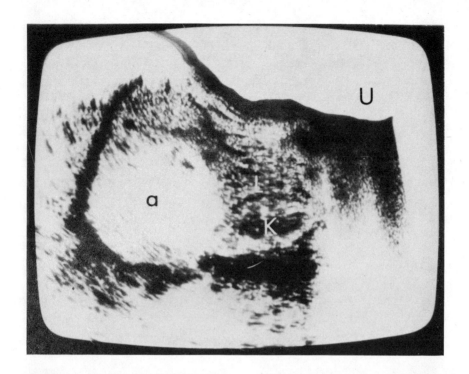

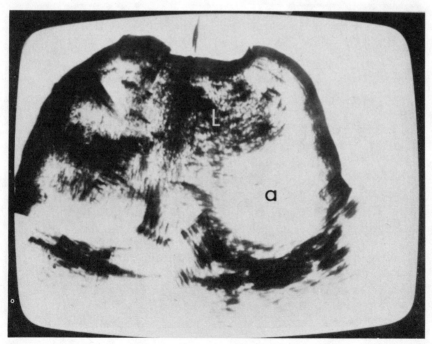

Fig. 3.12a. Longitudinal (upper) and transverse (lower) gray scale scan images of the liver. A large abscess is seen in the right lobe of the liver.

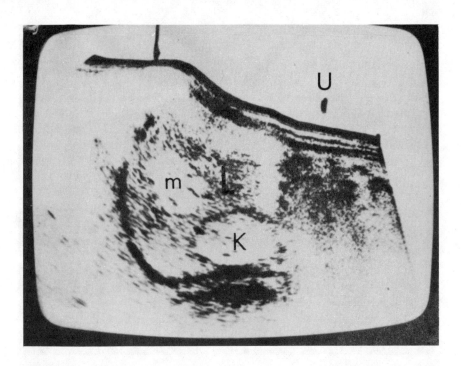

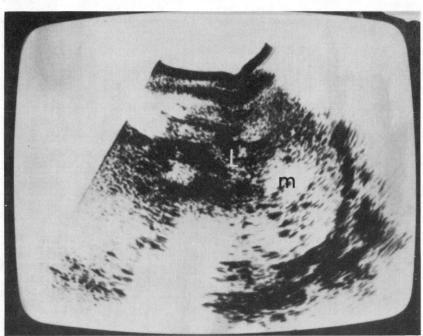

Fig. 3.12b. Longitudinal and transverse gray scale scan images of the liver show-ing multiple solid masses in the liver due to lung metastases. k = kidney; m = metastasis; u = umbilicus.

established. Its applications have been recently expanded to include visceral organs, including the liver. Primary and secondary neoplasms of the liver have been demonstrated by this technique in preliminary reports.[29,30] Further experience and technological refinements should establish the diagnostic technique in the evaluation of liver morphology. Because of its cost, the test will probably be limited to large medical centers.

REFERENCES

1. Gelfand DW: The liver: Plain film diagnosis. *Semin Roentgen* 10:177–186, 1975.
2. Clemmet AR: Radiology of the liver and bile ducts, in Margulis AR, Burhenne HJ (eds.): *Alimentary Tract Radiology.* St. Louis, C V Mosby, 1973, pp 1200–1258.
3. Miller RE, et al: Hypotonic roentgenography with glucagon. *Amer J Radiol* 121:264–274, 1974.
4. Eaton SB, Ferrucci JT Jr: Radiology of the pancreas and duodenum. Philadelphia, W B Saunders, 1972, pp 88–132.
5. Hodgson JR: The technical aspects of cholecystography. *Radiol Clin North America* 8:85–98, 1970.
6. Eaton SB, Ferrucci JT Jr, in Ref No. 4, pp 51–87.
7. Whitehouse WW: Examination of the gallbladder, in Ref No. 2, pp 1259–1263.
8. Stanley RJ, et al: A comparison of three cholecystographic agents. *Radiology* 112:513–517, 1974.
9. Wise RE: Intravenous cholangiography, in Ref No. 2, pp 1291–1302.
10. Evans JA: Transhepatic cholangiography, in Ref No. 2, pp 1339–1358.
11. Weiner M, Hanafee WN: A review of transjugular cholangiography. *Radiol Clin North America* 8:53–68, 1970.
12. Redeker AG, et al: Percutaneous transhepatic cholangiography: An improved technique. *JAMA* 231:386–387, 1975.
13. Sugawa C, et al: Peroral endoscopic cholangiography and pancreatography. *Arch Surg* 109:231–237, 1974.
14. Ogoshi K, et al: Endoscopic pancreatography in the evaluation of pancreatic and biliary disease. *Gastroenterology* 64:210–216, 1973.
15. Vennes JA: Peroral retrograde cholangiography and pancreatography, in Ref No. 2, p 1635–1653.
16. Viamonte MM Jr, Warren WD, Fomon JJ: Liver panangiography in the assessment of portal hypertension in liver cirrhosis. *Radiol Clin North America* 8:147–168, 1970.
17. Reuter SR, Atkin TW: High dose left gastric angiography for demonstration of esophageal varices. *Radiology* 105:573–578, 1972.
18. Athanasoulis CA, et al: Control of acute gastric mucosal hemorrhage. *New Eng J Med* 290:597–603, 1974.
19. Pollard JJ, Fleischli DJ, Nebesar RA: Angiography of hepatic neoplasms. *Radiol Clin North America* 8:31–42, 1970.

20. Ruzicka FF Jr: Portography, in Ref No. 2, p 1359–1390.
21. Lunderquist A, Vang J: Transhepatic catheterization and obliteration of the coronary vein in patients with portal hypertension and esophageal varices. *New Eng J Med* 291:646–649, 1974.
22. Maynard CD: Liver scanning in clinical nuclear medicine. Philadelphia, Lea and Febiger, 1969, pp 114–129.
23. Ludbrook J, Slavotinik AH, Ronai PM: Observer error in reporting on liver scan for space-occupying lesions. *Gastroenterology* 62:1013–1019, 1972.
24. James O, Wood EJ, Sherlock S: [67]Ga scanning in the diagnosis of liver disease. *Gut* 15:404–410, 1974.
25. Johnston G, Benua R, Teates CD: [67]Ga citrate in untreated Hodgkins: Preliminary report of a cooperative group. *J Nucl Med* 15:399–403, 1974.
26. Eaton SB, Ferrucci JT Jr, in Ref No. 4, pp 169–202.
27. Rasmussen, SN, et al: Ultrasound in the diagnosis of liver disease. *J Clin Ultrasound* 1:220–226, 1973.
28. Taylor KJW, Carpenter DA, McCready VR: Ultrasound and scintigraphy in the differential diagnosis of obstructive jaundice. *J Clin Ultrasound* 2:105–116, 1974.
29. Alfidi RJ, et al: Computed tomography of the thorax and abdomen; A preliminary report. *Radiology* 117:257–264, 1975.
30. Siegel S, Stanley RJ, Evans RG: Early clinical experience with motionless whole-body computed tomography. *Radiology* 119:321–330, 1976.

IMMUNOLOGIC ASPECTS

4

Recent advances in immunology have provided fresh insights into the mechanisms of disease and new diagnostic techniques. The immunologic perspective broadens our understanding of how liver injury starts and is perpetuated. Before considering the immunologic abnormalities in liver disease, a brief discussion of terminology and background facts is presented.

Hypersensitivity reactions are defined as antigen-antibody responses which damage tissues or cells. Four general types are recognized:[1]

	Type	Antigen	Antibody	Transfer to normal subject	Disease example
I.	Anaphylactic	Usually exogenous	IgE	Serum antibody	Hay fever
II.	Cytotoxic	Cell surface	Humoral	Serum antibody	RH incompatibility
III.	Immune complex	Extracellular	Humoral	Serum antibody	Serum sickness
IV.	Cell-mediated	Cell surface	Bound to T-lymphocytes	Lymphocytes	Skin graft rejection

Since type I, II, and III reactions depend on antibodies generated by B (bursa-dependent)-lymphocytes, they form the humoral immune system. Responses in these categories are immediate, hence immediate hypersensitivity occurs. In contrast, type IV response, also known as delayed hypersensitivity or cellular immunity, has a longer period involving antibodies bound to T (thymus-dependent)-lymphocytes.

Lymphocytes and the Transfer Factor

Tissue and circulating lymphocytes contain two subgroup populations—T- and B-lymphocytes—which differ in their maturation, life span, function, and final residence.[2] Both cell types are, however, derived from bone-marrow precursors. T-lymphocytes require thymus conditioning for maturation, form the majority of the recirculating lymphocytes, are long-lived, and appear in the paracortical area of the lymph node. B-lymphocytes do not require thymus conditioning, number less than T-cells in the recirculating pool, are short-lived, and populate the medullary area of the lymph node. T-lymphocytes sensitized by a specific antigen elaborate soluble mediators known as lymphokines, which commit other cells to react in the immune process. Among the well-documented lymphokines are migration inhibition factor (MIF), lymphotoxin, lymphocyte transforming factor, proliferation inhibition factor, and skin reactive factor. T-cell function is activated by transfer factor.[3] This small nonantigenic (MW 2000–4000 daltons), heat-stable, and dialyzable substance is liberated promptly from sensitized leukocytes by antigen or by chemical extraction. Transfer factor initiates cellular immunity by converting T-lymphocytes to an antigen-responsive state. Transfer factor differs from lymphokines, the effector molecules of the immunologic arc, in terms of latency, specificity, composition, and in vivo function. Transfer factor has been used to treat certain malignancies and T-cell deficiencies. The rationale is to increase the host's cellular immunity. It is also under trial for the treatment of liver diseases, such as chronic active hepatitis. There is no clear-cut evidence that transfer factor is efficacious in improving liver function.

Hypersensitivity Reactions in Liver Disease

Immunologic abnormalities in liver disease fall predominantly into type IV but also involve types II and III hypersensitivity reactions. Type I reaction is not encountered. Type II, cytotoxic-mediated injury, is probably uncommon but may account for some cases of drug-induced liver injury, acute viral hepatitis, and chronic active hepatitis. Immune complex (type III) and cell-mediated (type IV) mechanisms are implicated in the pathogenesis of acute viral hepatitis, chronic active hepatitis, some cases of cryptogenic cirrhosis, alcoholic hepatitis, and primary biliary cirrhosis. In addition, the presence of autoantibodies in these disorders, although considered epiphenomena, indicates a disturbance of autoimmunity, involving both T- and B-cell function. The persistence and high titers of autoantibodies in chronic active hepatitis, primary biliary cirrhosis, and cryptogenic cirrhosis has led to the concept of autoallergic hepatitis as the underlying disease entity.[4] In the subclinical stage all three conditions present similar hepatic lesions, presumably the result of a common pathway of tissue destruction. These hepatic disorders often share their serological abnormalities with other commonly accepted autoimmune syndromes such as Sjögren's disease, Hashimoto's disease, pernicious anemia, and collagen diseases. The hepatitis in autoimmune disorders and collagen diseases is often subclinical and overshadowed by other systemic manifestations.

Type III reactions. Immune complex-mediated hypersensitivity has been demonstrated in acute and chronic viral hepatitis associated with skin rashes and arthralgia, with membranous glomerulonephritis, and in patients with polyarthritis and vasculitis who have hepatitis. Serum sickness-like manifestations such as urticaria and arthritis appear in 5–20% of patients with acute viral hepatitis. Circulating immune complexes with HB_sAg are detected in cryoprecipitates from patients with arthritis.[5,6] The complement-fixing complexes are associated with activation of both classical and alternative complement pathways. Immune complexes are also found in the liver, kidney, skin, joints, and other organs. The tissue localization of these complexes would account for the cellular damage encountered in acute and chronic viral hepatitis.

Type IV reactions. Evidence for cell-mediated hypersensitivity has been sought in liver disease by studying the lymphokine production of lymphocytes, particularly macrophage migration inhibition factor (MIF). The rationale and techniques of the MIF test are detailed elsewhere.[4] MIF production indicates the presence of lymphocytes sensitized to specific antigens, a finding thought to represent in vivo cellular immunity. In contrast to tests for autoantibodies (see below), tests for cellular immunity, such as MIF and lymphocyte transformation (LT), are not standard laboratory procedures because they are complex and time-consuming. The clinical application of MIF and LT tests is limited. They may be useful in predicting response to steroid therapy in chronic active hepatitis and in the diagnosis of obscure drug reactions and infections.

A wide range of antigens has been employed in the MIF test, including autologous liver, pooled adult or fetal livers, liver-specific lipoprotein antigen, HB_sAg, and purified Mallory body extract. Two liver-specific antigens can be isolated from a fresh postmortem liver: a microsomal protein and an unstable lipoprotein from liver cell membranes. Both antigens, mixed with Freund's adjuvant, produce chronic hepatitis in rabbits after repeated injections over a five-month course.[7] The experiment represents the first successful animal model of chronic hepatitis induced by immunization with specific, well-delineated liver antigens.

In general, cell-mediated responses are often abnormal in acute viral hepatitis, chronic active hepatitis, and primary biliary cirrhosis, and to a lesser degree in alcoholic hepatitis (Table 4.1).[8,9,10,11,12] Recovery in these diseases is associated with the decline of abnormal immune responses and improvement in hepatic tests.

Progressive liver damage in chronic active hepatitis may be due to an autoimmune reaction directed against hepatocyte surface (lipoprotein) antigen.[13] In virus hepatitis-B infection, the T-cell recognizes the viral determinants on infected hepatocytes and destroys the cell. Some viral particles escape to enter uninfected hepatocytes. In most patients, sufficient antibody production prevents significant hepatocellular reinfection. Lack of antibody response may lead to persistent infection and HB_sAg-positive chronic active hepatitis. T-cells may also activate B-cells (the helper effect) to produce antibodies (autoantibodies) to the altered hepatocyte surface antigen. In this situation, for unknown reasons, K (killer) cells may be mobilized to kill the antibody-coated hepatocytes. K-cells are B-lymphocytes with special antibody receptors which become cytotoxic when bound to antibody-coated cells. B-cell production of autoantibodies is normally inhibited by suppressor T-cells. In HB_sAg-negative, chronic active hepatitis, liver damage proceeds because of defective suppressor T-cell function. In HB_sAg-positive disease continuous activation of helper T-cells may also increase the K-cell killing effect in the presence of normal suppressor T-cell activity.

Not only is cellular immunity responsible for tissue damage and perpetuation of hepatic lesion, it may also account for injury to other organs. Similar abnormal T-cell responses are directed against salivary gland and kidney antigens only when features of Sjögren's disease and renal tubular acidosis are present in CAH and PBC. This indicates that common surface antigens are shared by the liver and other organs. Hypersensitivity to the specific liver lipoprotein in both chronic active hepatitis and primary biliary cirrhosis reinforces the hypothesis that both entities have a common origin, as the early clinical and histological features of both disorders would suggest. The similar cellular hypersensitivity elicited in some cases of cryptogenic cirrhosis supports the theory that the disease evolves from chronic active hepatitis.

Nonorgan Specific Autoantibodies

Serum autoantibodies found in patients with liver disease are neither species nor organ specific.[4] They are directed against subcellular organelles or soluble proteins shared by the liver and other organs. The autoantibodies are not pathogenic in terms of tissue destruction, but are important mainly in diagnosis. They include primarily antinuclear, smooth muscle, and mitochrondrial antibodies. All three are usually detected by their immunofluorescent staining. Other less defined or less useful an-

Table 4.1 Migration inhibition factor in liver diseases.[8,9,10,11,12]

	Antigen						
	Autologous liver HBsAg −	Autologous liver HBsAg +	Fetal and adult liver	HBsAg	Liver-specific lipoprotein	Bile protein (biliary epithelial antigen)	Tamm-Horsfall glycoprotein
Acute viral hepatitis HBsAg positive	0	90%	10% transient	95%	?		
HBsAg carriers				?30%	50% transient		
Chronic persistent hepatitis	0	0		10%			
Chronic active hepatitis HBsAg positive	70%	40%	50%	100%	70%	80%	90%*
Alcoholic hepatitis	60%		0	0	?		
Cirrhosis: Alcoholic	0	0	10%	0	0		
Cryptogenic	0	0	30%		?		
Primary biliary cirrhosis	50%		64%		50%	30%	
Hemochromatosis	0		0		0		90%*
Extrahepatic obstruction	0		0		?	0	

* Abnormal responses obtained in patients who also had renal tubular acidosis.

tibodies described in liver disease include bile duct antibody, bile canalicular antibody, and antireticulum antibody.

Antinuclear antibodies. Antinuclear antibodies are detected by indirect immunofluorescence on fresh rat liver sections or human buffy coat smears (Table 4.2).[4] These antibodies occur in collagen and drug-induced diseases not affecting the liver, which limits their usefulness in diagnosing hepatic disorders. Occasionally, antinuclear antibodies arise and persist in patients with acute viral hepatitis who progress to chronic liver disease. In such cases, the presence of these autoantibodies may indicate genetically susceptible individuals.

Smooth muscle antibodies. Smooth muscle antibodies are usually detected in fresh unfixed rat stomach (Table 4.2).[4] This marker has its greatest usefulness in diagnosing chronic active hepatitis, but it is not specific nor are high titers common. Smooth muscle antibodies consist of a family of antibodies directed against contractible fibers in various other tissues. The autoantibodies are also commonly found in infectious mononucleosis.

Mitochondrial antibodies. Mitochondrial (M) antibodies are detected by immunofluorescence in unfixed frozen sections of rat or human stomach, thyroid, and kidney (Table 4.2).[4,14] The autoantibodies are not confined to any immunoglobulin class and can fix complement. M antibodies are directed against lipoproteins along the inner mitochondrial membrane of distal renal tubules, newborn brown fat, and other tissue. Over 90% of the cases of primary biliary cirrhosis give a positive M test. The antibodies may also be found in some patients with cryptogenic cirrhosis, usually middle-aged females, with cholestasis and histological features similar to PBC. Some patients with chronic active hepatitis resemble PBC clinically, and show comparable high-titered M antibodies. The reaction must be differentiated from that produced by the liver-kidney-microsomal antibodies which stain the proximal renal tubules of the rat.[15,16] Patients with liver-kidney-microsomal antibodies form a subgroup different from patients with chronic active hepatitis and positive M antibodies. They are younger, the sex incidence is equal, cholestasis is absent, and both antinuclear and smooth muscle reactivity is lacking. Positive M antibodies have been reported in chronic, prolonged, extrahepatic biliary obstruction in one study.[17] Almost all other authors, however, record negative M reactivity or a very low positive frequency in chronic extrahepatic cholestasis.[18,19] M antibodies are useful serological markers of primary biliary cirrhosis. A high titer excludes chronic extrahepatic duct obstruction.

Table 4.2 Autoantibodies commonly detected in liver disease.[4]

Groups	Autoantibodies		
	Antinuclear	Smooth muscle	Mitochondrial
Normal population	5%*		1%
Acute viral hepatitis	Rare	60%, low titer, transient	2%
Chronic active hepatitis	70-80% high titer, diffuse pattern, Ig class	70%, high titer in 25%, usually persistent	20%, low titer
Cirrhosis	Same as PBC	40%	25%, low titer
Primary biliary cirrhosis	25%, usually low titer, ½ speckled pattern	50% low titer	>90%, 50% high titer unaffected by therapy, persistent
Extrahepatic biliary obstruction			1%
Collagen diseases			1-8%
Drugs	Variable high incidence, high titer		Very low incidence, transient

*Positive cases.

Other autoantibodies. These are described in Table 4.3. None of the autoantibodies in this group are detected on a clinical basis in contrast to the above three autoantibodies.

T- and B-Lymphocytes

T- and B-lymphocytes bear different surface markers which allow for serological differentiation. T-lymphocytes are identified by reaction with theta-antibody and spontaneous formation of rosettes with sheep erythrocytes. B-lymphocytes bear surface receptors for C3 complement, Fc portion of IgG, and other immunoglobulins. Immunofluorescent conjugates of immunoglobulins and complement stain B- (but not T-) lymphocytes.

T-cells are decreased in acute viral hepatitis, fulminant hepatitis, chronic persistent and chronic active hepatitis, and alcoholic hepatitis.[20]

Table 4.3   Other autoantibodies in liver disease.

Autoantibody	Type	Disease association
Antiductular antibody	?	75% of cases with primary biliary cirrhosis; 70% of acute viral hepatitis; 10% of normal population
Antireticulum antibodies[39]	5 types described	Chronic heroin addicts with liver disease; dermatitis herpetiformis; celiac disease
Bile canalicular antibody[40]	Resembles SMA	30% of patients with primary biliary cirrhosis or viral hepatitis; small proportion of chronic active hepatitis and cryptogenic cirrhosis; not limited to liver disease
Antihuman albumin antibody[41]	IgA	40% of cases of alcoholic cirrhosis
Antiglomerular antibody[42]	?	Found in chronic active but not chronic persistent hepatitis
Rheumatoid factor[43]	IgM, IgG, IgA	60% of patients with acute liver disease; elevated titers also occur in various chronic liver diseases
Mallory body antibody[44]	?	Found in severe alcoholic hepatitis; preceded by appearance of serum Mallory body antigen

The decrease is transient in viral hepatitis and alcoholic hepatitis.[21] A reduction of smaller magnitude is also observed in alcoholic fatty liver. The percentage of T-lymphocytes remains unchanged in alcoholic cirrhosis and HB_sAg carriers.

B-lymphocytes are increased in acute viral hepatitis and in chronic persistent and active hepatitis.

T-cells predominate in the livers of patients with alcoholic liver disease, but in nonalcoholic liver disorders T- and B-cells are found in similar proportions.[22] Low circulating T-cells correlate with the increased hepatic content of T-cells, especially in alcoholic hepatitis.

Immune Globulins

Cryoglobulinemia and paraproteins.   Cryoglobulinemia of more than 100 mg/dl occurs in less than 10% of sera tested.[23,24] The association between cryoglobulinemia and liver disease is even rarer. Over 60% of the patients with cryoglobulinemia and liver disease have paraproteins.[23] In acute viral hepatitis, the monoclonal spikes consist of free and bound immunoglobulin chains, with antibody activities directed against IgG and alpha-1-fetoprotein. Concurrently, smooth muscle antibodies and HB$_s$Ag may appear in these cases; both paraproteins and antibodies usually disappear. In chronic active hepatitis the paraproteins, of similar range, persist unchanged over several years. In primary biliary cirrhosis, lasting paraproteins are mainly limited to the IgMK class, with antibody activity directed against mitochondria. The association between cryoglobulinemia and other types of cirrhosis is also recorded. The paraprotein production represents disturbed synthesis by clones of uncontrolled plasma cell proliferation. Monoclonal antibodies are directed against the autoantigens that are similar to the polyclonal antibodies encountered in liver disease. What pathogenic function these monoclonal antibodies may perform is obscure at present.

Serum gamma globulin and immunoglobulin. The hypergamma-globulinemia of liver disease includes all classes of immunoglobulin except IgD. The increase in IgE is frequently out of proportion to other immunoglobulins.[25] Over 50% of the patients with acute and chronic liver disease show an elevation of serum IgE level. The cause is not known. The development of a monoclonal pattern for a polyclonal increase may herald the onset of a lymphoma or multiple myeloma. Abnormalities of serum immunoglobulin values are regularly present in chronic liver disease. There is no correlation between a specific pattern of immunoglobulin alteration and the disease type (Table 4.4).

Hepatitis

Acute viral hepatitis.   High IgM levels are common, particularly in the first two weeks of illness. Raised IgM values are more frequent in type A hepatitis than in type B hepatitis. Unresolved hyperglobulinemia indicates evolution into chronic active hepatitis.

Chronic persistent hepatitis.   Slight to moderate elevation of gamma globulin may persist for months and decline with resolution of the disease.

Chronic active hepatitis.   Marked hyperglobulinemia and mild hypoalbuminemia are characteristic features. High IgG levels predominate, although IgA and IgM also are usually increased. The degree of hyperglobulinemia correlates with the severity of the disease. An increase in IgM is reported during corticosteroid treatment. Response to therapy may be gauged by following gamma globulin levels.

Table 4.4 Immunoglobulin levels in liver disease.[45,46]

	IgG	IgA	IgM	IgD	IgE
Acute viral hepatitis:					
HB$_s$Ag positive	N or ↑	N or ↑	N		↑↑↑
HB$_s$Ag negative	N or ↑	N or ↑	↑		
Chronic active hepatitis	↑↑↑	N or ↑	N	N	↑↑↑
Cryptogenic cirrhosis	↑ or ↑↑	N or ↑	N or ↑	N	↑↑↑
Primary biliary cirrhosis	N or ↑	N or ↑	↑↑↑	N	
Alcoholic cirrhosis	↑ or ↑↑	↑↑ or ↑↑↑	↑ or ↑↑	N	↑↑↑
Drug-induced cirrhosis	N	N	N		
Chronic extrahepatic cholestasis	N	↑	N	N	
Wilson's disease	N	N	N or ↑	N	
Hemochromatosis	N	N	N or ↑	N	

↑ , ↑↑ , ↑↑↑ = mild, moderate, marked elevation; N = normal levels.

Cirrhosis

Alcoholic cirrhosis. The main finding is a significant reduction in serum albumin with raised gamma globulin. The gamma globulin elevation characteristically obliterates the beta and gamma globulin gap, leading to beta-gamma fusion. The hyperglobulinemia is due to a predominant rise of IgA.

Cryptogenic cirrhosis. The pattern of increased immunoglobulin is similar to that of chronic active hepatitis, but the increments are smaller.

Primary biliary cirrhosis. Marked IgM hyperglobulinemia distinguishes this disease from drug-induced liver disease or early extrahepatic biliary obstruction. The IgM increase occurs early in the course of the illness.

Hyperglobulinemia in Liver Disease[26]

The liver is not a site for large-scale gamma globulin production. Hepatocytes do not synthesize the protein, nor is the population of immunoglobulin-secreting cells in liver disease large enough to account for the hypergammaglobulinemia. There is evidence that the increased antibody production occurs elsewhere in the RE system. Both spleen and lymph nodes undergo hyperplasia and hyperactivity in acute and chronic liver injury.[27] Cirrhotic patients react to immunization with tetanus toxoid and other antigens with enhanced antibody response. High-titered antibodies to naturally occurring antigens associated with dietary proteins (gluten), and gastrointestinal bacteria (notably *Escherichia coli* and bacterioides) are also found in cirrhosis. Chronic active hepatitis is associated with elevated antibody titers to measles and rubella, but antibody levels are normal in alcoholic cirrhosis or primary biliary cirrhosis.[28] Cytomegalovirus antibodies appear to increase in patients with all three conditions. Antibody levels to herpes simplex, varicella/zoster, parainfluenza 1, and *Mycoplasma pneumoniae* in all three forms of chronic liver disease do not differ from controls. These findings suggest that the antigenic stimulus for hyperimmunoglobulinemia is unrelated to the cause of the liver disease.

The liver may influence antibody production by the following mechanisms: (1) Failure of Kupffer cells to sequester antigens. The liver normally receives antigens from the gastrointestinal tract in the portal blood flow. Liver damage and portacaval shunting render ineffective the normal sequestration function of the Kupffer cells. These antigens bypass the liver to reach other RE sites where stimulation leads to antibody production. The inverse relationship of increased gamma globulin and decreased serum albumin in chronic liver disease is reproduced in normal rats with end-to-side portacaval shunts.[29] In this model the fall in albumin value may be attributed to malnutrition, as the animals fail to gain weight and survive a shorter length of time, as compared to controls. The rise of gamma globulin cannot be explained on this basis. Antibody titer to *E. coli* liposaccharide also shows an increase in the shunted group. Induction of cirrhosis in rats leads to reduced capacity of the liver to trap antigen and an increase in antigen in the spleen. These experiments support the thesis that gamma globulin rises in chronic liver disease as a result of the reduced trapping capacity of the liver. Kupffer cell dysfunction also leads to failure to detoxify bacterial endotoxins from the gastrointestinal tract. This could account for the low-grade endotoxinemia encountered in cirrhosis.[30] The extrahepatic manifestations of cirrhosis such as fever, intravascular coagulation, and depressed cardiac function may be due to the endotoxin effect. (2) Release of sequestered antigen by injured Kupffer cells. This would also result in excessive antibody synthesis. (3) Decreased immunological surveillance associated with abnormal cell-mediated T-cell function and hyperreactivity of B-cell antibody function. Cooperation between T- and B-cells is important for production of certain antibodies. Loss of T-cell control is inversely related to overcompensation by B-cell reactivity. This is seen in collagen diseases, lepromatous leprosy, and sarcoidosis, in which defective cell-mediated immunity is accompanied by increased immunoglobulin levels. A similar mechanism may occur in chronic active hepatitis and primary biliary cirrhosis where both impaired T-cell function and hypergamma-globulinemia are observed.

Immunoglobulins in Liver Tissue[31]

By using immunofluorescent staining, IgA-containing cells are found to predominate in acute viral hepatitis. A shift from IgA to IgG occurs when acute hepatitis progresses to chronic active hepatitis. Immunofluores-cence is seen mainly in periportal areas associated with piecemeal ne-crosis. In primary biliary cirrhosis, contrary to expectations, fluorescent staining is low but IgM-containing cells are more frequent than in other liver diseases. Alcoholic cirrhosis, alcoholic fatty liver, and cryptogenic cirrhosis, as well as normal liver, show little or no immunoglobulin staining. Complement-containing cells are not present in normal or dis-eased livers. There is no correlation between serum levels and hepatic contents of immunoglobulins.

Serum Complement[32,33,34,35]

The complement system consists of nine (C1 to C9) protein components which, once activated, act in a well-defined, cascading sequence. The end effect is to produce cell lysis by creating holes in the cell membrane. Immune adherence, chemotaxis, and anaphylatoxin activity are other side effects of this reaction. Serum complement activity may be quanti-tated by the measurement of serum C3 (beta lC), or serum C4, or by the hemolytic assay for total complement (CH_{50}). The latter two tests are considered more sensitive indicators of in vivo complement abnormalities than the test for C3. The liver produces C3 and C6; C7 is apparently not produced by the liver, although it may have a role in its catabolism.

In acute viral hepatitis serial determinations of C3 complement levels reveal an initial drop during the first week of illness, then a rise above normal during the second to fourth week, followed by a decline to normal complement activity by the sixth week.[32] In chronic liver disease, hypocomplementemia is not uncommon. The low-complement activity is due to decreased hepatic synthesis or increased consumption by immune complex formation, or both. Hypocomplementemia is generally as-sociated with decrease of synthesis of coagulation factors (II, V, VII, and X) but not with HB_sAg, smooth muscle and mitochondrial antibodies, and rheumatoid factor.

Histocompatibility Antigen

The association between HL-A (human leukocyte antigen) antigens and disease would indicate that certain immune responses are genetically determined. In autoimmune thyroiditis in the mouse, the degree of tissue damage and antibody response to thyroglobulin are dependent on the presence of a particular histocompatibility antigen. In humans, among liver diseases, only chronic active hepatitis has shown a strong association with HL-A antigens.[36,37] The frequency of HL-AI and HL-A8 in patients with chronic active hepatitis, especially the cryptogenic group,[37] is significantly higher than in two control groups: other liver diseases and normal Caucasians. In primary biliary cirrhosis, the distribution of HL-A antigens does not differ from that of the control group.[38]

REFERENCES

1. Roitt I: *Essential Immunology*. Oxford, Blackwell Scientific Publications, 1974, pp 129–132.
2. Craddock CG, Longmire R, McMillan R: Lymphocytes and the immune response. *New Eng J Med* 28:324–331, 1971.
3. Lawrence HS: Mediators of cellular immunity. *Transplant Proc*. 5:49–58, 1973.
4. Doniach D, Walker G: Immunopathology of liver disease, in Gen Ref No. 9, pp 381–402.
5. Wands JR, et al: The pathogenesis of arthritis associated with acute HB$_s$Ag-positive hepatitis: Complement activation and characterization of circulating immune complexes. *J Clin Invest* 55:930–936, 1975.
6. McIntosh RM, Koss NM, Gocke DJ: The nature and incidence of cryoproteins in hepatitis B antigen (HB$_s$Ag) positive patients. *Quart J Med* 45:23–38, 1976.
7. Meyer zum Büschenfelde KH, Kössling EK, Miescher PA: Experimental chronic active hepatitis in rabbits following immunization with human liver proteins. *Clin Exp Immunol* 11:99–108, 1972.
8. Miller J, et al: Cell-mediated immunity to a human liver-specific antigen in patients with active chronic hepatitis and primary biliary cirrhosis. *Lancet* 2:296–297, 1972.
9. Smith, MGM, et al: Cell-mediated immune responses in chronic liver disease. *Brit Med J* 1:527–530, 1972.
10. Gerber MJ, et al: Cell-mediated immune response to hepatitis B antigen in patients with liver disease. *Amer J Dig Dis* 19:637–643, 1974.
11. Newble DI, et al: Immune reactions in acute viral hepatitis. *Clin Exp Immunol* 20:17–28, 1975.
12. Howlett SA, McGuigan JE: Inhibition of macrophage migration in response to hepatitis B$_s$ antigen. *Gastroenterology* 69:960–964, 1975.

13. Eddleston ALWF, Williams R: Inadequate antibody response to HBA$_g$ or suppressor T-cell defect in development of active chronic hepatitis. *Lancet* 2:1543–1545, 1974.
14. Doniach D, Walker G: Mitochondrial antibodies (AMA). *Gut* 15:664–668, 1974.
15. Rizzetto M, Swana G, Doniach D: Microsomal antibodies in active chronic hepatitis and other disorders. *Clin Exp Immunol* 15:331–344, 1973.
16. Rizzetto M, Bianchi FB, Doniach D: Characterization of the microsomal antigen related to a subclass of active chronic hepatitis. *Immunology* 26:589–601, 1974.
17. Lam KC, Mistilis SP, Perrott N: Positive antibody tests in patients with prolonged extrahepatic biliary obstruction. *New Eng J Med* 286:1400–1401, 1972.
18. Kaplowitz N, et al: Hepatobiliary diseases associated with serum antimitochondrial antibody (AMA). *Amer J Med* 54:725–730, 1973.
19. Richer G, Viallet A: Mitochondrial antibodies in extra-hepatic biliary obstruction. *Amer J Dig Dis* 19:740–744, 1974.
20. Dehoratius RJ, Strickland RC, Williams RC Jr: T and B lymphocytes in acute and chronic hepatitis. *Clin Immunol Immunopath* 2:353–360, 1974.
21. Williams RC Jr, et al: Reduction in circulating T lymphocytes in alcoholic liver disease. *Lancet* 2:488–490, 1974.
22. Husby G, et al: Localization of T and B cells and alpha fetoprotein in hepatic biopsies from patients with liver disease. *J Clin Invest* 56:1198–1209, 1975.
23. Roux MEB, et al: Paraproteins with antibody in acute viral hepatitis and chronic autoimmune liver diseases. *Gut* 15:396–400, 1974.
24. Florin-Christensen A, Roux MEB, Arana RM: Cryoglobulins in acute and chronic liver diseases. *Clin Exp Immunol* 16:599–605, 1974.
25. Van Epps DE, et al: Liver disease—a prominent cause of serum IgE elevation. *Clin Exp Immunol* 23:444–450, 1976.
26. Triger DR, Wright R: Hyperglobulinaemia in liver disease. *Lancet* 1:1494–1496, 1973.
27. Thomas HC, MacSween RNM, White RC: Role of the liver in controlling the immunogenicity of commensal bacteria in the gut. *Lancet* 1:1288–1291, 1973.
28. Triger DR, Kurtz JB, Wright R: Viral antibodies and autoantibodies in chronic liver disease. *Gut* 15:94–98, 1974.
29. Keraan M, et al: Increased serum immunoglobulin levels following portacaval shunt in the normal rat. *Gut* 15:486–472, 1974.
30. Nolan JP: The role of endotoxin in liver injury. *Gastroenterology* 69:1346–1356, 1975.
31. Husby G, et al: Detection of immunoglobulins in paraffin-embedded liver biopsies: Studies in 100 patients with special regard to immunological findings in active chronic hepatitis. *Scand J Gastroenterol* 8:621–629, 1973.
32. Kosmidis JC, Leader-Williams LK: Complement levels in acute infectious hepatitis and serum hepatitis. *Clin Exp Immunol* 11:31–35, 1972.
33. Potter BJ, Trueman AM, Jones EA: Serum complement in chronic liver disease. *Gut* 14:451–456, 1973.

34. Thompson RA, et al: Serum immunoglobulins, complement levels and autoantibodies in liver disease. *Clin Exp Immunol* 14:335–346, 1973.
35. Kourilsky O, Leroy C, Peltier AP: Complement and liver cell function in 53 patients with liver disease. *Amer J Med* 55:783–798, 1973.
36. Page AR, et al: Genetic analysis of patients with chronic active hepatitis. *J Clin Invest* 56:530–535, 1975.
37. Lindberg J, et al: Trigger factors and HL-A antigens in chronic active hepatitis. *Brit Med J* 4:77–79, 1975.
38. Galbraith RM, et al: HL-A antigens in active chronic hepatitis and primary biliary cirrhosis. *Digestion* 10:304–305, 1974.
39. Rizzetto M, Doniach D: Types of "reticulum" antibodies detected in human sera by immunofluorescence. *J Clin Path* 26:841–851, 1973.
40. MacSween RNM, et al: Bile canalicular antibody in primary biliary cirrhosis and in other liver diseases. *Lancet* 1:1419–1421, 1973.
41. Hauptman S, Tomasi TB Jr: Antibodies to human albumin in cirrhotic sera. *J Clin Invest* 54:122–127, 1974.
42. Levy RL, Hong R: Antiglomerular antibody in chronic active and chronic persistent hepatitis. *J Ped* 85:155–158, 1974.
43. Markenson JA, et al: The interaction of rheumatoid factor with hepatitis B surface antigen-antibody complexes. *Clin Exp Immunol* 19:209–217, 1975.
44. Kanagasundaram N, et al: Occurrence of serum alcoholic hyalin antigen (AHAg). *Gastroenterology* 70:(A-127)985, 1976.
45. Feizi T: Immunoglobulins in chronic liver disease. *Gut* 9:193–198, 1968.
46. Bevan G, Baldus WP, Gleich GJ: Serum immunoglobulin levels in cholestasis. *Gastroenterology* 56:1040–1046, 1969.

JAUNDICE AND CHOLESTASIS

5

Jaundice and cholestasis represent the liver's inability to excrete organic anions. Although jaundice and cholestasis commonly occur together, they are separate pathological processes. Jaundice often develops in the absence of cholestasis, but cholestasis without jaundice is infrequent. Jaundice results from a disturbance of bilirubin metabolism, whereas the primary defect in cholestasis appears to involve the metabolism of bile salts. Consult Chapter 1 for a discussion of normal bilirubin and bile salt metabolism.

JAUNDICE (ICTERUS)

Yellow pigmentation of the sclera and skin is detectable when total serum bilirubin exceeds 2 mg/dl. Both tissues are rich in elastin, which has a strong affinity for bilirubin. This may account for the disparity between bilirubinemia and the depth of jaundice. It is not unusual for a patient to remain yellow after the serum bilirubin has returned to normal. The severity of jaundice is dependent on the rate of production and excretion of bilirubin. In total bile duct obstruction, jaundice may be variable due to enhanced renal excretion of the bile pigment. Serum bilirubin concentration in this case does not exceed 40 mg/dl. Conjugated bilirubin penetrates tissue easily because of its water solubility, and thus produces a more intense jaundice than a comparable rise in unconjugated bilirubin. Hemolytic jaundice is often less intense than hepatocellular or obstructive jaundice. Carotenemia and the yellowish discoloration due to atabrine treatment may be confused with jaundice. Both conditions produce little or no scleral pigmentation.

Disorders associated with jaundice can be classified on the basis of pathophysiological mechanisms or disease etiology. In the former approach bilirubin metabolism may be deranged at the following steps: (1) overproduction of bilirubin, (2) defect in hepatic uptake, (3) decreased conjugation of bilirubin, (4) intrahepatic impairment of biliary excretion, and (5) disturbance of the extrahepatic bile duct passage.

Clinically the term hemolytic jaundice would encompass a defect in step 1; hepatocellular jaundice, steps 2, 3, and 4; and obstructive jaundice, step 5. A useful classification of jaundice is presented in Table 5.1.

Jaundice in the Newborn

For a full discussion of liver disorders in the newborn see Chapter 15.

Heritable, Congenital Disorders of Bilirubin Metabolism

Functionally, three groups can be recognized: disorders due to impairment of hepatic uptake, those due to impairment of conjugation, and those due to impairment of hepatic excretion (Table 5.2).[1] The first two groups produce an unconjugated hyperbilirubinemia; the third group, an

Table 5.1   Classification of jaundice.[1]

 I. Overproduction of bilirubin (unconjugated fraction predominates)
   1. Hemolysis
   2. Ineffective erythropoiesis
 II. Defect in hepatic uptake (membrane transport or cytosol binding with Y or Z proteins)
   1. Inheritable: Gilbert's disease
   2. Drugs: flavaspidic acid, bunamiodyl
   3. Prolonged fasting
   4. Hepatocellular disease: cirrhosis, viral hepatitis
III. Decreased conjugation (decreased glucuronyl transferase)
   1. Inheritable deficiency: Crigler-Najjar syndrome, types I and II
   2. Physiologic jaundice of newborn
   3. Acquired transferase deficiency
      a. Drugs: pregnanediol, novobiocin
      b. Hepatocellular disease: cirrhosis, viral hepatitis
IV. Intrahepatic impairment of biliary excretion
   1. Inheritable disorders: Dubin-Johnson syndrome, Rotor syndrome
   2. Drug-induced: estradiol, methyltestosterone, oral contraceptives, chlorpromazine
   3. Hepatocellular disease: cirrhosis, viral hepatitis
   4. Rare conditions: cholestasis of pregnancy, recurrent intrahepatic cholestasis
 V. Extrahepatic blockage of bile ducts
   1. Stone
   2. Postoperative stricture
   3. Primary or secondary tumor

Table 5.2 Heritable, congenital disorders of bilirubin metabolism.

I. Impaired hepatic uptake
   ? Gilbert's disease
II. Impaired bilirubin conjugation (decreased glucuronyl transferase deficiency)
   1. Gilbert's disease
   2. Crigler-Najjar syndrome, types I and II
   3. Physiological jaundice of newborn (normal delayed development of glucuronide conjugating enzyme)
   4. Transient familial neonatal hyperbilirubinemia (inhibitory effect of maternal serum on bilirubin conjugation)
III. Impaired hepatic excretion
   1. Dubin-Johnson syndrome
   2. Rotor's syndrome
   3. Cholestasis of pregnancy
   4. Recurrent intrahepatic cholestasis

elevated conjugated bilirubinemia. Gilbert's disease is the most common disorder in the third group, affecting some 5% of the male population.

Gilbert's Disease

This benign condition, also known as constitutional hepatic dysfunction, comprises a heterogeneous etiology. The underlying defect in some cases is due to impaired hepatic uptake of bilirubin; in others, a decrease in glucuronyl transferase is found. Reduction of the cytosol-binding Y and Z proteins for bilirubin has also been proposed. Mild jaundice is the presenting and only manifestation. Except for a low-grade increase of serum unconjugated bilirubin (rarely exceeding 3 mg/dl), biochemical tests and hepatic histology are normal. In some cases the liver biopsy shows excess deposition of lipofuscin pigment in the centrolobular area. The jaundice may often go unrecognized but is usually chronic and intermittent. Intercurrent infection, drugs such as novobiocin and chloramphenicol, and prolonged fasting deepen the icterus. Gilbert's disease is to be distinguished from other disorders causing mild hemolysis, such as hereditary nonspherocytic disease, ineffective erythropoiesis, and posthepatitis hyperbilirubinemia. Family studies indicate an autosomal dominant mode of inheritance, with patients showing heterozygosity for a single mutant gene. Diagnosis is primarily made by the exclusion of other liver disease and hemolytic state. Prognosis is excellent, and treatment is usually unwarranted. Occasionally, the unconjugated bilirubinemia reaches 10 mg/dl. Phenobarbital may be given to induce activity in the conjugating enzyme system and thereby reduce the bilirubin level.

Crigler-Najjar Syndrome

Two forms of Crigler-Najjar syndrome (congenital nonhemolytic jaundice) are described. Type I, the clinically more severe and rarer form, is due to an absence of glucuronyl transferase. Affected infants show serum unconjugated bilirubin concentrations of 20-40 mg/dl. Other liver function tests and hepatic histology are not abnormal. Death usually occurs in the first year of life as a result of kernicterus. Absence of the conjugating enzyme precludes a therapeutic response to phenobarbital. The disease is inherited as an autosomal recessive trait. Type II Crigler-Najjar syndrome, relatively more benign, differs from type I in three respects: (1) There is only partial absence of glucuronyl transferase. Jaundice is milder, with unconjugated hyperbilirubinemia less than 20 mg/dl. Neurologic complication is rare. (2) The mode of inheritance is one of autosomal dominance. (3) Type II deficiency is cured by phenobarbital and other microsome-inducing drugs.

Dubin-Johnson Syndrome

Dubin-Johnson syndrome (chronic idiopathic jaundice) is a chronic, benign, and intermittent form of conjugated hyperbilirubinemia; it has a comparable animal disorder in mutant Corriedale sheep. In humans and sheep the main diagnostic feature is the presence of black pigment in centrolobular liver cells. Formerly considered lipofuchsin, this nonbilirubin pigment represents polymerized melanin derivatives stored in lysosomes. Inherited as an autosomal recessive trait, patients display no symptoms, or may have vague liver tenderness. Serum bilirubin ranges 3-10 mg/dl. The functional defect in hepatic excretion extends to other organic anions, such as BSP, porphyrins, and iodinated dyes. Failure to excrete the latter accounts for nonvisualization of the biliary system by cholecystogram. The BSP excretion test reveals a characteristic though not specific pattern: The serum level falls initially, but rises again at 90 and 120 minutes to exceed the 45-minute value. Another diagnostic abnormality is the urinary excretion of coproporphyrin. Total urinary coproporphyrin is normal but 80% or greater is coproporphyrin isomer I (normal 25%). This pattern contrasts with the finding in patients with Rotor's syndrome, and in those with extrahepatic or intrahepatic cholestasis, all of whom excrete increased amounts of total urinary coproporphyrin and coproporphyrin I. Anabolic steroids, oral contraceptives, hemolysis, and pregnancy may accentuate the disorder by overloading the excretory process. This might produce the clinical and laboratory features of mild intrahepatic cholestasis.

Rotor's Syndrome

This is considered a genetic variant of Dubin-Johnson disease. There are several differences, including the absence of black pigment in the liver, and the excretion of cholecystographic agents. Rotor's syndrome can be differentiated from Dubin-Johnson syndrome and from normal persons on the basis of urinary coproporphyrin excretion.[2] Coproporphyrin I is excreted in larger amounts in Rotor's syndrome than in normal persons but not in as large amounts as in Dubin-Johnson syndrome. Increased urinary excretion of coproporphyrin III is also found in the patient with Rotor's disease. On the other hand, the patient with Dubin-Johnson syndrome excretes much less or no isomer III coproporphyrin. Prognosis in both Rotor and Dubin-Johnson disorders is excellent.

CHOLESTASIS

Cholestasis, the accumulation of bile in the liver, arises when bile flow into the intestine is interrupted (Table 5.3).[3] Manifestations vary with the severity and duration of the lesion interfering with the normal excretory pathway of the bile. Clinical recognition of cholestasis depends on the effect of bile (and its components) on the liver (Fig. 5.1), its accumulation

Table 5.3   Clinical and pathological features of cholestasis.

Clinical features	Pathological features
1. Changes due to accumulation of bile in the blood	
a. Jaundice	Increased conjugated bilirubin, may fall after 3 weeks
b. Pruritus	Increased bile salts
c. Xanthosis	Increased total serum lipids
2. Changes due to failure of bile to reach duodenum	
a. Light-colored stool	Decreased fecal stercobilinogen and sterobilin
b. Steatorrhea	Hypoprothrombinemia; malabsorption of vitamins A, K, E, D and calcium
c. Malnutrition	
d. Skin pigmentation	Increased skin melanin deposition
3. Changes in the liver due to bile deposition	
a. Hepatomegaly	
b. Hepatic tenderness	
c. Biliary cirrhosis	Bile deposition, ductal proliferation, fibrosis

From F. L. Iber, in W. T. Foulk (ed.), *Diseases of the Liver,* 1968; used with permission of the author and McGraw Hill Book Co.

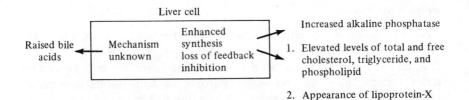

Fig. 5.1. Changes in the serum associated with cholestasis.

in the blood, and its absence in the intestinal tract. The toxic effects of bile salts in tissue (Table 5.4)[4] and the metabolic consequence of biliary obstruction are widespread. Cholestasis is generally divided into two types: extrahepatic and intrahepatic.

Extrahepatic Cholestasis

Extrahepatic cholestasis follows mechanical blockage of the major bile ducts (Table 5.5). Occlusion of the small intrahepatic ducts in experimental animals does not produce jaundice unless a major segmental branch is involved. In acute obstruction, the normal common bile duct pressure of 15–25 cm rapidly ascends to 35 cm or more. At this level bile flow ceases in the major ducts. The translocation of bile into blood occurs from leakage of ruptured ductules and retrograde movement in damaged cells. Evidence of liver cell injury, including centrolobular bile pigmentation, edema or portal triads, and ductular proliferation, develops within hours to days. Portal fibrosis is a later event, requiring 2–3 weeks for its

Table 5.4 Toxic effects of bile salts.[4]

	Hemolytic and pyrogenic effect	Effect on bile flow and bile salt secretion	Cirrhogenic (in lower animals)	ATPase inhibition (sodium transport)	Cytochrome P-450 binding (increased formation of monohydroxy bile acid?)
Lithocholate	Yes	Decrease	Yes	—	—
Chenodeoxycholate	Less than lithocholate	Decrease	No	Yes	Yes
Cholate	—	Increase	No	No	Less than chenodeoxycholate

Table 5.5 Causes of extrahepatic cholestasis.

1. Obstruction of common bile duct and ampulla
   Malignant:
   a. Carcinomas at the head of the pancreas, common bile duct, ampulla of Vater; and gallbladder carcinoma
   b. Metastatic tumors
   Benign:
   a. Stone, most common cause
   b. Parasitic infestation: *Clonorchis sinensis, Ascaris lumbricoides, Schistosomiasis japonicum*
   c. Benign polyp
   d. Chronic pancreatitis
   e. Perforated peptic ulcer
   f. Peritonitis in lesser omentum
   g. Diverticulum of duodenum
2. Obstruction at bifurcation of common hepatic duct and other hepatic ducts
   a. Carcinoma, primary or secondary
   b. Stricture
   c. Stone
3. Common in infants and childhood age
   a. Biliary atresia
   b. Ductal agenesis
   c. Choledochal cyst
4. Sclerosing cholangitis

appearance. Secondary biliary cirrhosis may follow a protracted obstructive course. This complication is found in 10% of patients who die of prolonged extrahepatic obstruction.

Clinical presentation. Deepening and persistent jaundice, pruritus, xanthoma, hepatomegaly, right-upper-quadrant tenderness, or a mass in the liver are among the features suggestive of extrahepatic cholestasis.

Diagnosis. Clinical and laboratory findings confirm the presence of cholestasis but often do not distinguish extrahepatic from intrahepatic causes (Table 5.6). The differential diagnosis can be difficult. The early histologic changes in both extrahepatic and intrahepatic cholestasis appear to be similar. Liver biopsy during this stage cannot reliably differentiate the two conditions (Table 5.7) (Fig. 5.2). Errors in interpretation may reach as high as 40% of the cases. The various tests become more accurate when used in conjunction repeatedly. Not infrequently an observation period of 2–4 weeks allows the disease process to manifest itself more clearly.

Table 5.6 Diagnostic tests in cholestasis.

Test	Comment
1. Increased conjugated bilirubin; marked rise in alkaline phosphatase; little or no elevation of aminotransferase activity	First evidence of cholestasis; normal values do not exclude diagnosis
2. Lipoprotein X	Does not distinguish extrahepatic from intrahepatic causes
Liver biopsy	At least 40% error in interpretation
Decrease or absent fecal urobilinogen	Confirms extrahepatic obstruction
3. Mitochondrial antibody	Negative test makes PBC unlikely
Serum bile acid profile, with or without cholestryamine challenge	Sensitive and specific indicator of extrahepatic vs intrahepatic cholestasis
4. Upper GI series, hypotonic duodenography, and duodenal sweep	For evaluation of periampullary lesions
Occult blood in stool	Malignancy more likely if positive
Alpha-fetoprotein	Positive in hepatoma, but also other diseases
Hepatic scintillation scan	Positive lesions must be > than 2 cm
Intravenous cholangiogram	Usefulness dependent on intact liver function
5. Endoscopic cholangiography	Single most useful test for diagnosis and location of lesion; technically difficult
Transhepatic cholangiography	Usefulness not dependent on liver function
Laparotomy	The definitive test of last resort
6. Response to corticosteroids (cause serum bilirubin to fall in viral hepatitis)	Limited usefulness
Duodenal intubation with secretin test	Limited usefulness
Hepatic arteriogram	Useful in delineating anatomy for surgery or drug perfusion

Table 5.7 Differentiation between intrahepatic and extrahepatic cholestasis by liver biopsy.[17]

| | Cholestasis | |
Changes	Intrahepatic	Extrahepatic
Bile deposition:		
Centrolobular	Early	Early
Ductular	Absent or late	Late
Infarcts or lakes	Absent	Late
Portal triads:		
Edema	Not striking	Prominent
Polymorphs	Few	Conspicuous
Eosinophiles	May be conspicuous	Inconspicuous
Bile ducts:		
Dilation	Absent	Early
Margination	Absent	Often present
Proliferation	Mild	Prominent
Periductal fibrosis	Absent	Late
Bile staining of duct cells	Absent	May be present
Polymorphs in lumen or between duct cells	Absent	May be present
Hyperplasia of duct cells	Absent	May be present
Hepatocellular:		
Focal injury	May be early	Late
Acidophilic bodies	Often present	Absent

Treatment and prognosis. This depends on the underlying disorder. Surgical intervention is required in most instances.

Intrahepatic Cholestasis

Anatomical blockage of the extrahepatic bile ducts is not demonstrable in intrahepatic cholestasis. The cause lies in the liver itself (Table 5.8). Bilirubin and bile salt compartments, the major solutes of bile, become altered. At the ultrastructural level the bile canaliculus dilates and loses its villi. The pericanalicular ectoplasm thickens. Neighboring Golgi apparatus enlarges with an increase in membrane and vacuole formation. Other organelle changes are seen but these are variable. Bile plugs accumulate at a later stage. The electron microscopic features of intrahepatic and extrahepatic cholestasis are virtually identical. In contrast to jaundice wherein the abnormality is confined to bilirubin metabolism, the

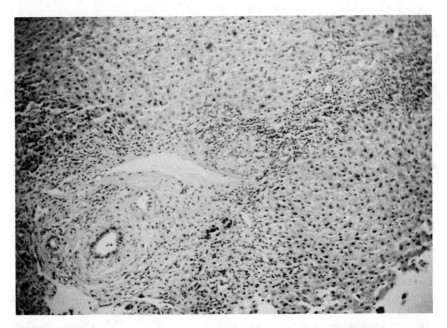

Fig. 5.2. Extrahepatic cholestasis. Numerous, slightly distorted bile ducts show periductular fibrosis and inflammation in a portal triad. H and E X200.

primary defect in intrahepatic cholestasis involves the secretory pathways of bile salt metabolism.[5] It has been theorized that virus, alcohol, and drugs damage the smooth endoplasmic reticulum (SER), resulting in formation of a hypertrophic but hypoactive SER.[6] This leads to incomplete hydroxylation of bile acids (Fig. 5.3) and relative predominance of the mitochondrial oxidative reactions. Formation of the less soluble monohydroxy bile acids and lithocholic acids is enhanced. These bile acids cause cholestasis in experimental animals by altering micelle formation. Monohydroxy bile salts exist in a liquid crystalline phase that is too viscous and large to cross the canalicular membrane. Interference with bile secretion is the end result. Other mechanisms, including decreased bile flow and direct impairment of micellar functions, are considered likely abnormal processes accounting for drug-induced cholestasis. A recent proposal invokes microfilament dysfunction as a pathogenic mechanism.[7] The various injurious agents disrupt the microfilament system leading to canalicular ectasia and reduction of bile flow. The attractive hypothesis presupposes that microfilaments are involved in bile salt translocation, a function which has not yet been proved.

Table 5.8 Causes of intrahepatic cholestasis.

1. Inheritable disorders of bilirubin metabolism
   a. Dubin-Johnson syndrome
   b. Rotor's syndrome
2. Hereditary and congenital diseases
   a. Neonatal hepatitis
   b. Alpha-1-antitrypsin deficiency
   c. Galactosemia
   d. Tyrosinemia
   e. Hereditary fructose intolerance
   f. Cerebrohepatorenal syndrome
   g. Leprechaunism (Donohue's syndrome)
3. Drug-induced liver injury (see also Chapter 12); secondary to therapeutic regimen such as intravenous hyperalimentation
4. Alcoholic fatty liver, hepatitis, and cirrhosis
5. Cryptogenic cirrhosis
6. Viral hepatitis, chronic persistent and chronic active hepatitis
7. Association with other diseases
   a. Primary and secondary carcinoma
   b. Extrahepatobiliary Hodgkin's disease
   c. Septicemia
   d. Pyogenic and amebic abscess
   e. Hemolysis and passive congestion
   f. Severe bacterial infections
8. Rare conditions
   a. Cholestasis of pregnancy
   b. Recurrent intrahepatic cholestasis
   c. Familial intrahepatic cholestasis (Byler's disease)

Clinical presentation. The clinical picture varies with the disease. Jaundice is frequently present. Hepatomegaly, fever, and pruritus may or may not occur. The constellation of onset, habits, associations, previous history, and drug abuse often provides valuable clues to the diagnosis. Cholestasis is observed in about 25% of the patients with acute viral hepatitis and cryptogenic cirrhosis, and in about 33% of cases with alcoholic fatty liver and alcoholic hepatitis. In these cases, biliary stasis usually forms a minor component of the disease, but it may become severe and be confused with extrahepatic obstruction.

Treatment and prognosis. Specific treatment is not available for most of these diseases and prognosis is variable.

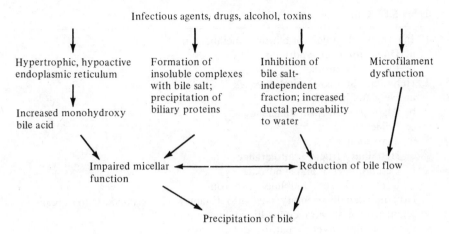

Fig. 5.3. Pathogenic mechanisms in intrahepatic cholestasis.

Disturbance of Lipid Metabolism in Cholestasis[8]

A pervading feature of cholestasis is the increase of almost all fractions of serum lipids: triglycerides, nonesterified cholesterol, choline phosphoglycerides, phospholipids, and lipoproteins. Concentrations of cholesterol esters and lysolecithin are, however, decreased. This is in contrast to the rise of cholesterol ester in the hypercholesterolemia of renal disease. Phospholipid elevation exceeds the rise in total cholesterol, so that the ratio of cholesterol to phospholipids is characteristically low. The hypercholesterolemia results not only from increased hepatic synthesis but also from enhanced small intestine synthesis. The cause for the increased hepatic synthesis is not clear. Loss of negative feedback inhibition by biliary cholesterol, decreased LCAT activity, and stimulation by regurgitated biliary lecithin are among possible pathogenic factors. The increase of nonesterified cholesterol and phospholipids is due in part to the presence of abnormal low-density lipoprotein, lipoprotein-X (LP-X). Antigenically unique, LP-X consists of a small amount of protein, cholesterol ester, and triglycerides, with larger amounts of phospholipids and free cholesterol. It also has a small amount of lithocholic acid. The protein moiety contains albumin and apolipoprotein C with a trace of apolipoproteins A and B. Structurally, LP-X appears as a disk-shaped particle about 400–600 Å in its major axis, with a lipid bilayer wall.[9] Such particles can be visualized in the liver of bile-duct-ligated rats on ultrathin sections.[10] LP-X accumulates in both intrahepatic and extrahepatic cholestasis.

CHOLESTATIC DISEASES

Postoperative Cholestasis

Jaundice is apt to follow major operative procedures, with many contributing factors including hypoxia, hypoperfusion of the liver, sepsis, anesthetic agent, and hemolysis of transfused red blood cells.[11,12] The multiple causes are grouped in Table 5.9.

Increased bilirubin load. Hemolysis resulting from congenital erythrocytic defect and drug-induced injury are rare. Hemolysis due to breakdown of aging erythrocytes in blood transfusion provides a considerable pigment load during surgery. The hemoglobin in 500 ml whole blood contains about 250 mg bilirubin, equivalent to the normal daily production. About 10% of the erythrocytes in a unit of two-week-old stored blood undergoes hemolysis within 24 hours of transfusion. The bilirubin load derived from hematomas is usually minor.

Impaired hepatocellular function. Jaundice due to halothane, hepatitis B virus, and cytomegalovirus is discussed elsewhere. Bacterial infections due to gram-negative organisms and pneumococcus are nowadays uncommon due to the liberal use of antibiotics. Postoperative shock causes jaundice in about 20% of patients. Typically, the serum bilirubin rises to 5-20 mg/dl within a week of surgery accompanied by an elevation of aminotransferases up to 500 IU/l and a modest rise of alkaline phosphatases. Recovery is the rule unless other complications, such as renal failure, intervene. Benign postoperative intrahepatic cholestasis occurs in patients who have undergone long, difficult surgery, with a period of shock, extensive blood transfusion, and other complications. These patients often suffer from heart failure prior to operation. Jaundice appears on the first or second postoperative day, reaches its height by the fourth to tenth day, and remits by the second week. Hyperbilirubinemia ranges 15-40 mg/dl, alkaline phosphatases increase to striking levels, and aminotransferases do not exceed 100 IU/l. Liver biopsy shows centrizonal cholestasis with minimal hepatocellular necrosis or inflammation. The cause is uncertain, but hypotension, hypoxia, and bilirubin overload are among contributing factors. Prognosis is good. Surgical intervention is contraindicated.

Extrahepatic biliary obstruction. Bile duct injury may occur during a cholecystectomy, common bile duct exploration, or other surgical procedure in the upper abdomen. Bile duct ligation or transection produces jaundice within a week of surgery. Unless promptly repaired, biliary

Table 5.9 Causes of postoperative cholestasis (jaundice).

---

1. Increased bilirubin load
   a. Hemolysis, due to glucose-6-phosphate dehydrogenase deficiency, sickle cell anemia, drugs such as sulfonamides and nitrofurantoin
   b. Hemolysis of transfused red blood cells
   c. Resorption of hematomas or hemoperitoneum
2. Impaired hepatocellular function
   a. Drugs and anesthetic agents (halothane)
   b. Shock
   c. Sepsis
   d. Infections such as hepatitis B virus, cytomegalovirus, and bacterial
   e. Benign postoperative intrahepatic cholestasis
3. Extrahepatic biliary obstruction
   a. Bile duct injury
   b. Choledocholithiasis

From J. T. LaMont and K. J. Isselbacher, *New Eng J Med* 288:305–307, 1973.

fistula, cholangitis, or subphrenic abscess may follow. Choledocholithiasis is a rare cause of postoperative jaundice.

Cholestasis of Pregnancy

Recurrent jaundice of pregnancy is a benign and self-limited complication which occurs in the last trimester of pregnancy and disappears spontaneously 1–2 weeks postpartum. The underlying cause is probably an idiosyncratic and cholestatic response to the hormonal change in pregnancy. In normal pregnancy slight increases in BSP, placental alkaline phosphatases, and serum bilirubin are common. These altered hepatic functions become exaggerated for unknown reasons in this disease. Clinically, jaundice and pruritus are the main symptoms. Serum bilirubin rarely exceeds 6 mg/dl. Both alkaline phosphatases and cholesterol show marked elevation. Liver histology confirms the cholestatic picture with little or no hepatocellular damage. Prognosis is good, although recurrence with subsequent pregnancies is the rule. The condition is more commonly seen in Europe and Scandinavia, suggesting a genetic susceptibility. A strong resemblance exists between this disorder and the cholestasis secondary to oral contraceptive ingestion.

Sclerosing Cholangitis[13]

In this liver disorder both intrahepatic and extrahepatic ducts undergo progressive fibrosis and stenosis. A rare disease, it may occur alone as the primary form, or secondarily in association with ulcerative colitis (30% of the secondary causes) or retroperitoneal fibrosis. Other rare secondary causes include Riedel's thyroiditis, cryptococcal hepatitis, gallstones, and familial immunodeficient syndrome.[14] Patients present with intractable biliary obstruction and eventual biliary cirrhosis. Signs and symptoms for the primary and secondary types merge into the general pattern of extrahepatic cholestasis: jaundice, right-upper-quadrant pain, pruritus, fever, hepatomegaly, and liver tenderness. The outstanding laboratory finding is a high serum alkaline phosphatase. Diagnosis is established by an exploratory laparotomy and a cholangiogram. Criteria for inclusion as primary sclerosing cholangitis should include (1) progressive obstructive jaundice; (2) finding of generalized thickening and stenosis of the walls of the biliary duct system; (3) absence of biliary stones, primary biliary cirrhosis, and malignancies; and (4) absence of associated diseases such as ulcerative colitis. Treatment consists of duct reconstruction or drainage if possible, or medical management with antibiotics.

Recurrent Intrahepatic Cholestasis[15]

This rare familial disorder usually starts in adolescence and is characterized by recurrent attacks of jaundice, pruritus, weakness, dark urine, and light stools. The episodes are accompanied by an obstructive liver profile with high serum bilirubin and markedly elevated alkaline phosphatases. The liver biopsy reveals centrolobular cholestasis without significant parenchymal inflammation or necrosis. Fibrosis is not seen. During symptom-free periods both biochemical functions and hepatic histology return to normal. There is no progression toward chronic liver disease. Other cholestatic diseases such as alcoholic liver disease, drug-induced hepatitis, and the inherited hyperbilirubinemias must be excluded. The familial occurrence and early onset suggest a genetic defect, but the exact cause is not known. Prognosis is excellent. Treatment is symptomatic, primarily involving relief from itching.

Familial Intrahepatic Cholestasis[16]

The first cases of this condition, described in 1969, were descendants of Jacob Byler who settled in the Amish counties of Ohio and Pennsylvania. Familial intrahepatic cholestasis (Byler's disease) is inherited as an autosomal recessive trait.

Symptoms appear in the first week of life; these include diarrhea, gastrointestinal hemorrhage, deepening jaundice, weight loss, and fever. Hepatosplenomegaly is present. The laboratory findings are those of severe biliary obstruction with marked increases of serum bilirubin and alkaline phosphatases. Characteristically, a bromsulphalein infusion study shows abnormal transport but normal storage of the organic anion. Bile acid kinetic studies reveal delayed plasma disappearance of labeled cholic acid and CDCA, with urine rather than fecal excretion. The elevated plasma bile acids contain abnormal percentages of lithocholic acid and other unknown derivatives. These findings suggest defective excretion of conjugated bile acid across the canalicular membrane. Liver histology reveals large bile plugs in ducts with severe diffuse cholestasis and cirrhosis. Affected males all bear a small Y chromosome, the significance of which is not known. The disease is usually fatal.

REFERENCES

1. Arias IM: Inheritable and congenital hyperbilirubinemia: Models for the study of drug metabolism. *New Eng J Med* 285:1416-1421, 1971.
2. Wolkolf AW, et al: Rotor's syndrome: A distinct inheritable pathophysiologic entity. *Amer J Med* 60:173-179, 1976.
3. Iber FL: Cholestasis, in Gen Ref No. 5, pp. 29-37.
4. Palmer RH: Bile acids, liver injury, and liver disease. *Arch Intern Med* 130:606-617, 1972.
5. King JE, Schoenfield LJ: Lithocholic acid, cholestasis, and liver disease. *Mayo Clinic Proc* 47:725-730, 1972.
6. Popper H, Schaffner F: Pathophysiology of cholestasis. *Human Path* 1:1-24, 1970.
7. Phillips MJ, et al: Microfilament dysfunction as a possible cause of intrahepatic cholestasis. *Gastroenterology* 69:48-58, 1975.
8. McIntyre N, Harry DS, Pearson AJG: The hypercholesterolaemia of obstructive jaundice. *Gut* 16:379-391, 1975.
9. Hamilton RL, et al: Cholestasis: Lamellar structure of the abnormal serum. *Science* 172:475-478, 1971.
10. Stein C, Alkan M, Stein Y: Obstructive jaundiced lipoprotein particles studied in ultra thin sections of livers of bile duct-ligated mice. *Lab Invest* 29:166-172, 1972.
11. LaMont JT, Isselbacher KJ: Postoperative jaundice. *New Eng J Med* 288:305-307, 1973.
12. Morgenstern L: Postoperative jaundice, in Gen Ref No. 14, pp 1353-1366.
13. Meyers RN, Cooper JH, Padis N: Primary sclerosing cholangitis: Complete gross and histologic reversal after long-term steroid therapy. *Gastroenterology* 53:527-538, 1970.
14. Record CO, et al: Intrahepatic sclerosing cholangitis associated with familial immunodeficiency syndrome. *Lancet* 2:18-20, 1973.
15. Lesser PB: Benign familial recurrent intrahepatic cholestasis. *Amer J Dig Dis* 18:259-264, 1972.
16. Linarelli LG, Williams CN, Phillips MJ: Byler's disease: Fatal intrahepatic cholestasis. *J Ped* 81:484-492, 1972.
17. Christoffersen P, Poulsen H: Histological changes in human liver biopsies following extrahepatic biliary obstruction. *Acta Pathol Microbiol Scand* 76A:150-157, 1970.

PORTAL HYPERTENSION

6

Portal hypertension encompasses increased resistance and flow states in the portal venous system. The normal portal pressure depends on the (1) resistance of the intrahepatic vasculature, (2) portal venous tone, (3) magnitude of blood flow, and (4) pressure transmitted from the mesenteric arteries to the portal bed.[1] Alterations in any of these variables will raise the normal portal vein pressure of 5–10 mm Hg, or wedged hepatic vein pressure above 4 mm Hg (with vena caval pressure as baseline), or intrasplenic pressure over 17 mm Hg unless other factors compensate for the shift. Portal hypertension is a major sequela of chronic liver disease, notably cirrhosis. The complication of hemorrhage from esophageal varices represents one of the frequent modes of exitus in liver disease. Portal hypertension is also involved in the pathogenesis of the other major manifestation of chronic liver disease—ascites.

Diseases Associated with Portal Hypertension

Portal hypertension is conventionally classified according to the presumed site of vascular involvement. In most instances, the locus of increased vascular resistance is not established, for example, cirrhosis. The classification presented here follows traditional lines (Tables 6.1 and 2).[2,3]

Cirrhosis

All cases with cirrhosis demonstrate portal hypertension at one stage or another. Corrosion cast studies of cirrhotic livers show a widespread reduction and deformity of intrahepatic vasculature, affecting radicles of the portal vein, hepatic vein, and sinusoids.[4] In addition, shunts are commonly visualized between the portal vein and hepatic veins and often between the portal vein and hepatic artery. The third possible type of shunt, between the hepatic artery and hepatic vein, is either very rare or not present. Both portahepatic venous and portaarterial shunts occur normally, but to a lesser degree. Portahepatic shunts develop from persisting sinusoids in fibrous septa. Portaarterial shunts are represented by

Table 6.1. Causes of portal hypertension.[2,3]

I. Prehepatic
  1. Portal vein (extrahepatic) or splenic vein obstruction
    a. Thrombosis: polycythemia vera; myelofibrosis; paroxysmal nocturnal hemoglobinurina; traumatic; recurrent, diffuse venous thrombosis; cryoglobulinemia
    b. Congenital anomalies: stenosis
    c. Pylephlebitis: appendiceal abscess
    d. Tumor encroachment: adjacent malignancies
    e. Pancreatic lesions: pseudocyst, chronic pancreatitis
II. Intrahepatic
  1. Cirrhosis
  2. Alcoholic hepatitis
  3. Cystic disease of the liver
  4. Infiltrative diseases: sarcoidosis, myeloproliferative diseases, Gaucher's disease
  5. Schistosomiasis
  6. Congenital hepatic fibrosis and partial nodular transformation of the liver
  7. Veno-occlusive disease
  8. Rarely: severe fatty liver and acute viral hepatitis
III. Posthepatic
  1. Hepatic vein obstruction (Budd-Chiari syndrome)
    a. Idiopathic in 70% of cases
    b. Secondary to tumor invasion, particularly renal cell carcinoma, adrenal carcinoma and hepatoma; to diseases with increased clotting tendency, polycythemia vera, paroxysmal nocturnal hemoglobulinuria, and myeloproliferative syndromes; to drug therapy, oral contraceptives; to radiation hepatitis, blunt traumas, graft vs host reaction; and to congenital webs
  2. Veno-occlusive disease
IV. Hepatoportal sclerosis (idiopathic primary portal hypertension)

---

arterial enlargement and dilation. Regenerative nodules apparently add to the increased vascular resistance by compressing hepatic veins. The reduction in portal flow is partly compensated by an increase in arterial flow, although portal inflow still constitutes the main vascular supply to the cirrhotic nodule. The prominence of hepatic arterioles can be observed around the proliferated bile ducts in portal scar tissue.

Alcoholic Hepatitis

This precursor of alcoholic cirrhosis is marked by centrolobular deposition of collagen in the early phase. Distortion of the hepatic central veins results in the outflow block type of portal hypertension.

Table 6.2. Hemodynamic changes in diseases associated with portal hypertension.[2,3]

	Site of vascular obstruction				Pressures	
	Sinusoidal fibrosis c̄/s̄ destruction	Presinusoidal block	Outflow (hepatic vein) block	Intrahepatic shunts	Wedged hepatic vein pressure	Intrasplenic pressure
Cirrhosis	+++		+++	++	↑	↑
Alcoholic hepatitis	+		+++	+	↑	N
Veno-occlusive disease, partial nodular transformation			++		↑	↑
Congenital hepatic fibrosis		++			N	↑
Schistosomiasis		++			N	↑
Sarcoidosis		?		?	V	V

N = normal: V = variable.

Hepatoportal Sclerosis

Hepatoportal sclerosis (idiopathic primary portal hypertension) embraces at least four separate entities reported from different areas of the world, all of which lack the usual features or etiologies associated with cirrhosis. In the portal hypertension associated with "idiopathic tropical splenomegaly" reported from Uganda, the increased blood flow is explainable on the basis of an increased splenic flow. Patients in Japan, India, and the United States with similar obscure portal hypertension and a grossly nonnodular liver, all reveal varying degrees of portal venule fibrosis on liver biopsy. The hemodynamic pattern is variable, with normal or slightly elevated wedged hepatic vein pressure and normal, increased, or depressed hepatic blood flow. In some instances, the disease is recognized as a sequela of an old pylephlebitis. In reports from India, significant presinusoidal resistance is found.[5] Patients usually present with recurrent but well-tolerated variceal hemorrhage and marked splenomegaly.

Portal Vein Occlusion

Thrombosis of the portal vein occurs more frequently than hepatic vein occlusion because of its greater length and exposure to contiguous structures. The thrombosis is usually secondary to another disease process, such as hypercoagulable disorders, low flow states, encroachment or invasion by adjacent tumor growth, and infection following umbilical or intraabdominal sepsis. Occlusion of the portal vein does not frequently cause a gross area of liver necrosis. Hepatic infarction more commonly results from hepatic artery obstruction. Less than 5% of cirrhotic cases shows portal vein thrombosis. Clinically, the occlusion is accompanied by sudden deterioration with shock, hematemesis, and increasing ascites. Partial occlusion may heal with vascular calcification, which can be visualized radiographically.

Hepatic Vein Occlusion

In hepatic vein occlusion (Budd-Chiari syndrome) obstruction is usually due to a thrombosis formed locally or by extension from the inferior vena cava. The cause is unknown in 70% of the cases. In the other 30% tumor, hematological diseases with clotting tendency, and oral contraceptives are the leading causes (Table 6.1). Hepatic vein thrombosis is becoming increasingly prevalent in young women on cyclic hormone therapy.[6] The liver becomes enlarged, tender, and congested. On biopsy there is marked centrolobular hemorrhage with infarction. In the acute form, upper abdominal pains, tender hepatomegaly, splenomegaly, ascites, esophageal varices, and mild jaundice are the presenting symptoms. In the chronic form, the onset is slower. The caudate lobe is usually spared and may undergo hypertrophy because its venous drainage empties directly into the vena cava. Characteristic vena caval collaterals (dilated superficial veins in the lumbar region or abdominal wall with ascending blood flow) appear on the abdominal wall. Hepatic or splenic venography confirms the diagnosis. In Japan, the Budd-Chiari syndrome is most frequently caused by membranous obstruction (web) in the hepatic portion of the inferior vena cava.[7] The appearance of abdominal wall collaterals precedes the abdominal pains, and the course is chronic in contrast to the experience in the West. Furthermore, conservative management permits long-term survival (an average of 10 years), although 40% of the patients develop hepatocellular carcinoma. Differential diagnosis includes heart failure and constrictive pericarditis. Prognosis is usually poor. Treatment is symptomatic and directed toward the underlying condition.

Veno-occlusive Disease

Ingestion of plants belonging to the genera *Senecio* (ragwort) and *Crotalaria* (rattlebox) produces, in humans and cattle, thrombosis and fibrosis of the hepatic venous system. The condition is common in

Jamaica, where patients take *C. fulva* (bush tea) for medicinal purposes. It occurs predominantly in children who, in the acute form, present with sudden hepatomegaly, ascites, abdominal pains, and vomiting. More commonly, the course is prolonged and portal hypertension becomes prominent. Fifty percent of patients die within several months. No specific therapy is available.

Cruveilhier-Baumgarten Syndrome

The term applies to cirrhotic patients with portal hypertension, who as a result develop prominent paraumbilical and deep epigastric veins communicating with the iliac veins and vena cava. Because of the large blood flow in these channels, a murmur is frequently heard. Chronic hepatic coma is the usual complication.

Diseases with Noncirrhotic Portal Hypertension

This group of disorders with portal hypertension lacks the usual histological features of cirrhosis (Table 6.3). Regenerative nodules are not seen on liver biopsy. Clinically, patients in this group contrast with those who have cirrhosis and portal hypertension in one important therapeutic aspect: portacaval shunting often leads to long-term survival. The preservation of hepatocellular function accounts for the favorable outcome.

Table 6.3.   Causes of noncirrhotic portal hypertension.

  I. Presinusoidal portal hypertension
  1. Congenital hepatic fibrosis
  2. Hepatoportal fibrosis
  3. Schistosomiasis
  4. Sarcoidosis and other hepatic granulomas
  5. Myeloproliferative syndrome
  6. Chronic arsenical intoxication
  7. Vinyl chloride toxicity
  8. Arteriovenous fistula in splanchnic bed
  9. ? Wilson's disease
 II. Postsinusoidal portal hypertension
  1. Alcoholic hepatitis, early stage
  2. Hypervitaminosis A
  3. Early Budd-Chiari syndrome
  4. Veno-occlusive disease
  5. Myxedema of the liver
  6. Partial nodular transformation

Clinical Presentation in Portal Hypertension

The clinical picture is largely due to the underlying liver disease. The portal hypertension itself causes the following conditions:

Development of collateral circulation. As much as 85% of the normal portal blood flow may be diverted to these shunts. There are anastomoses between portal or other venous drainages, as shown below.

Site	Drainage	
	Portal	*Systemic*
1. Lower esophageal submucosa (varices)	Coronary vein	Azygous → superior vena cava
2. Rectal submucosa (hemorrhoids)	Middle and superior hemorrhoidal veins	Inferior hemorrhoidal veins
3. Paraumbilical veins (anterior abdominal wall)	Left portal vein	Epigastric vein → superior vena cava
4. Parietal peritoneum	Veins of Retzius	Veins of Sappey
5. Left renal vein	Splenic vein	Renal vein

Rarely, ileal or mesenteric varicosities develop, particularly in relationship to postoperative fibrous adhesions.[8] These varices, which may account for obscure GI bleeding, are not visualized on conventional radiologic studies. Angiography would demonstrate these shunts.

Ascites. Ascites is partly due to increased lymph formation resulting from sinusoidal hypertension. The ascitic fluid escapes from the surface of the liver and splanchnic bed. Other factors are also involved.

Splenomegaly. Splenic enlargement is probably due to both passive congestion and a real increase of RE cells. Chronic liver injury stimulates the RE system. Splenomegaly accounts for the secondary hypersplenism with anemia, leukopenia, and thrombocytopenia. Banti's syndrome refers to the splenomegaly and hypersplenism associated with portal hypertension. The syndrome may result from extrahepatic portal block, eg, portal vein thrombosis, or from intrahepatic causes. More recently Banti's syndrome has been described as occurring in vinyl chloride workers.

Hypervolemia. Portal hypertension is regularly accompanied by an increase in plasma volume, presumably due to the expansion of the portal venous bed collateral system and splanchnic bed. The hyperdynamic state of cirrhosis itself with increased cardiac output and hypervolemia is an added factor. Increase of the plasma volume elevates portal hypertension and may lead to rupture of esophageal varices.

Laboratory Assessments

Examinations are directed to finding the cause of portal hypertension, to documenting the sequelae, and to assessing the nature and extent of the hepatic disease.

Hepatic tests. Serial determinations of standard tests, including liver biopsies, are required to assess the severity of hepatic lesion and the reserve capacity for possible surgery.

Investigations of the intrahepatic vasculature and mesenteric bed. These procedures (Table 6.4) are not mandatory for diagnosis but should form part of the preoperative workup. It is not clear if any of the preoperative hemodynamic studies has any value in predicting response to portosystemic shunt surgery.[9] However, radiologic visualization of the portal tree is helpful in establishing anatomic variations prior to surgery.

Assessment of the sequelae of portal hypertension. The principle sequelae of portal hypertension are the following:

1. Esophageal varices. They occur in at least 30% of cirrhotics with portal hypertension. Varices are detected by esophagoscopy with an accuracy approaching 90%. Radiological examination with barium administration is another diagnostic procedure, though its accuracy is only 50% at best. It should be remembered that varices are not pathognomonic of cirrhotic portal hypertension; varices may also be observed in hiatus hernia, acute viral hepatitis, normal pregnancy, and agnogenic myeloid metaplasia. Bleeding varices are the major cause of upper gastrointestinal hemorrhage in alcoholic liver disease.

2. Ascites. In most cases fluid accumulation in the peritoneal cavity is easily recognized. Ascites may be detected on physical examination with either the fluid wave or the shifting dullness maneuver. The latter technique is the more sensitive of the two, although in either test at least two liters of ascitic fluid must be present for a positive response. Paracentesis is required for definitive confirmation. The needle is inserted into the peritoneal cavity in an area dull to percussion, usually in the flanks (see Chapter 7).

3. Hepatic coma. The incipient precoma stage often occurs imperceptibly. Slight mental confusion, slurred speech, inattention to personal appearance, and disturbance of the sleep pattern are among the early signs. A blood ammonia determination and EEG test should be done for diagnosis (see Chapter 8).

Table 6.4. Assessment of hepatic vascular system.[3]

Technique	Comments	Contraindications	Complications
1. Percutaneous splenic manometry and portography	1. Measures portal vein pressure 2. Visualizes splenic and portal veins, and collaterals	1. Low platelets or co-agulation defects 2. Primary spleen dis-eases	1. Technical failure in 5% of cases 2. Hemorrhage uncommon
2. Operative portal manometry and portography	1. Largely replaced by proce-dure 1 2. Considerable hemodynamic artifacts		
3. Umbilical catheterization	1. Useful for hemodynamic studies 2. Requires operative team	1. Coagulation or bleed-ing problem	1. High technical failure rate 2. Sepsis not uncommon
4. Hepatic vein catheterization	1. Measures wedged hepatic vein pressure 2. Confirms postsinusoidal and sinusoidal hypertension 3. Does not exclude presinusoi-dal or extrahepatic hyperten-sion 4. Wedged hepatic vein pressure is equivalent to free portal venous pressure in normal subjects and cirrhotics 5. Free hepatic vein pressure minus wedged hepatic vein pressure reflects portohepatic gradient or sinusoidal pres-sure		1. Almost nil

Treatment

Management is primarily concerned with bleeding esophageal varices. Ascites is usually relieved by salt restriction and diuretic therapy and rarely requires surgical intervention. Hypersplenism commonly abates on portal decompression even without a splenectomy. Acute bleeding varices are treated either by medical or surgical procedures. Medically, three methods are available: the tamponade technique with the Sengstaken-Blakemore tube; gastric-esophageal cooling; and vasopressin or octapressin infusion to lower portal venous pressure. In many institutions, tamponade intubation is adopted as the initial therapy. Gastric-esophageal cooling is generally ineffective, providing only temporary relief. Vasopressin lowers portal hypertension by vasoconstricting the splanchnic bed and causing a decrease of portal inflow. About 75% of hemorrhages from varices are controlled by intraarterial administration of vasopressin.[10] The drug is also effective for stopping gastrointestinal bleeding from nonvariceal lesions and significantly reduces transfusion requirements. Intraarterial administration of vasopressin may be complicated by mesenteric venous thrombosis, small bowel infarction, decrease of portal pO_2, reduction of cardiac output, and coronary blood flow.[11] Vasopressin therapy does not decrease the mortality rate in ruptured varices. The severity of the underlying disease and the recurrent nature of most bleeding episodes account for the failure to improve survival.

The surgical treatment of varices includes ligation of the varices, sclerosing techniques, and portacaval shunt surgery. The first two methods have the drawback of not decompressing the portal system. In contrast, shunt surgery is highly effective in reducing portal pressure. Transesophageal varix ligation is not widely employed since it offers only temporary hemostasis. Sclerosing techniques are not popular, but a recent variation involving transhepatic catheterization of the portal vein has stimulated renewed interest. A catheter is passed to the coronary vein, followed by injection of a 50% glucose and thrombin solution.[12] This produces sclerosis of the esophageal varices. The procedure appears promising, although its general applicability remains to be evaluated.

The role of portacaval shunt surgery in the management of varices is a controversial issue in hepatology. The question is whether the increased morbidity of hepatic encephalopathy and failure after portacaval shunts is preferable to the high risk of variceal hemorrhage in nonshunted patients. Shunts may be performed as a prophylactic measure to prevent hemorrhage in a patient who has not bled, as a therapeutic measure to avoid recurrent hemorrhage, or in the acute emergency situation of rupture.

Basically, four types of portosystemic venous shunts are used: end-to-side portacaval, side-to-side portacaval, end-to-side splenorenal, and superior mesenteric caval or mesocaval (Fig. 6.1). Although decompression of the portal system is achieved, the shunting procedures may produce several undesirable effects: hepatic encephalopathy, peptic ulcer disease, increased hepatic iron deposition, and diabetes mellitus (Table 6.5).[13,14] Deterioration of the liver status results from two nonphysiological changes introduced by the operation: bypass of hepatic function by intestinal blood flow and deprivation of the portal inflow to the liver.

Loss of hepatotropic factors present in the portal blood, such as insulin and glucagon, affects the hepatic synthetic capacity and reduces liver size.[15] Encephalopathy as a complication appears to be more common after shunting than in medically treated patients, in terms of severity and type. Close analysis of the data reported in previous investigations reveals that the overall incidence of hepatic encephalopathy in patients after shunting may not be significantly different from the control group.[13] The severity and type of encephalopathy do differ for the two groups. Severe, recurrent, and spontaneous coma occurs rarely in unshunted patients (2%) but is about five times more common in the shunted patients.[13] Sporadic encephalopathy induced by an identifiable precipitating event (gastrointestinal hemorrhage, sedation, diuretics) occurs almost equally in both groups. The most frequent cause of coma in the shunted patients is dietary protein, in contrast to gastrointestinal hemorrhage for the unshunted group. Liver function tests do not identify those among the shunted series who will develop encephalopathy. According to some studies, postshunt development of peptic ulcer does not differ for the two groups,[16] while others report an increased incidence in the shunted patients. The ulcers are predominantly duodenal in the operated group and gastric in the control series.

Histamine bypassing the liver via shunts stimulates gastric acid secretion. The hyperacidity presumably accounts for the occurrence of peptic ulcer. Hemosiderosis does not complicate the postshunted liver more frequently than in the unshunted liver. However, when hemosiderosis occurs, the amount of iron deposition is about three times greater in the postshunt group. The increase of hepatic iron storage is usually asymptomatic but may potentiate chronic liver injury. Diabetes mellitus does not appear more frequently in the operated group as compared to the nonoperated group. Apparently all four problems—portosystemic encephalopathy, peptic ulcer, hemosiderosis, and diabetes mellitus—are related more to the cirrhotic process than to shunt surgery. To circumvent these side effects, variations such as hepatic arterialization of portacaval shunt,[17] selective distal splenorenal shunt in several forms,[18] and left gastric-inferior venal caval shunt are under current trial.

Hemodynamic studies of patients undergoing shunts indicate no correlation between portal flow and survival length postoperatively or the development of hepatic encephalopathy.[19,20] Furthermore, patients with

Collaterals in sclerosis

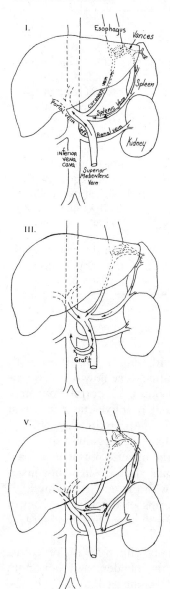

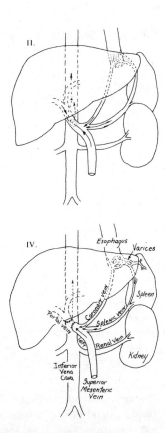

Fig. 6.1. I. The direction of blood flow and collateral circulation are indicated. II. Side-to-side portacaval shunt: 70 percent show reversal of portal flow; greater decrease in hepatic venous pressure and oxygen consumption; higher incidence of postoperative encephalopathy compared to procedure IV. III. Side-to-side mesocaval shunt: technically a simple procedure; indicated when portal vein is thrombosed. IV. End-to-side portacaval shunt: technically simple to perform; thrombosis of shunt rare; no complete protection against recurrent ascites, especially with retrograde portal flow. V. Distal end-to-side splenorenal shunt: technically very difficult to perform; relatively high operative mortality; contraindicated if there is retrograde portal flow or ascites; low incidence of postsurgical encephalopathy. (Gen Ref No. 12, pp. 301–302.)

Table 6.5. Sequelae of prophylactic shunt surgery.[13,14,16]

Complication	Not shunted	Shunted
1. Portosystemic encephalopathy (PSE)	20–30%	50% or more; overall incidence not significantly different from unshunted control; frequency of severe PSE significantly greater
2. Hemosiderosis	30%	50%; amount but not frequency different by threefold
3. Peptic ulcer	5–15%	15–20%; questionable greater incidence than unshunted series
4. Diabetes mellitus	10%	15%; not significantly different

the smallest portal flows do not do better with shunts than those with larger portal flows. Variable increases in hepatic artery flow follow surgical anastomosis. This variablity and its response to portal flow may influence the postoperative course. At present prophylactic portacaval shunts do not change the survival rate.[21,22,23] Approximately 50% of shunted patients are alive after five years, a figure distressingly similar to the unshunted control group. The status of therapeutic portacaval anastomosis is unsettled at this time. Several trials show a slight but insignificant enhancement of survival in patients with therapeutic shunts.[24,25] These studies, however, contain flaws in terms of the various control groups. Future trends may yet define a role for therapeutic shunt surgery in the decompression of portal hypertension.

Portosystemic shunt is, however, extremely effective in preventing recurring variceal bleeding. In one series, the incidence of postshunt variceal hemorrhage averaged less than 3% compared to 26% in the medically treated group.[21] Portacaval shunt surgery may have other uses besides controlling hemorrhage or ascites. The procedure reverses some of the metabolic disturbances associated with hepatic glycogen storage disease (types I, III, ?IV) and familial hypercholesterolemia (refractory type IIA and hyperlipoproteinemia).[26]

REFERENCES

1. Turcotte JG, Child CG III: Portal hypertension: Pathogenesis, management and prognosis, in Gen Ref No. 5, pp 97–106.
2. Sherlock S: The portal venous system and portal hypertension, and the hepatic artery and hepatic veins, in Gen Ref No. 15, pp 150–216, 217–233.
3. Reynolds TB: Portal hypertension, in Gen Ref No. 14, pp 330–367.
4. Mitra SK: Hepatic vascular changes in human and experimental cirrhosis. *J Path Bacteriol* 92:405–414, 1966.
5. Sama SK, et al: Noncirrhotic portal fibrosis. *Amer J Med* 51:160–169, 1971.
6. Langer B, et al: Clinical spectrum of the Budd-Chiari syndrome and its surgical management. *Amer J Surg* 129:137–145, 1975.
7. Nakamura T, et al: Obstruction of the inferior vena cava in the hepatic portion and the hepatic veins. *Angiology* 19:479–498, 1968.
8. Moncure AC, et al: Gastrointestinal hemorrhage from adhesion-related mesenteric varices. *Ann Surg* 183:24–29, 1976.
9. Charters AC III, et al: The influence of portal perfusion on the response to portacaval shunt. *Amer J Surg* 130:226–230, 1975.
10. Conn HO, et al: Intraarterial vasopressin in the treatment of upper gastrointestinal hemorrhage: A prospective, controlled clinical trial. *Gastroenterology* 68:211–221, 1975.
11. Millette B, et al: Portal and systemic effects of selective infusion of vasopressin into the superior mesenteric artery in cirrhotic patients. *Gastroenterology* 69:6–12, 1975.
12. Lunderquist A, Vang J: Transhepatic catheterization and obliteration of the coronary vein in patients with portal hypertension and esophageal varices. *New Eng J Med* 291:646–649, 1974.
13. Mutchnick MG, Lerner E, Conn HO: Portal-systemic encephalopathy and portacaval anastomosis: A prospective, controlled investigation. *Gastroenterology* 66:1005–1019, 1974.
14. Conn HO: Complications of portacaval anastomosis: By-products of a controlled investigation. *Gastroenterology* 59:207–220, 1973.
15. Starzl TE, Porter KA, Putnam CW: Intraportal insulin protects from the liver injury of portacaval shunt in dogs. *Lancet* 2:1241–1242, 1975.
16. Phillips MM, Ramsby GR, Conn HO: Portacaval anastomosis and peptic ulcer: A nonassociation. *Gastroenterology* 68:121–131, 1975.
17. Maillard JN, et al: Hepatic arterialization and portacaval shunt in hepatic cirrhosis. *Arch Surg* 108:315–324, 1974.
18. Warren WD, et al: Selective distal splenorenal shunt. *Arch Surg* 108:306–314, 1974.
19. Reynolds TB: The role of hemodynamic measurements in portosystemic shunt surgery. *Arch Surg* 108:276–281, 1974.
20. Reynolds TB: Promises! Promises! Hemodynamics and portal-systemic shunt. *New Eng J Med* 290:1484–1485, 1974.
21. Resnick RH, et al: A controlled study of the prophylactic portacaval shunt: A final report. *Ann Intern Med* 70:675–688, 1969.

22. Conn HO, et al: Prophylactic portacaval anastomosis: A tale of two studies. *Medicine* 51:27–40, 1972.
23. Editorial: Prophylactic portacaval shunt. *Lancet* 1:999–1000, 1972.
24. Resnick RH, et al: A controlled study of the therapeutic portacaval shunt. *Gastroenterology* 67:843–857, 1974.
25. Conn HO: The rational evaluation and management of portal hypertension, in Gen Ref No. 12, pp 289–306.
26. Editorial: Portacaval anastomosis for metabolic disease. *Lancet* 2:444–445, 1974.

RENAL DYSFUNCTION IN LIVER DISEASE AND ASCITES

7

Hepatic dysfunction and renal status are intimately linked though the interrelationship is not completely defined. Disorders with concurrent hepatic and renal components may be classified on the basis of disease association (Table 7.1) or altered renal physiology (Table 7.2). [1,2,3]

LIVER DISEASES WITH RENAL DYSFUNCTION

Acute Viral Hepatitis

Two types of renal disease may complicate this virus infection. The first is the rare occurrence of glomerulonephritis due to glomerular trapping of HB_sAg and HB_sAb immune complexes. The second nonspecific kidney change is more common, usually detected on urinalysis. Mild proteinuria and microscopic hematuria are found. Functionally, the kidney fails to excrete a dilute urine in response to a water load. On renal biopsy no specific pathological lesion is observed, although interstitial edema, granular tubular change, and glomerular swelling may be present. The renal lesion is self-limited.

Compensated Cirrhosis without Ascites

Renal hemodynamics in these patients are normal. However, there is evidence of tubular dysfunction. A water-load test reveals mild impairment of renal concentration and dilution capacities. Similarly, a salt load elicits a poor response in sodium excretion. About one-third of patients exhibit on renal biopsy nonspecific glomerular and tubular changes. The glomerular sclerotic alterations include increased cellularity, stromal fibrosis, and thickening of the basement membrane. Proximal tubular cells often contain hyaline droplets.

Decompensated Cirrhosis

The "true" hepatorenal syndrome, characterized by spontaneous development of azotemia, oliguria, hyponaturesis, and dilutional hypona-

Table 7.1.   Diseases involving both liver and kidneys.

I. Systemic disorders affecting both liver and kidney
  1. Infections: leptospirosis, yellow fever, fulminant meningococcemia
  2. Toxic: carbon tetrachloride, choline deficiency, mushroom poisoning
  3. Infiltrative: sarcoidosis, metastatic tumors, amyloidosis
  4. Circulatory: shock
  5. Drugs: tetracycline, methoxyflurane
  6. Unknown: systemic lupus erythematosus, periarteritis, nodosa, sickle
    cell anemia
II Primary renal diseases with secondary hepatic dysfunction
  1. Nephrogenic hepatosplenomegaly associated with renal cell carcinoma
  2. Toxemia of pregnancy
  3. Polycystic disease
III. Primary hepatobiliary diseases with secondary renal dysfunction
  1. With known antecedent cause
    a. Following trauma, bile duct surgery, or variceal hemorrhage
    b. Immunological alteration: viral hepatitis, primary biliary cirrhosis,
      chronic active hepatitis
    c. Metal poisoning: Wilson's disease
  2. Without known cause (hepatorenal syndrome)
    a. Spontaneous oliguria and azotemia in terminal chronic hepatic failure
      (decompensated cirrhosis) and in fulminant hepatic failure

tremia, occurs in approximately 50% of patients with terminal chronic liver disease. It is also common in acute fulminant hepatic failure. Kidney histology is surprisingly normal, with no constant tubular or glomerular abnormalities. The basic defect appears to be intrarenal vasoconstriction which is more severe in the cortex than in the medulla. This has been documented with [131]Xenon washout studies and cortical nephrograms obtained by renal angiography.[4] The cause(s) for this inappropriate rise of intrarenal vascular resistance is not known. Several hypotheses are offered (Fig. 7.1): (1) Decrease of effective plasma volume due to sequestration in splanchnic bed with portal hypertension, said to occur relatively infrequently. Infusion of plasma expanders is ineffective in ameliorating the hepatorenal syndrome in most cases. (2) Increased production of biogenic amines (false neurotransmitters), resulting in shunting of blood away from the kidneys. This attractive hypothesis finds support in reports that some patients respond to infusions of metaraminol, a sympathomimetic amine.[5] (3) Failure of intrarenal angiotensin production secondary to low circulating renin substrate levels (angiotensinogen). Cirrhotic patients have high plasma renin concentrations but low renin substrate levels due to defective hepatic synthesis.[6] The decreased angiotensin production affects afferent arteriolar vasoconstriction and leads to reduced cortical

Table 7.2. Types of renal dysfunction in hepatic disorders.

Renal dysfunction or disease	Mechanism	Hepatic disorders
1. ? none	Antiglomerular antibody	Chronic active hepatitis
2. Glomerulonephritis	$HB_sAg\text{-}HB_sAb$ immune complexes	Acute viral hepatitis
3. Glomerulosclerosis	Unknown	Alcoholic cirrhosis
4. Acute tubular necrosis	Shock	Hepatic trauma; hepatobiliary surgery; variceal hemorrhage
5. Tubular nephropathy	Hypokalemia	Overtreatment with diuretics
6. Oliguric, azotemic renal failure (hepatorenal syndrome)	Unknown, renal cortical vasoconstriction	Decompensated cirrhosis; fulminant hepatic failure
7. Renal tubular acidosis	? immune destruction[16]	Primary biliary cirrhosis; chronic active hepatitis
	Copper poisoning	Wilson's disease
8. Defective tubular acidification	? excess tubular reabsorption of sodium[17]	Alcoholic cirrhosis
9. Impaired renal concentrating capacity	Renal cortical hypoperfusion with shunting of blood to deep medullary nephrons and washout of medullary sodium and/or urea gradient[18]	Alcoholic cirrhosis
10. Hyperuricosuria (and hypouricemia)	? impaired tubular urate reabsorption	Alcoholic cirrhosis

perfusion. The alteration of renin substrate activity was corrected in three patients who underwent orthotopic liver transplantation with recovery from the hepatorenal syndrome.[7] (4) Circulating vasoactive substance(s). Ferritin, catecholamines, and endotoxins have been postulated to cause renal hypoperfusion. None, however, is generally accepted as the primary factor in the pathogenesis of hepatorenal syndrome. Whatever the

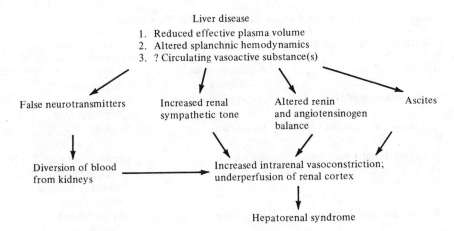

Fig. 7.1. Pathogenesis of hepatorenal syndrome. (Adapted from P. Baldus and W. H. J. Summerskill, Gen Ref No. 14, p 458.)

cause, the vasoconstrictive process affects the afferent arteriolar bed predominantly, giving rise to glomerulotubular imbalance,[8] and accounting for the oliguria, azotemia, and decreased salt excretion. Ascites and hepatic coma invariably accompany the development of hepatorenal syndrome. The onset of azotemia is usually slow, followed later by oliguria, hypotension, and not infrequently hypothermia. Urinary sediments are not unusual. Determinations of the glomerular filtration rate and effective renal plasma flow reveal low values. The high urine osmolality and very low sodium content make it possible to discriminate hepatorenal syndrome from acute renal tubular necrosis (Table 7.3). Precipitating factors such as gastrointestinal hemorrhage and vigorous diuretic treatment may be identified in some instances. Death within six weeks is invariable. No satisfactory treatment is available. Administration of mannitol or hypertonic sodium chloride and hemodialysis or peritoneal dialysis are all ineffective. Restriction of fluid and salt is advisable in the presence of oliguria.

ASCITES

Ascites, the accumulation of excess fluid in the peritoneal cavity, represents a major sequela of chronic liver disease. At least 60% of the patients with cirrhosis have ascites. It usually occurs in conjunction with esophageal varices and hepatorenal syndrome since all three share common pathogenic pathways. Variceal hemorrhage is uncommon in the

Table 7.3. Comparison between hepatorenal syndrome and acute tubular necrosis.

	Hepatorenal syndrome	Acute tubular necrosis
Antecedent course	None	Yes
Liver function	Severely impaired	Variable
Ascites, hepatic coma	Usually present	May be present
Precipitating factors	Sometimes present	Hypotension
Course	Usually slow	Rapid
Hypotension, oliguria	Late	Early
Urine sodium	Very low	Moderately low
Urine sediment	Normal	Abnormal
Urine osmolality	Greater than normal	Low, fixed
GFR and ERPF*	Low	Very low
Renal pathology	No abnormalities	Abnormal

*GFR = glomerular filtration rate; ERPF = effective renal plasma flow. From W. P. Baldus, in H. Popper and F. Schaffner (eds.) *Progress in Liver Diseases,* 1972; used with permission of author and Grune & Stratton, Inc.

patient without ascites, and likewise hepatorenal syndrome does not develop in the absence of ascites. Exception to these associations may occur in the patient with presinusoidal portal hypertension.

Pathogenesis

The development of ascites is dependent on both hepatic and extrahepatic factors (Fig. 7.2).

Hepatic factors. Two major hemodynamic changes are involved. First, hepatic venous outflow block regularly causes rapid onset and often intractable ascites, rich in protein content (>2.5 g/dl).[9] This occurs in the Budd-Chiari syndrome (hepatic vein thrombosis, tumor compression), and may be simulated to a lesser degree by severe chronic constrictive pericarditis. The transmitted increase of sinusoidal pressure forces fluid out into the perisinusoid lymphatic space and across the capsular surface of liver. Second, intrahepatic sinusoidal hypertension produces high thoracic lymph flow (the latter occurs in cirrhosis with or without ascites), and ascites low in protein content (<1 g/dl). The resultant portal venous inflow block gives rise to splanchnic congestion and exudation of fluid. The composition of ascitic fluid (<2.5 g/dl protein) in cirrhosis suggests that both hepatic venous outflow and portal inflow disturbances are involved in the production of this fluid.

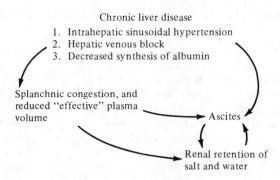

Fig. 7.2 Factors in the production of ascites. (Adapted from W. H. J. Summerskill and W. P. Baldus, Gen Ref No. 14, p. 424.)

Extrahepatic factors. These may be considered in two groups. First, there is decreased intravascular osmotic pressure secondary to hypoalbuminemia. Decreased albumin synthesis by the damaged liver, possible increased catabolism of albumin, loss of albumin into the peritoneal cavity, and the presence of antihuman albumin antibodies in cirrhosis all contribute to the hypoalbuminemia. Loss of osmotic pressure favors fluid transudation into the extravascular (peritoneal) compartment. Second, the kidney does not handle salt and water excretion in an appropriate manner. Instead, there is decreased renal excretion of salt, increased salt retention, and secondary hyperaldosteronism.

These interrelated phenomena arise in the following sequence: portal hypertension → excessive lymph formation → ascites → decreased effective plasma volume → increased secretion of aldosterone → decreased renal excretion of salt. This traditional concept does not explain the observations that (1) plasma volume is not decreased in most cirrhotics, (2) paracentesis does not decrease plasma volume during reaccumulation of ascites, and (3) plasma volume does not increase after spontaneous diuresis. To incorporate these findings, the overflow theory of ascites formation has been proposed:[10] portal hypertension → splanchnic bed expansion → increased plasma volume → increased renal retention of sodium → ascites.

Compartmentalization of ascitic fluid.[11] Ascitic fluid forms a separate and slowly mobilized compartment of extracellular fluid compared to peripheral edema. The rate of reabsorption of fluid from the peritoneal cavity is limited. In the treatment of ascites, rapid weight loss does not indicate the sole mobilization of ascitic fluid, particularly in the presence of peripheral edema. In the absence of this second compartment, vigorous diuresis may promote renal failure by lowering plasma volume and renal perfusion. The presence of peripheral edema confers some degree of protection from renal failure during treatment of ascites. Fluid enters the abdominal cavity 10 times faster than it exits. Within 24 hours of paracentesis, 40–60% of the original volume reaccumulates. This underlines the futility of paracentesis in many cases. The absence of weight gain does not exclude the reformation of ascites as fluid may shift from intracellular spaces.

Diagnosis

Ascitic fluid is usually straw-colored or bile-stained and sterile, with a few reactive mesothelial cells. The amount is variable, sometimes as high as several liters. The intraabdominal pressure rarely exceeds 10 mm Hg. Protein concentration is generally less than 2.5 g/dl. Higher values can occur in uncomplicated cirrhosis.[12] The explanation lies in the higher protein concentration of hepatic lymph compared to splanchnic lymph. In early cirrhosis, postsinusoidal portal hypertension produces an ascites derived largely from hepatic interstitial fluid with high-protein content. With late cirrhosis, the predominantly presinusoidal portal hypertension leads to an ascitic fluid derived from splanchnic interstitial fluid with low-protein content. High-protein ascites also may indicate extrahepatic venous outflow occlusion or development of hepatoma. Tuberculous peritonitis and pancreatic ascites are other conditions which must be excluded. Leukocyte counts exceeding 300/mm³ indicate spontaneous bacterial peritonitis or other infectious peritonitis.

Low-sodium content is found if sodium intake is restricted or if the ascitic fluid has been repeatedly tapped. Ascites of hepatic origin must also be differentiated from that due to cardiac, renal, malignant, and infectious causes.

Control

The basis of management is salt restriction (<500 mg sodium/day) and diuretic therapy. Paracentesis is not a routine procedure but is reserved for diagnosis if that is in doubt and for relief of a painful tense abdomen. A diuretic of the spironolactone group, such as Aldactone, 200–400 mg/day, would be the drug of choice as it acts by inhibiting the renal effects of aldosterone, decreases sodium reabsorption in the distal tubules, and retains potassium. Furosemide and ethacrynic acid are also effective drugs for ascites. Both act like the thiazides by inhibiting sodium reabsorption. These potent drugs also produce kaliuresis. Other diuretics of the organomercurial and thiazide classes are used to potentiate spinonolactone. The thiazides are avoided as sole agents because of their kaliuretic properties. Potassium depletion must be avoided since patients with decompensated cirrhosis already have a 10–30% reduction of total body potassium. Surgical portosystemic anastomosis is rarely indicated for relief of ascites alone.

Complications

Aside from nonphysiological alterations denoted by ascites, complications may result from overtreatment and bacterial infection. Vigorous diuretic therapy or paracentesis can precipitate hepatic coma by the mechanism of hypokalemic alkalosis or hypovolemic shock. About 20% of the onsets in hepatic coma are produced in this manner. Hyponatremia is another common electrolyte problem that results from overtreatment. Secondary infection may arise from contamination introduced during the withdrawal of ascitic fluid. There is the interesting entity of spontaneous bacterial peritonitis, which is not related to therapy or paracentesis. About 10% of cirrhotic patients with ascites develop this serious and often unrecognized infection.[13] It is reported in epidemic proportions from one institution.[14]

The disease starts as contamination of preexisting ascites by transient bacteremia originating from the gut flora (? due to altered mucosal permeability) and followed by a septic course. *Escherichia coli, Klebsiella,* and pneumococcus are among the common bacteria identified in the infection. Blood cultures are positive in 60% of the cases. Prognosis is poor. The survival rate has been reported as less than 5%, and in another series as 20%.[14,15]

REFERENCES

1. Baldus WP: Renal failure in advanced liver disease, in Gen Ref No. 9, pp 251–267.
2. Conn HO: The rational management of ascites, in Gen Ref No. 9, pp 269–288.
3. Conn HO: A rational approach to the hepatorenal syndrome. *Gastroenterology* 65:321–340, 1973.
4. Epstein M, et al: Renal failure in the patient with cirrhosis: The role of active vasoconstriction. *Amer J Med* 49:175–185, 1970.
5. Fischer JE, James JH: Treatment of hepatic coma and hepatorenal syndrome. *Amer J Surg* 123:222–230, 1972.
6. Schroeder ET, et al: Plasma renin level in hepatic cirrhosis: Relation to functional renal failure. *Amer J Med* 49:186–191, 1970.

7. Iwatsuki S, et al: Recovery from "hepatorenal syndrome" after orthotopic liver transplantation. *New Eng J Med* 289:1155–1159, 1973.
8. Bradley SE: Hepatorenal and glomerulotubular imbalance. *New Eng J Med* 289:1194–1195, 1973.
9. Witte MH, Witte CL, Dumont AE: Progress in liver disease: Physiological factors involved in the causation of cirrhotic ascites. *Gastroenterology* 61:742–750, 1971.
10. Lieberman FL, Denison EK, Reynolds TB: The relationship of plasma volume, portal hypertension, ascites and renal sodium retention in cirrhosis: The overflow theory of ascites formation. *Ann NY Acad Sci* 170:203–206, 1970.
11. Editorial: Compartmentalisation of ascitic fluid. *Lancet* 2:599–600, 1970.
12. Editorial: Diagnostic ascitic tap in cirrhosis. *Brit Med J* 1:701, 1975.
13. Conn HO: Spontaneous bacterial peritonitis: Multiple revisitations. *Gastroenterology* 70:445–457, 1976.
14. Correia JP, Conn HO: Spontaneous bacterial peritonitis in cirrhosis: Endemic or epidemic? *Med Clin North Amer* 59:963–981, 1975.
15. Curry N, McCallum RW, Guth PH: Spontaneous peritonitis in cirrhotic ascites. *Amer J Dig Dis* 19:685–692, 1974.
16. Goldring PL, Mason ASM: Renal tubular acidosis and autoimmune liver disease. *Gut* 12:153–157, 1971.
17. Better OS, et al: Defect in urinary acidification in cirrhosis: The role of excessive tubular reabsorption of sodium in its etiology. *Arch Intern Med* 130:77–83, 1972.
18. Whang R, Papper S: The possible relationship of renal cortical hypoperfusion and diminished renal concentrating ability in Laennec's cirrhosis. *J Chron Dis* 27:263–265, 1974.

LIVER FAILURE AND HEPATIC COMA

8

LIVER FAILURE

Liver failure supervenes when there is a severe reduction of hepatocellular function. The extent of liver cell necrosis required to produce this effect in humans is not known. In dogs an estimated 75% destruction of the liver leads to hepatic coma, a component of the liver failure syndrome. The term liver failure is not as specific or as uniformly agreed upon as cardiac failure and renal failure.[1] This is in part due to the fact that practically all organ systems are involved in liver failure. The multiple disorders occur in various combinations and at various times, depending on the nature of the underlying disease. It is generally accepted that liver failure suggests a serious syndrome associated with a grave prognosis and evidence of severe hepatic dysfunction, involving jaundice, ascites, fetor hepaticus, hepatic coma, coagulation disorders, renal failure, endocrine changes, and circulatory disturbances. The symptoms and course are modified by the etiology and are either acute or chronic. Coma, jaundice, coagulopathy, and renal failure are common to both forms. Jaundice and fetor hepaticus are generally more severe in acute hepatic failure. In addition, a sudden decrease in liver size is common. By comparison, renal failure, ascites, endocrine abnormalities, and circulatory disturbances predominate in chronic liver failure.

Major Features of Liver Failure

Jaundice. Deep jaundice is a primary feature of acute liver failure, and generally reflects the severity of the disease process. In fulminant viral hepatitis, 80% of the cases are said to have bilirubin values of 20–40 mg/dl. This is not invariable, as patients may die with hyperbilirubinemia of 2–3 mg/dl. Reye's syndrome, acute fatty liver of pregnancy, and tetracycline-induced fatty liver are other examples of acute hepatic failure with mild hyperbilirubinemia (<5 mg/dl). In alcoholic hepatitis bilirubin levels correlate well with other clinical and laboratory indicators of disease severity. In chronic liver failure, especially due to chronic alcoholism, jaundice fluctuates and bears no constant relationship to the degree of parenchymal damage.

Ascites.   For a full treatment of ascites see Chapter 7.

Fetor hepaticus.   In acute liver failure fetor hepaticus may herald the onset of coma. It may occur in chronic liver disease with large portosystemic shunts, in which instance prognosis is not necessarily grave (see below).

Hepatic coma.   Hepatic coma is discussed below.

Coagulation defects.   The varied pattern of coagulation protein defects in liver disease is summarized in Chapter 1. The liver normally synthesizes factors II, VII, IX, and X (the prothrombin complex), V, fibrinogen, and XIII. The prothrombin time measures this complex, which is frequently depressed in both acute and chronic liver failure. Correlation with the severity of parenchymal disease is good. A value of 30% or less of the control value indicates a grave outlook. Prothrombin time is a useful index of prognosis in fulminant viral hepatitis. Intravascular coagulation with secondary local fibrinolysis is a common preterminal phenomenon in fulminant hepatic failure. It is recognized by the thrombocytopenia, decreased plasma fibrinogen and other clotting factors, appearance of fibrin/fibrinogen degradation products, decreased plasminogen activator and plasminogen (Table 8.1).[2] Fibrin deposition is found in 50% of liver sections within sinusoids and areas of necrosis.[3] The process of intravascular coagulation is usually not severe and cannot be

Table 8.1.   Mechanism of disseminated intravascular coagulation in liver disease.[2]

---

1. Triggering events:
     Release of hepatic "thromboplastic" substances; ↓ hepatic clearance of coagulant factors
2. Primary events:
     Generation of prothrombin activator
                        ↓
     Conversion of prothrombin to thrombin
                        ↓
     Thrombin action on fibrinogen conversion → fibrin; platelet aggregation → thrombin; plasminogen → plasmin
3. Secondary events:
     Secondary fibrinolysis → fibrin products X, Y, D, E
     Circulating fibrin monomer → soluble complexes

---

correlated with either hematological or hepatic findings. It bears no constant relationship to the severity of bleeding. For these reasons, heparin is not suggested in the routine management of fulminant hepatic failure. The added risk that heparin itself may cause massive bleeding is also against its use.

Renal failure. This refers to the hepatorenal syndrome occurring in cirrhosis and in fulminant hepatitis (see Chapter 7). Oliguria, azotemia, and especially high urine osmolality and very low sodium content indicate intact tubular function and differentiate this condition from acute tubular necrosis.

Endocrine abnormalities. Gynecomastia, spider nevi, and testicular atrophy are well-known endocrine hallmarks of the cirrhotic process in alcoholics. These abnormalities are attributable in part to hyperestrogenism. Liver failure under these conditions does not signify shortened survival (see Chapter 10).

Circulatory disturbances. These are detailed elsewhere (Chapter 10). The hyperkinetic circulation described for cirrhosis occurs also in acute fulminant hepatitis.

Fulminant Hepatic Failure

Fulminant hepatic failure describes a syndrome clinically manifested by an abrupt onset of jaundice, hepatic coma, often death, and functionally by profound hepatic dysfunction.[4,5] There is usually an abbreviated time course leading to a conclusion within 2-3 weeks of symptoms. Rarely, a prolonged course of 1-2 months ensues, which is more common among older patients. Fulminant viral hepatitis which complicates less than 1% of the cases of acute viral hepatitis is the leading cause. Other causes are listed in Table 8.2. Although minor variations are associated with each of these diseases, a common pattern of symptoms and biochemical disturbance is observed. The term fulminant hepatic failure is preferable to fulminant hepatitis or acute hepatic necrosis since a number of causative diseases show neither necrosis nor hepatitis.

Pathology

In the majority of cases massive hepatic necrosis is seen (Fig. 8.1). At times, particularly in drug-induced cases, there is both necrosis and inflammation simulating severe hepatitis. Less commonly, fatty change constitutes the primary finding, eg, Reye's syndrome. The severity of

Table 8.2.   Causes of fulminant hepatic failure.[4,5]

Cause	Incidence of failure	Fatality rate
Infections		
Acute viral hepatitis	1%; 10% in post-transfusion hepatitis	70–80% with grade IV coma
Disseminated herpes sim-plex in newborns and preg-nant mothers		
Marburg monkey disease		
Ischemia		
Hepatic artery ligation		
Acute Budd-Chiari syndrome		
Heatstroke		
Toxins		
CCl_4		<5%
Phosphorus		
Amanita phalloides (toadstool)		30%
Drugs		
Halothane	30%	80–90%
Methoxyflurane	60%	100%
Paracetacol overdosage		
Isoniazid		
Iproniazid		
Pyrazinamide		
Indomethacin		
p-Aminosalicylic acid		
Tetracycline (2 g IV)		75%
Unknown etiology		
Reye's syndrome	100%	50%
Acute fatty liver of pregnancy		85%

histologic alterations does not correlate with the likelihood of fulminant failure. The evolution of hepatic coma in this condition remains largely unknown. Possible pathogenic factors are discussed below.

Clinical Presentation

Progressive, deepening jaundice is usual but not invariable, preceding the appearance of hepatic coma. Coma increases in graded steps, easily distinguishable by four separate stages (see below), with corresponding EEG alterations. Fetor hepaticus is a prominent accompaniment. Abdom-

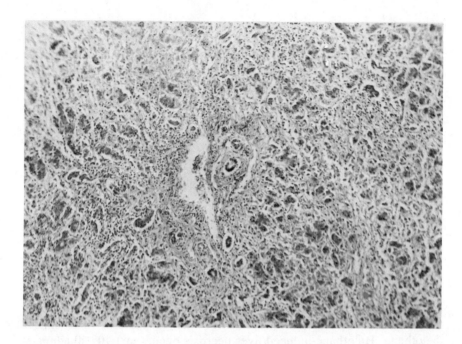

Fig. 8.1. Fulminant viral hepatitis. Fields of necrotic hepatocytes are interspersed with regenerative liver cells forming tubules. A triad is observed in the middle of the biopsy. H and E, X100.

inal pains may be common in poisoning cases, as in toadstool toxicity. A small liver is expected with massive hepatic necrosis. Tenderness of the liver rarely occurs in viral hepatitis. Systemic disturbances are usual; hypotension, high cardiac output, oliguria, hyponatremia, profuse sweating, hypoglycemia (particularly in children), and diffuse hemorrhage due to disseminated intravascular coagulation.

Hepatic tests document profound hepatic dysfunction. Serum aminotransferase levels are exceedingly high until the terminal stage, or moderate in cases of fatty change. Bilirubin concentrations generally are over 20 mg/dl. Serum alkaline phosphatase activity is normal or slightly raised. Typically, serum prothrombin values fall to 30%, more commonly to less than 5% of the control value. Serum albumin and globulin are maintained at the usual levels, but albumin may drop later. Blood ammonia elevation correlates with worsening coma, but a normal value is present in 10% of the cases. A respiratory alkalosis with low pCO_2 is the most common abnormality noted in acid-base studies.[6] This is ascribed to hyperventilation, resulting from stimulation of the respiratory center by cerebral toxins. Metabolic alkalosis also occurs frequently. Several factors may be responsible for the alkalosis: (1) a decrease of total body potassium, which has been described in hepatitis and cirrhosis; (2) movement of hydrogen ions into intracellular space; and (3) inappropriately high renal excretion of hydrogen ions. Metabolic acidosis is uncommon in fulminant hepatic failure. It is usually associated with cases of drug toxicity or with severe renal failure. In rare instances, the acidosis is due to lactic acid accumulation, occurring in the presence of peripheral circulatory failure. Other indicators of metabolic disturbances become abnormal as the terminal stage approaches. There are increased blood levels of lactate, pyruvate, acetoacetate, and citrate, and plasma free fatty acid concentrations.

Pathogenesis

Fulminant hepatitis is the commonest cause of this syndrome. Factors which might aggravate this type of attack are: old age (compared to a more benign course in children) and a questionable predilection for the female sex and for pregnancy. Positive or negative reactions for HB_sAg are not related to the likelihood of a fatal outcome in viral hepatitis. The next most frequent cause is halogenated anesthesia, particularly halothane. Halothane-induced liver necrosis occurs in 1:10,000 administrations for the first exposure, and in 7:10,000 administrations with multiple exposures to the anesthetic.

Prognosis

The mortality rate is high, 70-80% in adults, 50% in children. Adverse factors include age over 40, reduction of liver size, convulsions or decerebrate postures, prothrombin activity less than 30% of the control value, blood ammonia greater than 2 μg/ml, absence of AFP, and less than 35% intact hepatocytes as estimated by liver biopsy.[7] Favorable factors include an increase of AFP and coagulation proteins, measured as prothrombin activity. Low serum BUN or elevated creatinine are of no prognostic significance.

Treatment

Corticosteroids, exchange blood transfusion, hemodialysis, cross circulation, isolated pig perfusion liver, and transplantation have all been performed without proven efficacy. Steroids do not enhance survival of patients with fulminant viral hepatitis.[8] Steroids may in fact be harmful to those patients who are HB_sAg positive or who show bridging necrosis on liver biopsy. Therapy with heparin to control intravascular coagulation or infusion with HB_sAb immune serum have not been encouraging. Hemoperfusion on charcoal or other resin columns appears promising.[9] Further refinement and experience with the techniques are awaited. Depletion of platelets, leukocytes, and clotting factors is a major problem with these artificial liver systems.

HEPATIC COMA

Hepatic coma (portosystemic encephalopathy) is characterized neurologically by changing levels of consciousness, flapping tremors, and distinctive EEG findings, and biochemically by severe liver dysfunction. There may or may not be evidence of portosystemic shunts. The clinical course can be acute or chronic, self-limited, progressive or intermittent. Hepatic coma is one of the major manifestations of severe liver failure and a common mode of death in liver disease. At least 30% of the patients with alcoholic cirrhosis die in hepatic coma.

Clinical Presentation[10]

Several patterns are recognized, depending on the nature of the underlying hepatic disease (Table 8.3). The onset in the acute pattern is often

Table 8.3. Onset of hepatic coma.[1]

Type	Time interval	Precipitating factors	Pathology	Disease
Acute	Hours to days	Usually absent	Severe or massive cell necrosis	Fulminant viral hepatitis, Reye's syndrome, drug-induced liver necrosis (tetracycline, methyldopa)
	Up to weeks	Often present	Fibrosis and necrosis	Alcoholic hepatitis, chronic active hepatitis
Chronic	Weeks to months	Usually present	Fibrosis, necrosis, portacaval shunting	Cirrhosis

dramatic, with delirium, violent behavior, convulsions, and a clouding of consciousness which rapidly passes into coma in hours or days. This is usually seen in fulminant hepatic failure due to virus, drugs, and other toxins. The fatality rate in these cases is around 75%. An acute presentation may also occur in patients with alcoholic hepatitis and chronic active hepatitis. The patients are usually in the late stages of the disease with ascites, deep jaundice, or portal hypertension. A precipitating event is often noted. A second common pattern is characterized by a slow, insidious onset. Apathy, drowsiness, loss of intellectual function, and a deepening stupor are present. Precipitating causes are often implicated. The symptoms are largely reversible. A third, and infrequent mode of onset consists of gradual, progressive acquirement of basal ganglia and cerebellar disease-like features, along with mental disturbances. This disorder has been termed "acquired chronic hepatocerebral degeneration" because of its clinical and pathological similarities to Wilson's disease. The pattern may develop in patients who show little initial hepatic dysfunction or in patients who have relapsing hepatic coma. In the latter situation, the chronic liver disease is usually associated with evidence of large portosystemic shunting.

Pathogenesis

Two groups of factors are involved: Those which increase cerebral sensitivity, and those which affect cerebral activity (cerebral toxins). Factors heightening cerebral susceptibility of patients and experimental animals with liver injury are not well understood. Clinically, patients with seemingly well-compensated liver disease are precipitated into hepatic coma by factors (sedatives, diuretics) which normal patients tolerate. In experimental brain-liver perfusion models removal of the liver impairs brain function, suggesting a parabiotic relationship between the two organs. Among the various cerebral toxins implicated, amino acid imbalance,[11] ammonia,[10] short-chain fatty acids,[12] mercaptans,[12] and biogenic amines[13] rank among the serious contenders in the pathogenesis of hepatic coma (Fig. 8.2). Other toxic substances are proposed, but their importance is not established.

Amino acid imbalance.[11]   The toxicity of amino acids in brain transmission is suggested by the finding that phenylalanine, methionine, and tryptophan are elevated in the plasma of humans and animals in hepatic coma. In contrast, the branched-chain amino acids (leucine, isoleucine, and valine) and threonine are reduced. The abnormal plasma amino acid pattern is attributed to the hyperinsulinemia which results from impaired extraction by the cirrhotic liver.[11] The excess insulin enhances the in-

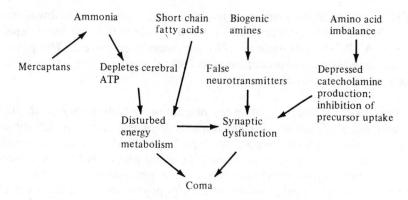

Fig. 8.2. Pathogenesis of hepatic coma.

creased uptake of the branched-chain amino acids by muscle tissue with subsequent reduction of the plasma levels of these amino acids. Since branched-chain amino acids, tryptophan, tyrosine, and phenylalanine, share a common transport system, the altered plasma pattern affects the entry of amino acids into the brain. A low level of branched-chain amino acids reduces the competitive action of these amino acids on the entry of tryptophan into the brain. This promotes excess buildup of cerebral tryptophan, acceleration of serotonin synthesis, and depression of catecholamine formation. The events are thought to bring on the hepatic coma state. The high concentration of phenylalanine may affect the hydroxylation-converting step to tyrosine. This could account for the depression of the adrenergic neurotransmitter, norepinephine, found in experimentally induced acute hepatic coma. The synthesis of norepi- nephrine starts with 3-hydroxylation of tyrosine. Excess phenylalanine in- hibits brain uptake of tyrosine and secondarily diminishes norepinephrine synthesis. The lack of norepinephrine production predisposes the brain to pick up false neurotransmitters (see below).

Infusions of essential and nonessential amino acids into patients with hepatic coma do not correct the abnormal plasma pattern of elevated phenylalanine and reduced branched-chain amino acids.[14] In the past the toxicity of methionine was emphasized but this is related to its degrada- tion to mercaptans and ammonia in the gut. Glutamine was also formerly held as an important cerebral toxin since it is found at high levels in the spinal fluid of comatose patients. At one time glutamine was thought to function as a neurotransmitter, but current thinking assigns it to the neuroglial compartment, without a role at the synaptic junction. Synthesis of glutamine is derived from a rapidly turning over pool of glutamic acid, rather than from alpha-ketoglutarate as was once assumed. Incorporation of NH_3 into the alpha-ketoglutarate-glutamic acid-glutamine pathway was thought to drain intermediates from Kreb's cycle with subsequent depletion of ATP. The postulate is no longer considered correct. The prominence once assigned to glutamine as a cerebral toxin appears less convincing at the present date.

Ammonia.[10] The importance of ammonia intoxication in the pathogenesis of hepatic encephalopathy remains generally accepted. Three clinical findings support the hypothesis. First, patients in hepatic coma generally have increased levels of blood and CSF ammonia. Second, creation of portacaval shunts leads to hyperammonemia and hepatic encephalopathy. Third, removal of factors producing ammonia reverses the coma state.

Ammonia interferes with brain function at several biochemical sites (Fig. 8.3),[15] causing the following:

1. Impaired oxidative decarboxylation of pyruvic acid
2. Decreased ATP production resulting from NADH depletion
3. Depletion of alpha-ketoglutarate
4. Utilization of ATP in glutamine formation
5. Stimulation of membrane ATPase
6. Decreased synthesis of acetylcholine

The net effect of impairment at sites 1–4 would result in decreased availability of ATP. Steps 5 and 6 would lead to depressed neuronal activity. Interference with cerebral energy metabolism is the most widely held hypothesis of ammonia's effect upon the brain.

Short-chain fatty acids (SCFA).[12] The important SCFA are the 5, 6, and 8 carbon chain fatty acids (butyric, valeric, and octanoic) derived from medium-chain fatty acids. Experimental liver injury in animals elevates the blood SCFA. Infusion of SCFA in high concentrations induces coma in animals. Although serum and CSF concentrations of SCFA are increased in patients with liver disease and in hepatic coma, correlation with experimental models is not exact, since the levels of SCFA reached in humans do not cause coma in animals. SCFA interferes with cerebral metabolism by uncoupling oxidative phosphorylation and inhibiting neuronal membrane activity.

Mercaptans.[12] Mercaptan derivatives—methanethiol, ethanethiol, and dimethylsulfide—can all experimentally induce coma in rats. Dimethylsulfide is less toxic by a 14,000-fold difference compared to methanethiol, suggesting that dimethylsulfide may be an important pathway of detoxification for methionine derivatives. Methanethiol enhances

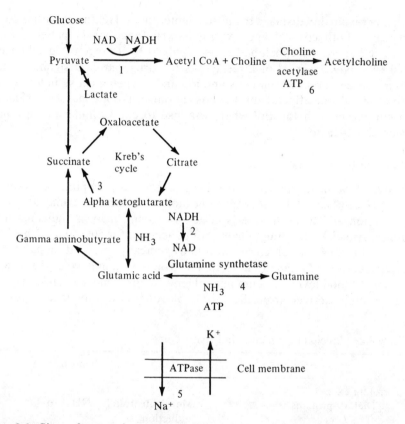

Fig. 8.3. Sites of ammonia cerebrotoxicity; see text for explanation. (Adapted from K. J. Breen and S. Schenker.[15])

the blood level of ammonia when the latter is administered to rats. The mechanism for the increase is unknown. Mercaptans act synergistically with ammonia or octanoate in producing experimental hepatic coma.

Biogenic amines.[13]   Octopamine and beta-phenylethanolamines are degraded from intestinal proteins by gut bacteria. They bypass the liver through portacaval shunts and accumulate in the brain to interfere with normal synaptic transmission as false neurotransmitters. Octopamine is found in increased levels in the urine and serum of patients with hepatic coma, and in the brain of animals with hepatic injury. The stage of encephalopathy in patients correlates well with serum-octopamine levels.[16] The cerebral excess mimics the findings in Parkinson's disease. This has led to the use of L-dopa in hepatic coma. L-dopa increases the brain content of dopamine and norepinephrine, normal neurotransmitters, which presumably displace the false counterparts. Treatment with L-dopa improves both cortical and extrapyramidal functions in patients with chronic hepatic encephalopathy, as adjudged by a range of speed-based tasks.[17] Over a period of three weeks the drug causes a significant increase in cerebral oxygen consumption and oxygen-glucose index. Gastrointestinal side effects limit the dosage range. L-dopa may be indicated in chronic encephalopathy when response to conventional therapy has been unsatisfactory.

Precipitating Factors

In over 50% of the patients with hepatic coma a precipitating factor is recognized (Table 8.4). More than one factor can occur at a time, and they may often add to each other's effect. A recent analysis indicates that drugs, especially the tranquilizer group, account for 50% and GI hemorrhage for 20% of all cases with iatrogenically induced hepatic encephalopathy.[18] Precipitating factors in groups 1, 2, and 3 (see Table 8.4) augment blood levels of ammonia, chiefly by three mechanisms: (1) Excess protein derived from diet or GI bleeding is metabolized to amino

Table 8.4. Precipitating factors in hepatic coma.[1,15]

Factor	Mechanism
1. Protein excess	
a. Dietary proteins	More substrate for NH_3 production
b. GI hemorrhage	Hypovolemia comprises renal and hepatic function (100 ml blood provides 20 g protein)
2. NH_3 overload	
a. Diuretics	Induces hypokalemic alkalosis
b. Hypokalemic alkalosis	↑ renal output of NH_3; ↑ diffusible NH_3 across cell membrane
c. Uremia	↑ enterohepatic cycle of urea
d. Frequent paracentesis	Hypovolemia and prerenal uremia
3. Cerebral depressants	
a. Sedatives, narcotics, anesthetics	Hypoxia
4. Increased tissue catabolism	
a. Infections	↑ endogenous nitrogen and NH_3 load
b. Acute pancreatitis	
c. Hepatoma	

acids which undergo deamination by the action of bacterial deaminase to form NH_3. (2) Metabolic alkalosis or hypokalemia increases renal production of NH_4 from glutamine by the action of glutaminase. (3) At an alkalotic pH the blood NH_4 equilibrium of $[NH_4]^+ + OH \leftrightharpoons NH_3 + HOH$ is shifted to the right favoring the un-ionized NH_3. The latter crosses the blood-brain barrier and cell membrane more rapidly than the ionized form $[NH_4]^+$. At the normal pH of 7.4 blood ammonia exists mostly as the poorly diffusible $[NH_4]^+$.

Hepatic Features

The hepatic features represent manifestations of the underlying acute or chronic liver disease. Varying degrees of jaundice, hepatomegaly, ascites, or portal hypertension are observed. Fetor hepaticus is usually present in patients with fulminant hepatitis or cirrhosis in hepatic coma. The odor is pungent and fetid, resembling that of feces and is a grave prognostic sign. The fetor is ascribed to mercaptan derivatives, principally dimethyl-sulfide, appearing on the breath. Normally, mercaptans are formed in the gut by bacterial degradation of methionine and metabolized in the liver. A small amount is exhaled in the normal breath, but impaired hepatic metabolism leads to mercaptan accumulation.

Stages of hepatic coma. Evaluating the stages in this condition allows for assessment of the patient's prognosis and status during treatment. The course need not be progressively downhill; it often fluctuates. Stage IV coma is associated with a 70–80% mortality rate (Table 8.5).

Neurological Features

The neurological features are summarized as follows.

Table 8.5. Stages of hepatic coma.

Stage	Sensorium	Tremor	EEG changes
I. Prodromal	Confusion, impaired mentation	Usually slight	Absent
II. Impending coma	Drowsiness, inappropriate behavior	Present	Present
III. Stupor	Sleeps mostly, but arousable	Present, if patient co-operates	Present
IV. Coma	Unconscious, may respond to deep stimuli	Usually absent	Generally present

Altered levels of consciousness.   Apathy, insomnia, increasing periods of sleep, delirium, and stupor are common symptoms.

Impaired intellectual functions.   Slurred, hesitant speech, visual agnosia, gross confusion, loss of memory, and constructional apraxia may appear. The latter is demonstrated by the five-star match or drawing test which patients are unable to master. Writing of sentences is also a test of motor performance function. The tests may be recorded periodically as a check of mental status and progress.

Flapping tremor or asterixis.   This is a characteristic though not specific sign of hepatic coma. The disordered extrapyramidal movement can also be seen in uremia, hypokalemia, hypoglycemia, cardiac failure, and pulmonary failure. The tremor is best elicited with arms outstretched, wrists extended, and fingers apart. In this posture there appears rapid, arrhythmic movement, 1–2/second, consisting of lateral deviations of the fingers, flexion-extension of the fingers, and a similar motion at the wrist. The same tremor may be observed in the feet, eyelids, tongue, and corners of the mouth. The abnormal movements disappear in the deep coma state.

Nonspecific cerebral disturbances.   They include hyperreflexia, increased muscle tone leading to rigidity, sucking and grasping reflexes, and appearance of extensor plantar reflexes at a late stage.

EEG pattern.   The change is characteristic but not specific. The normal alpha pattern of 8–12 cycles per second (cps) is replaced by symmetrical, high spikes of 3–5 cps (delta waves), appearing in the frontal regions initially. As the disturbances progress, this pattern spreads to the entire cerebral hemisphere. EEG changes not only aid diagnosis of the impending coma, but indicate therapeutic response.

Neuropathological changes.   In acute hepatic coma, brain changes are absent except for perhaps mild cerebral edema. In the chronic type of hepatic encephalopathy, diffuse increase in the number and size of astrocytes is observed.[19] The commoner of the astrocyte abnormalities is the Alzheimer type II change, in which the nuclei become greatly swollen and indented with prominent nucleoli. The rarer abnormality is the Alzheimer type I change. The nuclei become enlarged, deformed, often multilobular, with twice the normal DNA content. Alzheimer type II change can be readily induced in the brain of rats with portacaval anastomosis and hyperammonemia. The change is probably an expression of metabolic hyperactivity in which water shifts into the nucleus. There is evidence that astrocytes are normally involved in the detoxification of ammonia, which is produced as a byproduct of neuronal metabolism.

Laboratory Findings

Altered hepatic tests reflect the extent of parenchymal necrosis and portacaval shunts in the underlying liver disease. The primary finding consists of an elevation of blood ammonia (> 1 $\mu g/ml$). Ten percent of patients with hepatic coma lack this increase. Acid-base balance and electrolytes are often abnormal; the pattern is determined by the nature of the precipitating factor. A hypokalemic alkalosis is common. Increased levels of alpha-ketoglutaric acid and pyruvic acid, and hypoglycemia correlate with the disturbance in carbohydrate metabolism. Short-chain fatty acids are elevated, indicating impaired fat metabolism. Concentrations of spinal fluid glutamic acid, glutamine, and alpha-ketoglutaramate are high.[20] The CSF is otherwise clear, normal in pressure and free of cellular elements, although a mild increase of protein may be present. The EEG shows a delta-wave pattern which replaces the normal alpha rhythm.

Differential Diagnosis

The main diseases to be considered are those caused by acute and chronic alcoholism, such as the following.

Delirium tremens. Agitation, severe hallucinations, and a fine rapid tremor are characteristics of this state. The tremors become worse at rest.

Wernicke's encephalopathy. Ophthalmoplegia, nystagmus, and ataxia are the three diagnostic signs.

Korsakoff's psychosis. Memory defect and confabulation are components of this disease.

Wilson's disease. The tremor is choreoathetoid rather than flapping. The Kayser-Fleischer corneal ring is invariably found.

Brain injury. Subdural hematoma is particularly difficult to differentiate from hepatic coma, unless a history of trauma and localizing neurologic signs can be established.

Management

The aims of therapy are threefold: First, control of liver disease. In most instances, this means avoiding further damage to the liver. Second, control of precipitating factors. The measures are directed toward avoiding unwarranted use of sedatives, diuretics, and paracentesis, toward controlling GI hemorrhage and infection, and toward correction of electrolytes and fluid abnormalities. Third, reduction of nitrogenous substances in the blood. The aim of the various therapeutic regimens is to decrease ammonia absorption from the gut and its production in the intestine. For impending or acute hepatic coma, protein restriction, a cleansing colonic enema, and neomycin therapy are standard procedures. Dietary protein is eliminated for 2–4 days, and gradually increased by 10–20 g increments every day until tolerated. A cleansing enema is employed to evacuate the contents of the lower colon. Neomycin (4–8 g/day) is given to reduce the number of urease-producing bacteria. Although the antibiotic is considered essentially nonabsorbable, about 1% of the dose is reabsorbed from the gut, a small amount which can produce renal and ototoxicity.

For chronic or intermittent hepatic coma, a combination of a low-protein diet (about 25 g/day) and neomycin in small doses (2–4 g/day) is recommended. The amount of dietary protein should be tailored to the presence of neuropsychiatric symptoms. Lactulose, a synthetic disaccharide, may be added to the regimen or substituted for neomycin. The addition of lactulose allows for a lower dosage of neomycin to be used. Lactulose is not metabolized until it reaches the large intestine, where it is hydrolyzed by bacterial action to lactic and acetic acids.[21] The alkaline pH in the colonic lumen becomes acidic, below pH 5. Absorption of ammonia is reduced, although the mechanism by which lactulose acts is not completely understood. Lactulose is usually administered in doses of 60–160 g/day until a laxative effect is observed.

An interesting approach to the problem of improving protein tolerance involves oral supplementation with glucose. Hourly glucose ingestion increases insulin secretion but decreases the glucagon level.[22] The increased ratio of insulin to glycogen is attended by a slight fall in blood ammonia after protein meals supplemented by glucose. In contrast, blood ammonia rises after meals without extra glucose. The explanation is that insulin either suppresses hepatic ureagenesis or reduces amino acid availability for gluconeogenesis, or both. The effectiveness of glucose supplementation in the treatment of hepatic coma requires further documentation. For chronic encephalopathy unresponsive to conventional therapy, L-dopa may be given a trial.

Other unproved heroic methods employed in the treatment of hepatic coma are exchange transfusion, isolated perfusion of the liver, artificial liver systems, cross circulation with primates, hemodialysis, total body washout, and hepatic transplantation. These procedures are either technically difficult and impractical or offer a low success rate. However, there is a promising technique—hemoperfusion with activated charcoal or resin columns.[23] The method has not yet been fully developed and further confirmation is needed.

REFERENCES

1. Zimmerman HJ: Hepatic failure, in Gen Ref No. 6, pp 384–405.
2. Roberts HR, Cederbaum AI: The liver and blood coagulation: Physiology and pathology. *Gastroenterology* 63:297–320, 1972.
3. Hillenbrand P, et al: Significance of intravascular coagulation and fibrinolysis in acute hepatic failure. *Gut* 15:83–88, 1974.
4. Rueff B, Benhamou JP: Acute hepatic necrosis and fulminant hepatitis. *Gut* 19:805–815, 1973.
5. Redeker AG: Fulminant hepatitis, in Gen Ref No. 12, pp 149–155.
6. Record CO, et al: Acid-base and metabolic disturbances in fulminant hepatic failure. *Gut* 16:144–149, 1975.
7. Scotto J, et al: Liver biopsy and prognosis in acute liver failure. *Gut* 14:927–933, 1973.
8. Gregory PB, et al: Steroid therapy in severe hepatitis: A double-blind, randomized trial of methyl-prednisolone versus placebo. *N Eng J Med* 294:681–687, 1976.
9. Editorial: Progress with an artificial liver. *Lancet* 2:992–994, 1974.
10. Schenker S, Breen KJ, Hoyumpa AM Jr: Hepatic encephalopathy: Current status. *Gastroenterology* 66:121–151, 1974.
11. Munro HN, Fernstrom JD, Wurtman RJ: Insulin, plasma aminoacid imbalance and hepatic coma. *Lancet* 1:722–724, 1975.
12. Zieve L, Doizaki WM, Zieve FJ: Synergism between mercaptans and ammonia or fatty acids in the production of hepatic coma. *J Lab Clin Med* 83:16–28, 1974.
13. Fischer JE, Baldessarini RJ: False neurotransmitters and hepatic failure. *Lancet* 2:75–80, 1971.
14. Fischer JE, et al: Plasma amino acids in patients with hepatic encephalopathy: Effects of amino acid infusions. *Amer J Surg* 127:40–47, 1974.
15. Breen KJ, Schenker S: Hepatic coma: Present concepts of pathogenesis and therapy, in Gen Ref No. 9, pp 301–332.
16. Manghani KK, et al: Urinary and serum octopamine in patients with portal-systemic encephalopathy. *Lancet* 2:943–946, 1975.
17. Lunzer M, et al: Treatment of chronic hepatic encephalopathy with levodopa. *Gut* 15:555–561, 1974.
18. Fessel JM, Conn HO: An analysis of the causes and prevention of hepatic coma. *Gastroenterology* 62:191, 1972 (abstr).
19. Editorial: The astrocyte in liver disease. *Lancet* 1:1189–1190, 1971.

20. Vergara F, Plum F, Duffy TE: Alpha-keto-glutaramate: Increased concentrations in the cerebro-spinal fluid of patients in hepatic coma. *Science* 183:81–83, 1974.
21. Bircher J, et al: Treatment of chronic portal-systemic encephalopathy with lactulose: Report of six patients and review of the literature. *Amer J Med* 51:148–159, 1971.
22. Walker C, Petersen W Jr, Unger R: Blood ammonia levels in advanced cirrhosis during therapeutic elevation of the insulin: glucagon ratio. *New Eng J Med* 291:168–171, 1974.
23. Wilson RA: Acute fulminant hepatic failure: Potential therapeutic role of hemoperfusion. *Gastroenterology* 69:244–248, 1975.

HEPATIC FIBROSIS AND CIRRHOSIS

9

The magnitude and duration of liver damage determines the extent of hepatic fibrosis.[1] Collagen deposition follows cell necrosis and chronic inflammation in a well-defined sequence, although the mechanisms which govern collagen synthesis and degradation are poorly understood. Fibrosis may occur focally or diffusely. Focal fibrosis is often clinically silent. Diffuse fibrosis is a major feature in the clinical-pathologic entity of cirrhosis. Clinically, jaundice, ascites, portal hypertension, and hepatic coma present in a similar manner for the various types of cirrhosis. Morphologically, cirrhosis is characterized by nodular regeneration, diffuse fibrosis, inflammation, and necrosis. Grossly, the liver appears macronodular (nodules greater than 1 cm in size) or micronodular, or mixed macronodular-micronodular.

Cirrhosis is classified as follows: (1) alcoholic (Laennec's cirrhosis, the most common type in the United States), (2) cryptogenic cirrhosis, (3) biliary cirrhosis—primary and secondary, (4) hemochromatosis, (5) Wilson's disease (hepatolenticular degeneration), (6) cardiac cirrhosis, and (7) other rare forms. The causes and types of human cirrhosis are presented in Tables 9.1a and 1b. An increased incidence of cirrhosis occurs in hepatoma, diabetes mellitus, inflammatory bowel disease, and chronic pancreatitis. Biochemically, enzymes which participate in collagen synthesis such as prolyl hydroxylase[2] and an atypical amino oxidase[3] are elevated in the serum of patients with cirrhosis. Other enzymes engaged in the metabolism of acid mucopolysaccharides, beta-glucuronidase and beta-glucosaminidase, are similarly raised. Although sensitive indicators of hepatic fibrosis, they are not specific and are not widely employed in clinical practice. The enzymes do not improve diagnostic accuracy. A liver biopsy and standard liver function tests are still required for diagnosis. Collagen degradation products can also be detected in serum and urine. Serum levels of collagen-like protein, urinary excretion of hydroxyproline or hydroxyproline-containing peptides are increased in liver diseases (Table 9.2).[4] Chemical tests for these proteins are available but are cumbersome to perform and not generally used. Our recent under-

Table 9.1a.   Causes of human liver cirrhosis.

Infections:
  Viral hepatitis
  Cytomegalovirus
  Rubella
  ? Congenital syphilis
Metabolic disorders:
  Alpha-1-antitrypsin deficiency
  Cystic fibrosis
  Fanconi syndrome
  Galactosemia
  Glycogen-storage diseases (types III and IV)
  Hemochromatosis
  Hereditary fructose intolerance
  Hereditary tyrosinemia
  Porphyria cutanea tarda and erythropoietica
  Wilson's disease
Toxins and drugs:
  Pyrrolidizines (veno-occlusive disease)
  CCl_4, chloroform, phosphorus
  Arsenic, methotrexate, urethane
  Chlorpromazine, vinyl chloride
  Chronic hypervitaminosis A
Unknown etiology:
  Primary biliary cirrhosis
  Chronic extrahepatic biliary obstruction
  Hereditary hemorrhagic telangiectasia
  Hemosiderosis superimposed on malnutrition
  Sickle cell disease
  Thalassemia
  Jejunal shunt surgery
  Cryptogenic cirrhosis
  Indian childhood cirrhosis
  Atransferrinemia
  Pyridoxine-dependent anemia

standing of collagen metabolism has led to attempts to interrupt hepatic fibrosis with inhibitors or chelating agents.[5] These include corticosteroids which inhibit both ribosomal synthesis of collagen and prolyl hydroxylase activity; penicillamine, which interferes with cross-linkage of the collagen molecule; and colchicine which inhibits the extracellular secretion of the peptide precursor of collagen and stimulates collagenase activity. All three drugs have been employed in alcoholic hepatitis and acute cirrhosis but none has been established as a standard regimen.

Table 9.1b. Morphologic classification of cirrhosis.

Type	Synonyms	Anatomic substructure within nodule	Disease
Micronodular	Laennec's, portal cirrhosis	None	Alcoholism, hemochromatosis, Indian childhood cirrhosis, galactosemia, tyrosinemia, hereditary fructose intolerance
		With central veins	Primary and secondary biliary cirrhosis
	Cardiac cirrhosis	With portal triads	Budd-Chiari syndrome, chronic constrictive pericarditis, tricuspid insufficiency
Macronodular	Postnecrotic, coarsely nodular cirrhosis	With portal triads and central veins	Alcoholism, postviral hepatitis, posttoxic necrosis, Wilson's disease, alpha-1-antitrypsin deficiency, type IV glycogenosis
Mixed micro-nodular and macronodular	Mixed cirrhosis	—	Alcoholism

Table 9.2. Urinary hydroxyproline excretion in liver disease.[4]

Increased in:	Acute viral hepatitis
	Alcoholic hepatitis
	Chronic active hepatitis
	Cirrhosis
Normal in:	Alcoholism
	Intra- and extrahepatic cholestasis
	Metastatic hepatic carcinoma
	Granulomatous hepatitis

FIBROGENESIS IN EXPERIMENTAL AND HUMAN CIRRHOSIS[6]

Kinetic study of experimental cirrhosis has indicated a reversible and an irreversible phase. In CCl_4, ethionine, and choline deficiency models of cirrhosis, there is a dividing point during the developmental stage beyond which fibrosis continues or persists despite the cessation of hepatic injury. In rats given CCl_4 (0.15 ml twice weekly subcutaneously) the evolution of cirrhosis occurs in four stages:[7] (1) Necrosis and steatosis lasting 10 days. During this stage regeneration as determined by ^{3}H thymidine uptake is marked, particularly in hepatocytes, less in mesenchymal cells, and least in ductular cells. (2) The next phase, nonseptal fibrosis, dates approximately up to the sixty-fifth day. Connective tissue increases in the centrolobular areas and to a lesser degree around the portal tract. This is borne out by the increase of hydroxyproline, a marker for the collagen molecule. DNA labeling at this stage decreases. (3) In the third stage, septal fibrosis, collagen synthesis increases with septal formation. Early nodules are formed, and labeled hepatocytes once again are strikingly increased. This phase occurs up to 95 days after initiation of CCl_4 injections. (4) The final and fourth stage, cirrhosis, is marked by septal fibrosis increase, but cell uptake of ^{3}H thymidine has subsided. After 135 days, septal cirrhosis is well developed and established.

A similar staging applies to the ethionine model, in which young female rats are fed a synthetic diet low in protein, deficient in methionine, and supplemented by 0.5% DL-ethionine.[8] The resulting injury evolves as follows: (1) 0–3 weeks, with little fibrosis and cellular proliferation; (2) 3–7 weeks, marked by diffuse fibrosis and cell proliferation which increase progressively; (3) 7–12 weeks, stationary phase in which fibrosis and proliferated cells are maintained but do not increase; (4) after 12 weeks, development of cirrhosis with septum formation. During this period mortality among the animals is high.

A choline-deficient diet with 38% lard and low protein induces in rats a comparable cirrhosis.[9] The development of liver disease is recognizable in four stages: stage 1 (the first week), starting with centrolobular fat; stage 2 (second to third week), with panlobular fat; stage 3 (fourth to twelfth week), described as hypertrophic "cirrhosis," consisting of fatty cyst formation and fibrous trabeculation; and stage 4 (beyond the twelfth week) in which cirrhosis becomes established.

In all three models, the evolution of cirrhosis can be prevented at a given point. Reversal of cirrhosis is achieved in the CCl_4 model at the third stage of septal fibrosis on cessation of CCl_4 injection. For ethionine injury, restitution of methionine at the third stage, 12 weeks, prevents further hepatic lesions and leads to eventual healing. Replenishment of a choline-adequate diet at stage 3, the fourth week, interrupts progression toward cirrhosis. The reversible phases for the three toxins—CCl_4, ethionine, and choline deficiency—are approximately 12 weeks, 12 weeks, and 4 weeks, respectively. The ratio of collagen to cells (hydroxyproline to DNA) remains constant at this stage, in contrast to the irreversible phase in which the amount of collagen far exceeds the number of cells. Furthermore, in the CCl_4 model, the half-life of collagen is said to be 21–30 days in the reversible phase, while in the irreversible stage the half-life of collagen exceeds 240 days, a figure greater then the life span of the rat.[10] This would suggest that not only is there active synthesis of collagen during cirrhogenesis, but that a decrease of collagen degradation also occurs. In all three experimental models, irreversible cirrhosis is characterized by diffuse fibrosis and nodular regeneration. Fibrosis without regeneration, such as that induced in rats by repeated injections of heterologous serum, does not lead to cirrhosis with portal hypertension.[11] Human cirrhosis as a clinicopathological entity corresponds to the animal counterparts. In humans alcoholic cirrhosis is characterized by increased incorporation of ^{14}C or ^{3}H proline into salt-soluble collagen, expanded hepatic pool of free proline,[12] and raised concentration of prolyl hydroxylase.[2,13] These indices of active collagen synthesis account for the two to fourfold hepatic increase in total and neutral salt-soluble collagens encountered in alcoholic cirrhosis and alcoholic hepatitis.[14] The normal liver contains 5% or less of its weight as collagen. About 80% of the collagen is type I, and 20% type III. Both types are increased in alcoholic cirrhosis, although the increase in type III collagen is proportionately larger. The percentage distribution becomes reversed in the cirrhotic liver; type III collagen accounts for 55% of the total hepatic collagen.[15]

HUMAN CIRRHOSIS

Alcoholic Cirrhosis

For a full treatment of alcoholic cirrhosis see Chapter 10.

Cryptogenic Cirrhosis[16]

The disease may also be known as macronodular, postnecrotic, or toxic cirrhosis. The etiology has not been established. In some cases the disease represents the late effects of accepted antecedent causes which are not evident at the time of diagnosis. It is likely that hepatitis B virus (especially the anicteric form), alcoholism, drugs, chemical toxicity, metabolic conditions such as alpha-1-antitrypsin deficiency and Wilson's disease are among the unrecognized etiologic factors which initiate the development of the cirrhosis. Clinical and laboratory features in some female patients resemble the cryptogenic type of chronic active hepatitis, suggesting a shared pathogenesis for both diseases. The recognition of cryptogenic cirrhosis depends largely on investigative efforts which exclude the known causes of cirrhosis.

Clinical presentation.   This differs from alcoholic cirrhosis, the major differential diagnosis, in that:

1. The sex predominance is not male and all ages are affected.
2. Signs of malnutrition and folic acid deficiency are uncommon.
3. Feminizing changes and Dupuytren's contracture are rare.
4. Jaundice tends to persist and deepen rather than wax and wane.
5. Bleeding esophageal varices or hepatic coma may be the initial presenting manifestations and may appear abruptly.
6. Muscle wasting and ascites occur late in the clinical course.
7. Hepatomegaly may often be inconspicuous or even absent.
8. The complication of hepatoma in as many as 15% of the cases represents a common mode of exitus.

Laboratory findings.   Hypergammaglobulinemia is often more impressive and hypoalbuminemia is less constant than in alcoholic cirrhosis. The other liver function tests do not differ measurably. Serum autoantibodies are often elevated. Diagnosis is confirmed by a liver biopsy. Grossly, the liver appears deformed with macronodules, many of which exceed 1 cm in size (Fig. 9.1). Microscopically, the irregular regenerative nodules are interspersed with collapsed areas and surrounded by broad fibrous bands, dense inflammation, and bile duct proliferation (Fig. 9.2). The necrosis at the periphery of the nodules indicates the degree of disease activity.

Treatment.   Specific therapy is not available in most cases. Steroids do increase survival time in compensated female cirrhotics who are not alcoholics.[17] It is likely that this group represents cryptogenic chronic active hepatitis. Negative determinant factors are ascites and possibly alcoholism which is too closely linked to the male sex to be analyzed separately.

Primary Biliary Cirrhosis[18]

Primary biliary cirrhosis (PBC) or chronic nonsuppurative destructive cholangitis[19] represents a rare form of cirrhosis with several distinctive features. First, 90% of the cases appears in women 40–60 years old. Second, a strong immunologic bias exists so that a host of nonorgan-specific autoantibodies is found, although none is considered pathogenic (Table 9.3). Association with diseases with known immunologic abnormalities or with collagen disorder is common: rheumatoid arthritis, Sjögren's syndrome, autoimmune thyroiditis, systemic lupus erythematosus, ulcerative colitis, and CRST syndrome (calcinosis, Raynaud's

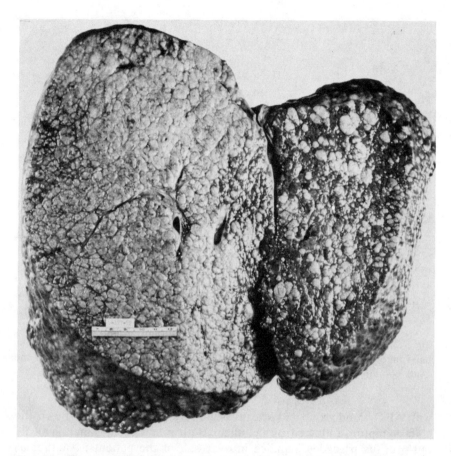

Fig. 9.1. The macronodular liver of cryptogenic cirrhosis. The large irregular nodules exceed 1 cm in size.

phenomenon, scleroderma, and telangiectasia). Third, the onset is insidious, preceded by a subclinical stage with a detectable autoantibody pattern that merges with chronic active hepatitis.[20] This suggests a similar genetic predisposition for the two diseases.

Rarely, the disease follows an attack of cholestatic acute viral hepatitis, or drug hepatitis due to the phenothiazines, or cholestatic jaundice of late pregnancy. The incidence of HB_sAg in PBC is not different from that in the normal population.[21] Recent epidemiological studies confirm the rarity of the disease. In England it is responsible for only about 2% of all deaths due to cirrhosis. It seems to have a predilection for those of European descent and is virtually absent in Orientals. A possible bimodal peak for mortality occurs at ages 50–54 and 70–74.[22] PBC is not correlated

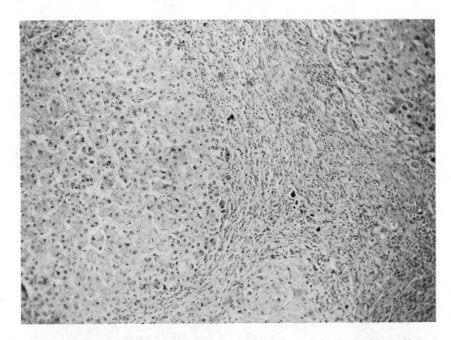

Fig. 9.2. Macronodular cirrhosis. A large cirrhotic nodule is rimmed by a fibrous band incorporating many small bile ducts and inflammatory cells. Some of the ducts contain bile plugs. H and E, X100.

with ABO blood group and Rhesus negativity.[23] Clinically, pruritus is the chief symptom followed by jaundice. Both may appear simultaneously but pruritus precedes jaundice in over half of the patients. Xanthomas appear late, and 40% of patients have gallstones.[24] Discrimination between this disease and the causes of extrahepatic cholestasis often leads to repeated laparotomies. Laboratory findings show a mild rise of serum total bilirubin (only 20% exceeds 5 mg/dl), very high elevation of alkaline phosphatases (50% of cases have three times normal value), simulating extrahepatic biliary obstruction; and high serum IgM concentration. Aminotransferase activity is usually low and serum globulin level is increased. Not unexpectedly, serum lipids and bile acids are raised. Among autoantibody tests, mitochondrial (M) fluorescence is detected in over 90% of the cases in most reported series. A positive M test confirms the diagnosis of PBC but does not exclude mechanical large duct obstruction.

Pathologically, four stages are recognized.[19] Histological diagnosis is predicated upon evaluation of a large number of bile ducts such as seen in

Table 9.3. Autoantibodies and other immunological abnormalities in PBC.[43,44]

Autoantibody	% Incidence
Mitochondrial	>90, ½ high titered
Smooth muscle	45, ⅘ low titered
Antinuclear	25, ⅔ low titered
Bile canalicular	30
Thyroid (CF) specific	15, ½ high titered

T-lymphocyte abnormality	Mechanism
↓ lymphocyte transformation to PHA and PPD	Serum inhibitory factor, intrinsic T-cell deficiency
↓ skin reactivity to PPD, DNCB, and hemocyanin (60% of cases)	↓ cellular immunity
MIF production with mitrochondrial antigen or biliary protein	↓ cellular immunity

a wedge biopsy of liver. In the first stage, the early lesions are characteristic. Focal interlobular ducts are either deformed or eroded by a chronic inflammatory exudate rich in histiocytes and plasma cells (Fig. 9.3). Granulomatous organization is present in about one-third of the specimens. The ducts undergo a variety of injury patterns without actual necrosis: crowding, pseudostratification, hyperchromatism, and nuclear deformation. There is no portal fibrosis. The second stage consists of further extension of the triadal lesion throughout the liver, with evidence that the damaged ducts have disappeared. In their place small ductules appear and proliferate. Slight periportal necrosis may occur. Cholestasis remains centrolobular in distribution. Portal fibrosis is evident in the third stage. The inflammation usually dampens down. Cholestasis becomes widespread and severe. Mallory bodies are evident in 20% of cases.[25] The final fourth stage is not easily differentiated from other types of cirrhosis. A decrease in the number or total disappearance of interlobular ducts suggests PBC. These somewhat artificial stages often merge imperceptibly, or occur at uneven paces in different parts of the biopsy. Copper accumulation in PBC generally exceeds 250 μg/g dry liver, a level comparable to that seen in Wilson's disease and chronic extrahepatic cholestasis (obstruction longer than six months).[26]

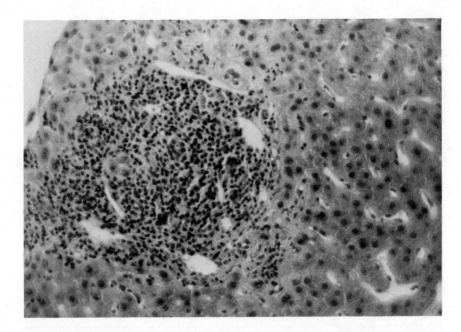

Fig. 9.3. Primary biliary cirrhosis. The early and characteristic lesion exhibits a dense mononuclear infiltrate destroying bile ducts in the portal tract. H and E, X400.

Diagnosis is based on exclusion of extrahepatic cholestasis, compatible hepatic tests, and liver biopsy findings. Abnormal laboratory findings, including elevated IgM level and positive M test, may precede the onset of symptoms during the asymptomatic stage of PBC.[27] Relatives of subjects with PBC have an incidence of M antibodies of 7–8%, about 10 times that found in the general population. Other causes of chronic intrahepatic cholestasis such as drugs (chlorpromazine, tolbutamide, arsenicals, and anabolic steroids) and conditions such as sarcoidosis,[28] scleroderma, ulcerative colitis, cryptogenic cirrhosis, and Hodgkin's disease may simulate the clinical and biochemical features of PBC. The history and serological studies would normally distinguish PBC from these diseases.

Specific treatment is not available. Cholestyramine affords relief from distressing pruritus and xanthomas. Steroids are not used because of their osteolytic side effects. Fat-soluble vitamins (D, A, K) may be required to correct the vitamin loss by malabsorption. Azathioprine suppresses the immunological disturbances in this condition but does not prolong survival. Prognosis is related to the frequency of exploratory laparotomy and duct surgery. Otherwise, the course is ultimately fatal, usually within five years of diagnosis. Hepatic coma and bleeding varices are common causes of death.

Secondary Biliary Cirrhosis

This disorder follows chronic extrahepatic cholestasis. It may develop in as short a period as six weeks. More typically, there is a longstanding history of extrahepatic biliary block and surgery. Abdominal pain, right-upper-quadrant tenderness, itching, fever, weight loss, deepening jaundice, and hepatomegaly are common symptoms which relate to the underlying disease. Hepatic tests show high elevation of excretory enzymes out of proportion to the indicators of cell death. Serum lipids, especially the free cholesterol fraction, and bile salts (trihydroxy bile acids) are accordingly raised. LP-X, the abnormal lipoprotein, is detected. Serum IgM and mitochondrial antibody are not increased, as in PBC. Radiologic evidence of biliary tract abnormality is usual.

Pathologically, the liver is swollen, greenish in color, and macronodular in configuration. Microscopic changes include widespread cholestasis with or without extracellular extravasation of bile, portal scarring, inflammation, duct reduplication, and nodular distortion of liver parenchyma. Not infrequently discrimination from intrahepatic cholestasis poses a major diagnostic challenge (see Chapter 5). Prognosis depends on the primary disease and relief of the mechanical block. Generally the outlook is poor. Patients usually succumb to hepatic coma, ruptured varices, or liver abscess.

Alpha-1-antitrypsin Deficiency [29,30]

Alpha-1-antitrypsin (A-1-AT), a serum glycoprotein with an MW of 54,000 daltons and a half-life of six days, is synthesized by the liver and appears in the circulation at the concentration of 200 mg/dl. The antienzyme inhibits various proteases, including trypsin and collagenase. Increased levels of A-1-AT are found in acute and chronic infections, neoplasms, pregnancy, and ingestion of oral contraceptives. Deficiency of A-1-AT, detectable by an absence of alpha-1-globulin band on serum electrophoresis, is associated with emphysema and/or cirrhosis. The lung disease is characterized by an early onset of panacinar emphysema (before the age of 40), predominance in females, and absence of chronic bronchitis. An estimated 2% of patients with severe obstructive emphysema show an absence of this antienzyme.

Antitrypsin variants constitute the Pi (protease inhibitor) system. At least 11 allotypes and 21 phenotypes have been identified. Most normal individuals are PiMM homozygous. Both lung and liver diseases in A-1-AT deficiency are essentially associated with the homozygous PiZZ phenotypes. Homozygous subjects show serum levels of A-1-AT that range 10–15% of the normal concentration. Heterozygous phenotypes have higher but still subnormal serum concentrations. Heterozygous PiMZ, PiSZ, and PiFZ individuals may develop emphysema, neonatal hepatitis, or cirrhosis. The estimated homozygote frequency for the PiZ gene varies from 1 in 1800 to 1 in 3410, depending on the population group surveyed. The chances of subjects with PiZZ phenotype developing cirrhosis are estimated at 20–30%, and pulmonary disease at 50–60%. In the childhood period, A-1-AT deficiency is associated with neonatal hepatitis, chronic active hepatitis, or cirrhosis. Fifteen to forty percent of all forms of neonatal hepatitis have the PiZZ phenotype.

The clinical picture of this hepatitis is not distinctive. Jaundice and cholestasis usually appear 1–2 weeks after birth. Bleeding may be prominent. Liver histology reveals variable features of necrosis, mononuclear cell infiltration, cholestasis, and portal bile duct proliferation. Giant cell formation is uncommon. Prognosis is quite variable.[31] Early manifestations of jaundice and cholestasis may disappear, although mild hepatic dysfunction could be detected. The clinical course need not be progressively downhill; on the contrary, it is often mild.

Juvenile cirrhosis with A-1-AT deficiency appears before the first year of life. All have hepatomegaly with or without obstructive jaundice. The disease progresses relentlessly with severe portal hypertension or hepatic coma. Hepatic disease in adults with PiZZ phenotype is characterized by rapidly progressive cirrhosis in nonalcoholics above 50 years of age, terminating in the complications of portal hypertension or hepatic coma.[31] Concomitant emphysema is usually subclinical. Hepatoma is another frequent complication, up to 30% in one study.[32] Absence of marked cholestasis, HB_sAg, or serum autoantibodies is characteristic of this cirrhosis. Other laboratory findings include high IgM levels and increased alpha-2-macroglobulin values. In heterozygous adults, partial deficiency of A-1-AT does not increase susceptibility to cirrhosis associated with other causes, such as alcoholism.[33]

Pathologically, the distinctive feature consists of intracytoplasmic globules in periportal hepatocytes. The acidophilic bodies stain with PAS but resist diastase digestion. Measuring 3–40 μ in size, the amorphous material at the ultrastructural level reveals a central osmophilic core and a surrounding radiolucent halo, usually bound by a single membrane. The inclusions are usually situated in the dilated cisternae of endoplasmic reticulum. By immunofluorescent staining, the globules are identified as A-1-AT material. Emphysematous patients with A-1-AT deficiency may have intrahepatocellular globules not associated with liver disease. The

PAS-positive inclusion bodies in liver differ from normal A-1-AT in the absence of a terminal sialic acid.[34] The defect may be due to a deficiency of sialyltransferase which is involved in the transfer of sialic acid groups. Decreased serum levels of this enzyme have been demonstrated in some patients. Hepatic A-1-AT disease may represent a specific defect in Golgi-membrane-bound sialyltransferase. This could account for the accumulation of unsialylated A-1-AT globules characteristic of the liver lesions.

Cardiac Cirrhosis[35]

This is a rare entity, as the underlying responsible cardiovascular diseases are either uncommon or often adequately controlled. Chronic constrictive pericarditis, severe chronic tricuspid insufficiency, cor pulmonale secondary to mitral valve disease, and protracted congestive failure may cause right heart failure and increase hepatic venous pressure. The raised venous pressure and decreased hepatic blood flow contribute to centrolobular hypoxia, which appears to be the primary pathogenic factor. Grossly, the liver is tense, somewhat tough, with a thickened capsule and an accentuated nutmeg pattern. Morphologically, the centrolobular areas are disrupted by hemorrhage, congestion, cell death, and septal fibrosis linking central veins (reverse lobulation). A rare variant shows diffuse nodular hyperplasia with considerable scarring. Clinically, the diagnosis is difficult. Cardiac cirrhosis cannot be differentiated from the congested liver in chronic heart failure, except by liver biopsy. Whether ascites and splenomegaly occur more frequently than in the congested liver remains unsettled. Portal hypertension is not a common sequela. The diagnosis of cardiac cirrhosis should be considered if hepatic pulsations are absent in tricuspid insufficiency, or when a small liver is found in a patient with ascites and no plausible cause of hepatic disease. Differential diagnoses include Budd-Chiari syndrome, veno-occlusive disease, central congestive hepatic fibrosis occurring in myxedema ascites, and hypervitaminosis A.

Liver dysfunction in heart failure.[35] This condition occurs prior to the development of cardiac cirrhosis. The basic mechanism of hepatic centrolobular anoxia is similar to that in the cirrhotic condition. The chief complaint is abdominal pain due to stretching of Glisson's capsule by the engorged organ. Tender hepatomegaly, ascites, and rarely splenomegaly are the main physical findings. The ascitic fluid contains protein in excess of 2.5 g/dl, analogous to that produced in hepatic venous block (exudate rather than transudate) in 30% of the patients. Serious signs of liver failure such as portal hypertension and hepatic coma occur rarely. Hepatic dysfunction correlates well with the degree of centrolobular congestion and damage. BSP excretion is the most sensitive test for liver congestion. Total serum bilirubin infrequently exceeds 2 mg/dl with a predominant unconjugated fraction. The aminotransferases are usually less than 100 IU/l. In 20% of the cases levels may reach 1000 IU/l when shock or centrolobular necrosis supervenes. A liver biopsy should be done if cardiac cirrhosis is also suspected. Treatment is directed toward the underlying cardiovascular condition and heart failure. A further therapeutic consideration should be taken into account: the fact that a congested liver alters the metabolism of drugs. Increased sensitivity to dicumarol and lidocaine but not to digitalis has been reported. This may require an adjustment of the drug dosage.

Cystic Fibrosis

Also known as mucoviscidosis, this common disorder of childhood affects 1 in 2000 Caucasian births but is rare among blacks and Orientals. The mode of inheritance follows that of an autosomal recessive trait. The disease represents a generalized exocrinopathy, in which exocrine glands secrete excessive, viscid but not qualitatively abnormal mucus, and sweat glands produce sweat with a high saline content. The fundamental defect is not known. However, a serum inhibitory factor of sodium transport, similar if not identical with the ciliary dyskinesis factor, has been recently identified. This would account for the decreased salt reabsorption in sweat glands and the secretion of excessively saline sweat. The main target organs are the lungs, resulting in bronchiectasis and chronic obstructive emphysema, and the pancreas, manifesting as meconium ileus and malabsorption. Focal biliary cirrhosis is found in 25% of surviving children and adolescents but is uncommon in infants with cystic fibrosis.[36] Excessive mucus in the biliary tree, bile duct proliferation, periportal inflammation and fibrosis, and cholestasis are common nonspecific hepatic changes which tend to disappear in infants after one year of age. Progression to diffuse biliary cirrhosis occurs in 5% of surviving patients. Clinically, hepatic disease is recognized by the development of portal hypertension with variceal hemorrhage, splenomegaly, and ascites.[36] Treatment is empirical and palliative. Control of respiratory complications ensures prolonged useful survival.

Galactosemia

Two disorders associated with inborn errors of galactose metabolism are described (Table 9.4). The first is galactokinase deficiency which pro-

Table 9.4. Major steps in galactose metabolism.

Galactose + ATP $\xleftrightarrow{\text{Galactokinase}}$ Galactose-1-phosphate + ADP

Galactose-1-phosphate + UDP $\xleftarrow{\text{Galactose-1-P}}$ UPD galactose
$\qquad\qquad\qquad\qquad\quad{\text{uridyl transferase}}$
$\qquad\qquad\qquad\qquad$ + Glucose-1-phosphate

UPD galactose $\xrightarrow{\text{2 steps}}$ UTP + Glucose-1-phosphate

---

duces juvenile cataract formation and galactosuria. The second, and more important, disease involves galactose-1-phosphate uridyl transferase deficiency. It is inherited as an autosomal recessive trait, with an incidence ranging from 1 in 18,000 to 1 in 100,000 births. Failure to thrive, vomiting, and diarrhea appear soon after birth. Hepatomegaly, jaundice, and other signs of hepatic dysfunction present after the first week of life. Increased serum galactose level, galactosuria, albuminuria, and aminoaciduria are found. The liver shows fatty change, parenchymal tubularization, cholestasis, and cirrhotic nodules. Experimentally, galactose itself does not damage the liver, but galactosamine, a possible by-product, causes a hepatitis-like injury. Diagnosis is proved by the demonstration of the enzyme deficiency in erythrocytes. Treatment consists of removing galactose or galactose-producing sugars from the diet. The galactose-free diet has improved symptoms and survival outlook. Failure of early detection leads to mental retardation and cataract development in the child.

DIFFUSE NONCIRRHOTIC FIBROSIS
OF THE LIVER

Portal hypertension is the chief problem in hepatic diseases with diffuse but noncirrhotic fibrosis (see Table 6.3 and Chapter 6). Morphologically, the fibrosis may appear striking but the other characteristic features of cirrhosis such as regenerative nodules, severe hepatocellular inflammation, and necrosis are absent. Portacaval shunt surgery often produces excellent results since liver function remains near normal in the patients.

Congenital Hepatic Fibrosis[37, 38]

This variant of the infantile polycystic kidney/liver complex is inherited as an autosomal recessive trait (see also Chapter 17). The hepatic changes consist of widespread portal fibrosis incorporating enlarged and proliferating ducts but not macroscopic cysts, absence of cholestasis, and a normal parenchyma. The ductal disturbance affects all branches from the hilum to ducts draining a functional liver unit. Congenital hepatic fibrosis is usually associated with renal cysts but the changes are much less severe than in polycystic kidneys. The infantile form may accompany infantile polycystic kidneys, in which case the renal symptoms predominate. Typically, the patient with congenital hepatic fibrosis presents with portal hypertension at 5–10 years of age. Bleeding varices, splenomegaly, and hypersplenism are common complications. A satisfactory response follows portacaval anastomosis since liver cell function remains preserved.

Fibrosis in Other Conditions

Hepatoportal fibrosis.   Hepatoportal fibrosis is discussed in Chapter 6.

Alcoholic hepatitis.   The early phase of this disease begins with fibrosis, among other alterations, in the centrolobular area. Blockage of the hepatic (central) venule may produce an outflow type of portal hypertension. In the later stages, cirrhosis becomes evident.

Schistosomiasis.   Schistosomiasis is discussed in the section on parasitic diseases in Chapter 16.

Arsenic-induced noncirrhotic portal hypertension.[39]   The cases of this condition follow prolonged chronic ingestion of arsenic compounds such as Fowler's solution (arsenic trioxide 1%). Hematemesis, splenomegaly, and other signs of portal hypertension develop slowly over a protracted period with little evidence of hepatocellular injury. Skin changes and other manifestations of arsenic poisoning may be present. Histologically, the hepatic lesions resemble hepatoportal fibrosis or idiopathic portal hypertension. The portal spaces are enlarged and fibrotic, containing portal veins which are greatly thickened with hypertrophied walls. The parenchyma is usually well preserved. Patients respond well to portacaval shunts.

Vinyl chloride exposure.   Industrial exposure to vinyl chloride may cause hepatic fibrosis and portal hypertension without cirrhosis, and Banti's syndrome. Liver histology reveals multifocal subcapsular fibrosis, concentric portal fibrosis, hyperplasia and atypia of sinusoidal lining cells, increased collagen deposition in sinusoidal spaces, and patchy sinusoidal dilation. In addition, there is the serious hazard of liver carcinogenesis (see also Chapter 17).

Other diseases.   Hypervitaminosis A (Chapter 18), early Budd-Chiari syndrome (Chapter 6), veno-occlusive disease (Chapter 6), and myxedema of the liver (Chapter 14) are discussed elsewhere.

DISORDERS WITH FOCAL HEPATIC FIBROSIS

Included in this group are two rare disorders: focal nodular hyperplasia and partial nodular transformation.

Focal Nodular Hyperplasia[40,41]

The many synonyms, eg, adenoma, hamartoma, solitary hyperplastic nodule, and focal cirrhosis, indicate the obscure nature of the lesion. It is clinically asymptomatic, detected as an incidental finding at autopsy, surgery, angiography, or by liver biopsy. Confusion with cirrhosis or hepatoma is the main diagnostic problem. Most of the lesions are located in the right lobe and are less than 5 cm in size. Histologically, the regenerative nodules involve a portion of the liver, generally in the subcapsular area. Thin or thick fibrous bands separate the nodules incorporating a variable amount of hyperplastic and fibrous vessels. A central stellate scar is a characteristic feature. An association with a cavernous hemangioma is not uncommon. Angiography reveals increased arterialization in the lesion. Animal experiments indicate that arterialization of a portion or all of the liver reproduces the changes seen in focal nodular hyperplasia. Localized vascular anomaly, resulting in an AV shunt or increased sinusoid pressure, may account for the observed focal injury and hyperplasia. Recent reports show an association with oral contraceptive therapy. The nodule is frequently resected as the result of confusion with more serious diseases.

Partial Nodular Transformation[42]

This rare disease, in contrast with focal nodular hyperplasia, involves the perihilar areas of the liver. Hepatic size is not enlarged, although up to two-thirds of the liver mass may be transformed. Compression of the hepatic venous outflow leads to postsinusoidal portal hypertension. Peripheral portions of the liver appear normal or atrophic. Histologically, the regenerative nodules are limited in extent, and there is little or no surrounding fibrosis. The cause is unknown and diagnosis is difficult. Hepatocellular function remains undisturbed even with the onset of portal hypertension. Hence, the prospects of long-term survival after portacaval shunt surgery are good. Differential diagnosis includes nodular regenerative hyperplasia encountered in Felty's syndrome and chronic hepatic congestion.

REFERENCES

1. Popper H, Udenfriend S: Hepatic fibrosis, *Amer J Med* 49:707–721, 1970.
2. Takeuchi T, Prockop DJ: Protocollagen proline hydroxylase in normal liver and in hepatic fibrosis. *Gastroenterology* 56:744–750, 1969.
3. Lin AWSM, Castell DO: Comparative studies on human plasma monoamine oxidase in normal subjects and in fibrotic liver disease. *Biochem Med* 9:373–385, 1974.
4. Resnick RH, et al: Urinary hydroxyproline excretion in hepatic disorders. *Amer J Gastroenterol* 60:576–584, 1973.
5. Hirayama C: Hepatic fibrosis: Biochemical considerations, in Gen Ref No. 12, pp 273–282.
6. Rubin E, Popper H: The evolution of human cirrhosis deduced from observations in experimental animals. *Medicine* 46:163–183, 1967.
7. Rubin E, Hutterer F, Popper H: Cell proliferation and fiber formation in chronic carbon tetrachloride intoxication. *Amer J Path* 42:715–728, 1963.
8. Rubin E, Hutterer F: Methods in the study of structural changes induced by experimental chronic hepatic injury, in Bajusz E, Jasmin G (eds.), *Methods and Achievement in Experimental Pathology,* vol 2, Basel, S Karger, 1967, pp 224–242.
9. Zaki FG, Bandt C, Hoffbauer FW: Fatty cirrhosis in the rat: III: Liver lipid and collagen content in various stages. *Arch Path* 75:648–653, 1963.
10. Hutterer F, Eisenstadt M, Rubin E: Turnover of hepatic collagen in reversible and irreversible fibrosis. *Experientia* 26:244–245, 1970.
11. Rubin E, Hutterer F, Popper H: Experimental hepatic fibrosis without hepatocellular regeneration: A kinetic study. *Amer J Path* 52:111–119, 1968.
12. Kershenobich D, Fierro FJ, Rojkind M: The relationship between the free pool of proline and collagen content in human liver cirrhosis. *J Clin Invest* 49:2246–2249, 1970.
13. McGee J O'D, et al: Collagen proline hydroxylase activity and ^{35}S sulphate uptake in human liver biopsies. *Gut* 15:260–267, 1974.
14. Galambos JT, Shapira R: Natural history of alcoholic hepatitis: IV: Glycosaminoglycuronans and collagen in the hepatic connective tissue. *J Clin Invest* 52:2952–2962, 1973.
15. Rojkind M, Martinez-Palomo A: Increase in type I and type III collagens in human alcoholic liver cirrhosis. *Proc Nat Acad Sci USA* 73:539–543, 1976.
16. Sherlock S: Hepatic cirrhosis, in Gen Ref No. 15, pp 425–444.
17. Juhl E, et al: A report from the Copenhagen study group for liver diseases: Sex, ascites and alcoholism in survival of patients with cirrhosis: Effect of prednisone. *New Eng J Med* 291:271–273, 1974.
18. Sherlock S, Scheuer PJ: The presentation and diagnosis of 100 patients with primary biliary cirrhosis. *New Eng J Med* 289:674–678, 1973.

19. Rubin E, Schaffner F, Popper H: Primary biliary cirrhosis: Chronic non-suppurative destructive cholangitis. *Amer J Path* 46:387–407, 1965.
20. Galbraith RM, et al: High prevalence of seroimmunologic abnormalities in relatives of patients with active chronic hepatitis or primary biliary cirrhosis. *New Eng J Med* 290:63–69, 1973.
21. MacSween RNM, et al: Australia antigen and primary biliary cirrhosis. *J Clin Path* 26:335–339, 1973.
22. Hamlyn AN, Sherlock S: The epidemiology of primary biliary cirrhosis: A survey of mortality in England and Wales. *Gut* 15:473–479, 1974.
23. Hamlyn AN, Morris JS, Sherlock S: ABO blood groups, Rhesus negativity, and primary biliary cirrhosis. *Gut* 15:480–481, 1974.
24. Summerfield JA, et al: The biliary system in primary biliary cirrhosis: A study by endoscopic retrograde cholangiopancreatography. *Gastroenterology* 70:240–243, 1976.
25. MacSween RNM: Mallory's ('alcoholic') hyaline in primary biliary cirrhosis. *J Clin Path* 26:340–342, 1973.
26. Smallwood RA, et al: Liver-copper levels in liver disease: Studies using neutron activation analysis. *Lancet* 2:1310–1313, 1968.
27. Fox RA, Scheuer PJ, Sherlock S: Asymptomatic primary biliary cirrhosis. *Gut* 14:444–447, 1973.
28. Rudzki C, Ishak KG, Zimmerman HJ: Chronic intrahepatic cholestasis of sarcoidosis. *Amer J Med* 59:373–387, 1975.
29. Brunt PW: Antitrypsin and the liver. *Gut* 15:573–580, 1974.
30. Feldmann G, Bignon J, Chahinian P: The liver in α-1-antitrypsin deficiency. *Digestion* 10:162–174, 1974.
31. Odievre M, et al: Alpha$_1$-antitrypsin deficiency and liver disease in children: phenotypes, manifestations, and prognosis. *Pediatrics* 57:226–231, 1976.
32. Eriksson S, Hagerstrand I: Cirrhosis and malignant hepatoma in α-1-antitrypsin deficiency. *Acta Med Scand* 195:451–458, 1974.
33. Morin T, et al: Heterozygous alpha$_1$-antitrypsin deficiency and cirrhosis in adults: A fortuitous association. *Lancet* 1:250–251, 1975.
34. Weiser MM, LaMont JT, Walker WA: α-1-antitrypsin deficiency—a defect of secretion. *New Eng J Med* 292:205–206, 1975.
35. Dunn GD, et al: The liver in congestive heart failure: A review. *Amer J Med Sci* 265:174–189, 1973.
36. Oppenheimer EH, Esterly JR: Hepatic changes in young infants with cystic fibrosis: Possible relation to focal biliary cirrhosis. *J Ped* 86:683–689, 1975.
37. Lieberman E, et al: Infantile polycystic disease of the kidneys and liver: Clinical, pathological, and radiological correlations and comparison with congenital hepatic fibrosis. *Medicine* 50:277–318, 1971.
38. Hodgson HJF, Davies DR, Thompson, RPH: Congenital hepatic fibrosis. *J Clin Path* 29:11–16, 1976.
39. Morris JS, et al: Arsenic and noncirrhotic portal hypertension. *Gastroenterology* 66:86–94, 1974.
40. Whelan TJ Jr, Baugh JH, Chandor S: Focal nodular hyperplasia of the liver. *Ann Surg* 177:150–158, 1973.

41. Blendis LM, et al: Nodular regenerative hyperplasia of the liver in Felty's syndrome. *Quart J Med* 169:25–32, 1974.
42. Sherlock S, et al: Partial nodular transformation of the liver with portal hypertension. *Amer J Med* 40:195–203, 1966.
43. MacSween RNM, Thomas MA: Lymphocyte transformation by phyto-haemagglutinin (PHA) and purified protein derivative (PPD) in primary biliary cirrhosis: Evidence of serum inhibitory factors. *Clin Exp Immunol* 15:523–533, 1973.
44. Fox RA, Dudley FA, Sherlock S: The primary immune response to hemocyanin in patients with primary biliary cirrhosis. *Clin Exp Immunol* 14:473–480, 1973.

ALCOHOLIC LIVER DISEASE

10

Alcoholic consumption induces in humans and animals widespread and profound metabolic upsets and structural changes, the pathogenesis of which is not completely understood. The liver is a primary target organ, but the brain, heart, peripheral nerves, and gastrointestinal tract are also affected. There is a controversy as to whether alcohol (ethanol), in causing liver lesions, acts as a direct hepatotoxin or as a secondary factor associated with malnutrition. Countless experiments conducted on animals, and some on humans, seem to support both viewpoints. However, in recent years the evidence tends to favor the hepatotoxic effect of ethanol in producing liver disease. This does not exclude the role that malnutrition may play in potentiating the ethanol effect in alcoholism.

GENERAL METABOLISM OF ALCOHOL[1,2]

Alcohol is readily absorbed from the stomach and the small and large intestines. About 90% of intake is completely oxidized, primarily by the liver. The small amount remaining is excreted by the kidneys and lungs. The extrahepatic metabolism of alcohol is insignificant. It is estimated that alcohol can be metabolized at the rate of 100–200 mg/kg body weight per hour (Fig. 10.1). Whether racial differences exist in the rates of metabolism and sensitivity to alcohol remains unsettled. Older studies reported that Caucasians had a faster blood clearance of ethanol than Eskimos and American Indians. Recent observations with refined techniques fail to confirm these findings.[3] However, sustained drinking does increase tolerance to alcohol.

Persons who drink over a long period of time have a greater capacity for accelerating blood ethanol clearance than those who do not. The first step in the hepatic disposal of ethanol is its oxidation to acetaldehyde, catalyzed by the cytosol enzyme alcohol dehydrogenase (ADH). Hydrogen is transferred from ethanol to NAD, converting the latter to NADH. The acetaldehyde produced loses another hydrogen to form acetate.

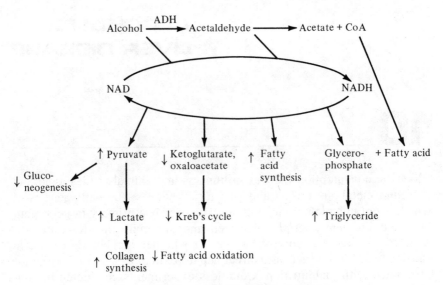

Fig. 10.1. Metabolic effects of ethanol.[1,2]

Thus,

$$\text{Ethanol} + \text{NAD} \xrightarrow{\text{ADH}} \text{Acetaldehyde} + \text{NADH}$$

$$\text{Acetaldehyde} + \text{NAD} \xrightarrow[\text{dehydrogenase}]{\text{Acetaldehyde}} \text{Acetate} + \text{NADH}$$

The net result is the generation of excess reducing equivalents, as NADH, in the liver. Metabolites dependent on the NADH/NAD ratio are accordingly changed. The initial reaction involving alcohol dehydrogenase is considered the rate-limiting step.

Acetaldehyde, the metabolite of ethanol, is potentially more toxic than ethanol itself. The toxicity of acetaldehyde is due to its greater lipid solubility and reactivity. Studies on volunteers with ethanol infusion have shown that the mean acetaldehyde blood level is significantly higher in alcoholic than in nonalcoholic subjects.[4] The high acetaldehyde concentration in alcoholics is attributed to the greater activity of the microsomal ethanol oxidizing system (see below) and mitochondrial damage. Acetaldehyde releases catecholamines, favors condensation reactions of biogenic amines (one of the possible mechanisms involved in addiction), reduces mitochondrial shuttle reactions, and impairs protein synthesis of myocardial cells. Thus, the pathological consequences of ethanol may, in part, be attributed to acetaldehyde.

Alterations in Lipid Metabolism[5]

Ethanol consumption increases the triglyceride content of the liver. The hepatic fat accumulates by four mechanisms: (1) decreased lipid oxidation, (2) enhanced hepatic lipogenesis, (3) decreased hepatic release of lipoproteins, and (4) increased mobilization of depot fat. Both decreased lipid oxidation and increased lipogenesis are linked to the generation of excess NADH. Lipogenesis is promoted by the mitochondrial elongation pathway, or transhydrogenation to NADPH. The increased NADH/NAD ratio also blocks citric acid cycle activity by decreasing oxaloacetate and alpha-ketoglutarate concentrations. This has the effect of supplanting the usual 2 carbon fragments derived from fatty acids which the mitochondria normally utilizes with hydrogen equivalents derived from alcohol.

The altered NADH/NAD level is also expressed by an increased lactate/pyruvate ratio which promotes hyperlactacidemia. The lactic acidosis adds to the general acidosis seen in alcohol consumption. The lactate effect also explains the secondary hyperuricemia because renal excretion of uric acid is decreased. The increased lactate concentration provides a link with collagen metabolism. Alcohol stimulates collagen synthesis by the mediation of lactate, as lactate is a known stimulant of fibroblast growth in culture. In the usual dose ethanol does not influence lipoprotein secretion and release, but with moderate and large doses lipoprotein production is enhanced and hyperlipemia occurs. Although all fractions of serum lipids are increased, the change is particularly striking with the low-density lipoprotein fraction and chylomicrons. Marked hyperlipemia following alcoholism is not all hepatic-mediated, as post-heparin lipoprotein lipase activity is decreased in some of these patients. The hyperlipoproteinemia resembles types I, IV, or V of the classification of D. S. Fredrickson et al. Extremely high doses of alcohol, however, depress lipoprotein synthesis and decrease serum lipids. Acute drinking bouts in chronic alcoholics are often accompanied by a rise in alpha-lipoproteins, which as a rule returns to normal values within two weeks.[6] The role of increased mobilization from the peripheral fat depot is not as prominent in the genesis of ethanol-induced fatty liver in humans as it is in rats. In humans, chronic ingestion of large doses of alcohol up to 300 g/day does not affect the free fatty acids (FFA) level. Acute alcoholism in humans as opposed to results obtained with rats has been shown to lower circulating FFA concentration and decrease FFA turnover. The effect is mediated by the acetate produced on ethanol oxidation. The fatty acids deposited in the liver are derived mainly from dietary fat.

Alterations in Protein Metabolism

Ethanol intake regularly produces an increased proliferation of smooth endoplasmic reticulum (microsomes). One source suggests that this is a microsomal linked oxidation system of ethanol.[2] The hepatic microsomal ethanol oxidizing system (MEOS) accounts for 20–25% of ethanol metabolism in liver slices and perfused isolated livers, and requires the cofactors NADPH-NADP:

$$\text{Ethanol} + \text{NADPH} + \text{H}^+ + \text{O}_2 \xrightarrow{\text{MEOS}} \text{Acetaldehyde} + \text{NADP} + 2\text{H}_2\text{O}$$

Controversy exists as to the identity of MEOS with the catalase system, and its physiological role in ethanol oxidation. Chronic ethanol consumption increases the rate of ethanol metabolism. Under these conditions alcohol dehydrogenase concentrations are not increased. MEOS activity is, however, increased along with the induction of smooth endoplasmic reticulum membrane, and could account for 33–66% of the increase in blood ethanol clearance. This would explain, at least partly, the increased tolerance to ethanol in chronic alcoholics. Other microsomal enzyme systems involved in reactions such as detoxification and conjugation are also induced, nonspecifically, by prolonged alcohol ingestion. The acceleration of drug metabolism, probably in conjunction with decreased sensitivity of the brain, accounts for the well-known tolerance of sober alcoholics to sedatives and other drugs. However, in the inebriated state ethanol acts differently, as it accentuates the drug effect.

Alterations in Carbohydrate Metabolism[7]

Ethanol inhibits glucose synthesis from various precursors: alanine, glutamate, glycerol, and lactate in human liver biopsy tissue. Infusion of labeled glucose or lactate with ethanol demonstrates inhibition of lactate conversion to glucose, glucose cycling, and glucose conversion to lactate. Blood glucose level and glucose turnover rate are not affected. The degree of lactate inhibition in the nonfasting state does not differ from that in the fasting state. Starvation is not necessary for ethanol inhibition of gluconeogenesis from lactate but is required for the appearance of hypoglycemia. The inhibition of lactate incorporation into glucose in nonfasting patients is probably masked by an increase in glycogenolysis preventing hypoglycemia. Alcoholic hypoglycemia does not appear unless the patient has fasted. Circulating insulin is not involved, as there is no detectable change in insulin synthesis after ethanol consumption.

Other Effects of Ethanol[8]

Acute alcohol ingestion producing blood levels between 100–150 mg/dl increases urinary excretion of catecholamines and elevates serum cortisol secretion and aldosterone production. Arterial pH does not change during the drinking of alcohol, but on alcohol withdrawal, arterial pH rises accompanied by a fall in pCO_2 and hypomagnesemia. The latter may be related to respiratory alkalosis and hyperventilation occurring after a debauch.

ALCOHOL-INDUCED HEPATIC LESIONS
IN ANIMALS

Experiments conducted on animals reveal varied patterns of hepatic injury, depending on the feeding schedules with alcohol.[9] Rats fed with an acute dose of alcohol (6 g/kg body weight) given as a 40–50% solution develop a fatty liver within two hours. Fat is deposited in the periportal hepatocytes initially. Hepatic triglycerides double at four hours, quadruple at eight hours, and return to normal at sixteen hours. The mitochondrial volume enlarges transiently at four hours; the smooth endoplasmic reticulum also increases at this time and decreases by the eighth hour. Serum enzymes are not altered in this acute model.

In the Porta-Hartroft model, rats consume 30% of their calories as alcohol in a diet with 20% of calories as protein and with a lipotropic value between 75–100 mg choline per 100 kcal. The regimen produces hepatic fatty change, fibrosis, and cirrhosis. The liver injury can be prevented if the diet is replenished with lipotrope and vitamins, which correct the deficiencies. Sucrose can substitue for the alcohol in the diet that produces the fatty fibrous liver. The results obtained by Porta and Hartroft seem to indicate that nutritional deficiency, and not alcohol, is toxic to the liver. On the other hand, the experiments of Lieber and Rubin demonstrate the direct hepatotoxicity of alcohol. In Lieber and Rubin's model, ethanol is given as 36% of the total calories, isocalorically replacing carbohydrate or fat in a totally liquid and nutritious diet.[2] At this concentration ethanol regularly increases triglycerides in rats five to tenfold over controls. During the first month of alcohol intake hepatic lipid accumulation develops progressively and persists for at least one year in the rat, and for three years in the baboon.[5] Lipotrope supplement does not reverse the effect of ethanol in these experiments.

Acute alcohol-induced fatty liver can be prevented or reduced in animals by the following: decreasing fat in the diet, replacing with medium-chain triglycerides, barbiturates, antihistamines, beta-sympatholytic agents, prostaglandin E_1, and large doses of ATP. Asparagine and chlorpromazine (an inhibitor of ADH activity) are not effective. Pyrazole, another ADH inhibitor, prevents some aspects of ethanol effects on lipid metabolism but does not affect the changes of chronic ethanolism. Anabolic steroids accelerate the mobilization of fat from an alcoholic fatty liver.

ALCOHOLIC LIVER DISEASE IN HUMANS

Damage to the liver in humans spans a spectrum which includes: alcoholic fatty liver (the early stage); alcoholic hepatitis (the intermediate stage); and alcoholic cirrhosis (the end stage).[10] Fatty change is a universal and invariable hepatic response to alcohol consumption. The factors which contribute to the chronic and destructive phase of cirrhosis are largely unknown. It is estimated that at least 10% of the population in the United States consumes alcohol on a regular basis. Out of this pool of 20,000,000 persons, 10% or 2,000,000 develop cirrhosis. Epidemiological studies indicate the duration and degree of alcohol abuse is important. Seventy-five percent of persons with a daily consumption of alcohol exceeding 160 g/day reveals severe liver injury, whereas less than 20% of those consuming a lesser amount shows similar liver damage. After 15 years of heavy alcoholism, the incidence of cirrhosis is eight times greater than after five years. The following table dramatically shows the relationship between the amount of alcohol consumed and the incidence of cirrhosis.[11]

	Cirrhosis. of liver (death/100,000), 1960	Absolute alcohol consumption (US gal/capita), 1960			
		Spirits	Wine	Beer	Total
USA	11.3	0.60	0.15	0.77	1.52
Canada	6.1	0.44	0.12	0.84	1.40
UK	2.9	0.22	0.08	0.78	1.06

In the past because of the lack of an experimental model for ethanol-induced cirrhosis, there has been reluctance to accept ethanol as a cirrhogenic toxin. More recently, primates have been used as a model resembling the human variant. Chronic feeding of alcohol (4.5–8.39 g/kg body weight as isocaloric replacement of carbohydrate in a nutritious diet) produced the whole spectrum of alcohol liver disease in baboons.[12] Fatty liver was seen as early as the first month, with fat droplets appearing in the centrolobular and midzonal hepatocytes. Except for a threefold rise in AsAT, hepatic tests were not altered. Alcoholic hepatitis, characterized by patchy inflammation, balloon degeneration, and Mallory body accumulation, was observed after nine months to four years of alcoholic consumption. Cirrhosis had developed in two baboons autopsied four years after the beginning of the experiment.

Alcoholic Fatty Liver

Pathogenesis. The development of alcoholic fatty liver is shown by an experiment designed to simulate heavy weekend social drinking.[13]

Under controlled conditions 270 g of alcohol (10 g = 1 oz or 30 cc whiskey) were fed to nonalcoholic volunteers for two days. The liver specimen showed a twofold increase of hepatic triglycerides over control values, and striking ultrastructural changes. The mitochondrial deformity and enlargement accounted for the decreased hepatic oxidation of fatty acids. The increase of vesiculated smooth endoplasmic reticulum was reflected by the increase of hepatic drug-metabolizing enzymes, enhanced lipoprotein secretion, and increased cholesterol biosynthesis. The liver function tests were essentially unchanged. Other drinking schedules in volunteers produced similar hepatic changes which were not prevented by a high-protein diet. The short-term experiments in which blood alcohol fluctuated 20–80 mg/dl indicated that alcohol, independent of nutrition, causes significant liver damage.

Clinical features. Most patients present with hepatomegaly, often with abdominal pain and liver tenderness. A variable percentage, depending on drinking and eating habits, has nutritional changes such as sore red tongue, peripheral neuritis, and edema. Features of mild jaundice, ascites, and hemodynamic evidence of portal hypertension are not unusual. Portal hypertension is due to mesenchymal cell hyperplasia, resulting in sinusoidal narrowing. Alcoholic fatty liver produces relatively few functional consequences. Ordinary hepatic tests are not remarkable except for mild BSP elevation and aminotransferase increase of less than 200 IU/l. Histologically, fat appears in the liver sections as vacuoles in cell cytoplasm. There is no lobular distribution that indicates an ethanolic etiology nor is the morphologic appearance distinctive for the disease (Fig. 10.2). The condition is self-limited on cessation of alcohol ingestion. Mobilization of fat occurs in 6–8 weeks on a nutritious diet or in 12 days on treatment with low-dosage anabolic steroids. This type of fatty liver does not normally predispose toward cirrhosis unless sustained injury and other factors intervene.

Alcoholic Hepatitis

This precursor stage of cirrhosis is defined as acute hepatocellular disease in a chronic alcoholic. Both clinically and morphologically there is evidence of acute liver necrosis and inflammation. The determining factors which promote the development of the disease are not understood. Alcohol abuse and malnutrition themselves are not precipitating causes since both appear equally in alcoholics with or without alcoholic hepatitis. Host susceptibility is a likely explanation. There is evidence that altered immune reactivity may be involved. Lymphocytes from patients with alcoholic hepatitis elaborate macrophage migration inhibition factor

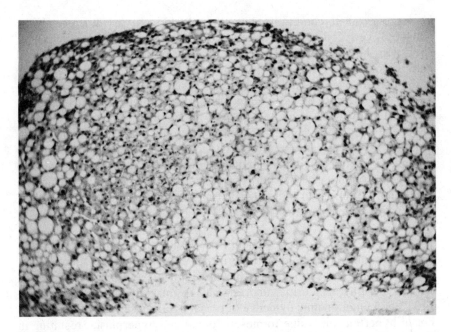

Fig. 10.2. Severe fatty liver. Fat vacuoles distend otherwise intact hepatocytes. H and E, X100.

(MIF) on contact with Mallory bodies, an intracellular neoprotein related to microfilaments.[14] Reactivity to Mallory bodies, prepared as a transfer factor, can be transferred to normal persons.[15] The alterations are highly suggestive that a peculiar sensitivity to alcohol-induced liver tissue component(s) initiates the disease process.

Clinical presentation.[16,17] Alcoholic hepatitis is somewhat more common among females, especially black women, in their early 40s. Common complaints are nausea, vomiting, abdominal pains, and weight loss, often accompanied by evidence of alcoholic gastritis and peripheral neuritis. Physical findings include hepatomegaly (90% of cases), jaundice (70%), ascites (50%), malnutrition (40%), encephalopathy and esophageal varices (10%). Fever, a characteristic sign, occurs in 60% of the patients but associated conditions such as infections, especially of the urinary tract, may be responsible for the fever in half of the cases. Laboratory studies commonly reveal: anemia and leukocytosis ($> 10,000/mm^3$, in 80% of cases), serum bilirubin (up to 30 mg/dl), aminotransferase elevation (< 300 IU/l), and mild rise of alkaline phosphatases (70% of cases). Diagnosis is facilitated by the serological finding of Mallory body antigen and autoantibody. Mallory body antigen appears during the early phase of alcoholic hepatitis, while the autoantibody rises as the disease progresses. Inadequate prothrombin time levels not infrequently preclude liver biopsy. Mild azotemia not due to intercurrent GI hemorrhage or organic renal disease is observed in 25% of cases.

Characteristic features on liver biopsy consist of centrolobular deposition of collagen, polymorphonuclear cell infiltration, hydropic swelling of hepatocytes, cell necrosis, variable but usually severe steatosis, and Mallory bodies (Fig. 10.3). The latter structures are absent in about 30% of the biopsies. None of the histological alterations, including Mallory bodies, can be correlated with prognosis. Other diseases with similar acute symptoms must be excluded, eg, acute viral hepatitis (especially with cholestasis), drug-induced hepatitis, and intraabdominal processes such as acute cholecystitis, gallstone obstruction, perforated peptic ulcer, and pancreatitis. Alcoholic hepatitis may simulate an abdominal crisis, with right-upper-quadrant pain, leukocytosis, fever, and raised serum alkaline phosphatases. Inadvertent surgery may kill the patient. A liver biopsy should be obtained to confirm the diagnosis and exclude other conditions.

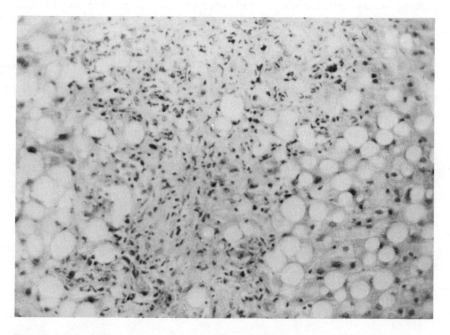

Fig. 10.3. Alcoholic hepatitis. The collapsed centrolobular area is obliterated by fibrosis and acute inflammation. H and E, X200.

Prognosis is variable; 5–30% mortality is described from several institutions. Long-term survival appears similar to that for cirrhosis. About 60% are alive five years after the onset of illness. Approximately 50% will progress to cirrhosis. Treatment is not specific, although supportive measures are indicated. Steroids have been used but their efficacy is doubtful.[18] They may be of some benefit in patients with alcoholic hepatitis and hepatic encephalopathy.[19]

Mallory bodies (alcoholic hyalin). Recently there has been increased interest in the nature of Mallory bodies and their role in alcoholic liver disease. Mallory bodies may also be found in hepatoma, Indian childhood cirrhosis, Wilson's disease, primary biliary cirrhosis, and rarely in cases of extrahepatic biliary obstruction, chronic active hepatitis, malnutrition (postileojejunal bypass),[20] and abetalipoproteinemia.[21] The only extrahepatic site reported so far is in the lung of asbestosis.[22] Although once considered as giant mitochondria (distinguished as ovoid globules within cells) or deformed endoplasmic reticulum, Mallory bodies are now believed to be neoproteins secreted by the endoplasmic reticulum and related to the microfilament system.

Histologically, Mallory bodies appear as spherical or irregular homogeneous, eosinophilic cytoplasmic masses, about 2–3 μm in size (Fig. 10.4).[23] Mallory bodies may be found in hepatocytes, ductular cells, Kupffer cells, or uncommonly in extracellular sites. They occur often with cholestasis, particularly of long duration. Centrolobular Mallory bodies in specimens without lobular destruction are most often observed in alcoholic liver injury; in the periphery of the lobule, without cirrhosis, their presence favors primary biliary cirrhosis over extrahepatic cholestasis.[24] When they are scattered throughout hepatic lobules, they are not specific and may indicate any of the diseases with which hyalin is associated. Histochemically, a glycoprotein composition rich in basic groups is detected. Electron microscope identification offers the only certain means of confirmation at present. Three ultrastructural forms are recognized (Fig. 10.5).[25]

Type	Arrangement of fibrils	Electron density	Size of fibrils (mean ± 1 SD, in Å)
I	Parallel	++	141 ± 42
II	Random	+++	152 ± 33
III	Clumpy; loss of fibrillar structure	++++	–

Our studies indicate that Mallory bodies may play a key role in the evolution of alcoholic hepatitis.[14] As neoantigens, these hyalin inclusions

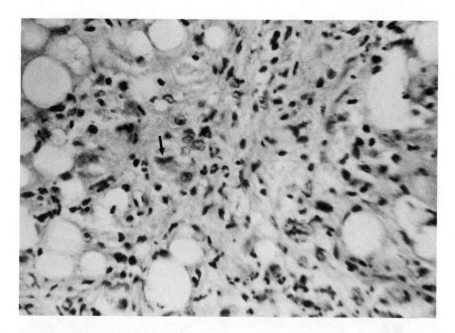

Fig. 10.4. Mallory body (alcoholic hyalin). The intracytoplasmic amorphous inclusion (arrow) is surrounded by leukocytes and swollen liver cells. H and E, X100.

induce both cellular and humoral mediated immune abnormalities encountered in the disease. Circulating antigen and antibodies to Mallory bodies are also present in patients with alcoholic hepatitis.

Alcoholic Cirrhosis

Cirrhosis of all types ranked seventh among the leading causes of mortality in 1973, accounting for 33,000 deaths. Cirrhosis due to alcoholism predominates in the United States (60–70% of all cirrhosis). There are no pathognomonic features which differentiate alcoholic cirrhosis from other types of cirrhosis. Diagnosis rests on clinical association with alcoholism, a constellation of clinical features, and laboratory findings.

Pathogenesis. Sustained and high alcoholic consumption is required to generate hepatic lesions. Nevertheless, it has been shown that abstinence from alcohol may neither completely reverse nor prevent disease once the process has started. The role of malnutrition in initiating or promoting the disease process has been subject to hot debate. In an urban

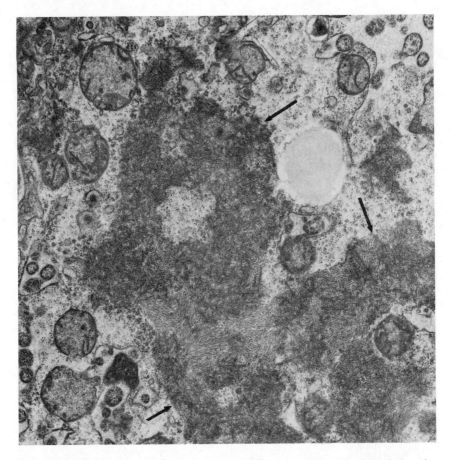

Fig. 10.5. Ultrastructure of the Mallory body (Type 1). The characteristic microfilaments (arrows) are arranged in parallel pattern in a hepatocyte. X27,000. Courtesy of Dr. F. G. Zaki (Squibb Institute for Medical Research).

setting where low-socioeconomic groups live, malnutrition does seem to be a cofactor; while in other socioeconomic groups, it does not.

Just how ethanol produces cirrhosis is not understood. Some antecedent events are known (Fig. 10.6). Although it is the first change, fat by itself does not appear to be necessary for the initiation of the cirrhotic process. Necrosis of liver cells is required, a finding based on both clinical and experimental observations. The destructive phase is followed by a cycle of regeneration and fibrosis. There is evidence that not only can alcohol influence fibroblast activity, but that necrotic liver elaborates a stimulator factor which activates collagen synthesis.

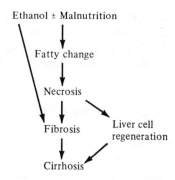

Fig. 10.6. Development of alcoholic cirrhosis.

Clinical presentation. The average age of onset is in the late 40s. Cirrhosis is more common in males, occurring in the ratio of 2 or 3 to 1 female. About 10–20% of the cases are latent, clinically silent, and detected only at autopsy. The early symptoms are not specific; anorexia, weight loss, abdominal distress and gas pains, and weakness occur in over 50% of the patients. Hematemesis from esophageal varices may present as the initial symptom in 10–20% of cirrhotics. It should be remembered that there are other causes of upper GI bleeding in the alcoholic, the three most common being esophageal varices (60% of cases), peptic ulcer (25%), and alcoholic gastritis (15%). The classical features of hepatomegaly, jaundice, ascites, edema, and splenomegaly appear relatively late. Physical findings are listed in Table 10.1. Overt signs of malnutrition such as beefy sore tongue, ankle edema, peripheral neuritis, perifollicular hemorrhage, and shark skin are found in at least 40% of the patients.

Table 10.1. Physical findings in alcohol cirrhosis.

	Incidence, %
Hepatomegaly	90
Splenomegaly	30
Jaundice	80
Ascites	75
Spider angiomas	50
Collateral veins	50
Esophageal varices	40
Malnutrition	40
Fever	20
Hydrothorax, usually right-sided	10

Other manifestations of alcohol injury such as gastritis, and acute and chronic pancreatitis occur with varying frequency, depending on host susceptibility. In the decompensated stage, ascites, hepatic coma, and portal hypertension become prominent, usually out of proportion to the jaundice.

Systemic features.   Some of the more important features are the following:

Fever: Generally, fever does not exceed 101°F; it occurs in up to 30% of cases in some series. It is present more often when signs of liver failure appear. Although the mechanism is not understood, three factors could be involved:

1. Bacteremia, found in 5–10% of patients with cirrhosis
2. Endotoxinemia
3. Metabolic abnormalities involving production of etiocholanolone and other pyrogenic steroids

The first two factors are related to Kupffer cell dysfunction (see Chapter 4). The last possibility is rarely documented.

Feminizing signs of cirrhosis:[26,27] Gynecomastia, loss of axillary and pubic hair, testicular atrophy, and appearance of vascular spiders are observed in up to 70% of cases (Table 10.2). These phenomena are attributable to altered hepatic metabolism of estrogen and testosterone. Normally, the gonads, and to a very small extent the adrenals, secrete estrogens. Peripheral conversion from androstenedione and testosterone also contribute to the estrogen pool. In the circulation both conjugated and unconjugated estrogens, the former bound to albumin and to a specific globulin (sex hormone binding globulin, SHBG), are found. Liver is the major metabolic site where hydroxylation and conjugation of the estrogens take place. About one-third of the circulating estrogens are excreted in the bile. Of this fraction 80% undergoes intestinal reabsorption. The remainder is disposed of by the kidneys.

   In cirrhosis, plasma androstenedione and its production rate are increased, whereas plasma testosterone is decreased.[27] The increased peripheral conversion of androstenedione to estrone, and testosterone to estradiol accounts for the elevated circulating level of estrogens in cirrhosis. The high plasma concentration of estradiol is sustained in the presence of an increased urinary excretion of the hormone. The presence of gynecomastia and spider nevi correlates with high plasma estradiol levels, but signs of androgen deficiency such as testicular atrophy, impotence, and hair loss are poorly related with low-testosterone levels. Reduced hepatic degradation of estrogen is not the primary cause of the

Table 10.2. Systemic alterations in alcoholic cirrhosis.

System	Functional	Clinical
Cardiovascular	Hyperkinetic state, ↑ cardiac output, ↑ peripheral flow, ↑ blood volume, ↓ peripheral vascular response[39]	Palmar erythema, vascular spiders Hypotension after trauma or surgery
Pulmonary	AV shunting, ↑ pulmonary arterial pressure, ↓ O_2 saturation	Cyanosis, clubbing
Gastrointestinal	? ↑ hemolysis, ? altered bile salt metabolism ↑ gastric acid secretion	Gallstones (twice normal), predominantly bilirubinate type Peptic ulcers
Endocrine	↓ retinal formation, ↓ plasma testosterone (total and unbound) and dihydrotestosterone ↑ plasma gonadotropins ↑ plasma and urinary estradiol ↓ serum somatomedin (sulfation factor; identical with nonsuppressible insulin-like activity), due to ? inhibition by ↑ estrogen and ? malnutrition[38] ↑ fasting concentration of growth hormone: exaggerated response to hypoglycemia and not suppressed by oral glucose, secondary to ↑ estrogen activity and ↓ metabolic clearance	Testicular atrophy Impotence Gynecomastia, spider nevi
Hematologic	↓ clotting factors ↓ folate absorption Uncompensated hemolysis LCAT deficiency	Purpura Macrocytosis Anemia Spur cells
Renal	See Tables 7.1 and 2	

elevated estradiol level. Both the increased plasma gonadotropin level found in most patients and the poor testicular output of testosterone after chorionic gonadotropin injection indicate that the hypogonadism in cirrhosis is primary. Other hormonal abnormalities include increased circulating SHBG; reduced estriol level, which is related to the cholestasis and interruption of the enterohepatic circulation; and impaired gonadotropin responses after clomiphene challenge.

The impotence, sterility, testicular atrophy, and diminished body hair encountered in alcoholics have also been attributed to alcohol itself rather than alcoholic liver disease.[28] One pathway affected is the retinol-retinal (vitamin A) oxidation required for spermatogenesis. Vitamin A is transported in circulation as retinol, but oxidation by alcohol dehydrogenase is required for retinal activity. Ethanol competitively inhibits testicular retinal formation and thereby produces aspermatogenesis. Several steps in the conversion of pregnenolone to testosterone are NAD-dependent. Excess NADH generated by the metabolism of ethanol might inhibit the conversion rates. It is assumed that ethanol provokes both aspermatogenesis and decreased testosterone production, which initially are reversible. With the superimposed liver disease, the changes become irreversible.

Infections: Impaired immunity may account for the increased incidence of tuberculosis, salmonellosis, and other gram-negative organisms (Table 10.3).[29] The entity of spontaneous peritonitis in cirrhotic ascites is described elsewhere (Chapter 7).

Hematologic changes:[30,31] Hematological abnormalities affecting all hemopoietic cell lines are common in alcoholic liver disease (Tables 10.2 and 4). The incidence of these complications is reported as megaloblastic erythropoiesis secondary to folic acid deficiency (40%), ring sideroblastic defect of marrow (30%), thrombocytopenia (20%), and leucopenia (10%). Many of the disorders involve folic acid metabolism. Both dietary deficiency and malabsorption of the vitamin are described. Folate storage in humans is on the order of 5-10 mg. Its availability in food is relatively limited because the cooking process destroys folic acid in vegetables and because the average American prefers a meat diet. Several months of dietary deprivation quickly leads to folate deficiency, a condition readily met in the chronic alcoholic. The role of LCAT in formation of acanthocytes and spur cells is discussed in Chapter 1.

Circulatory changes: The cause of the hyperdynamic circulation with decreased peripheral vascular resistance in cirrhosis is not known (Table 10.2). Anemia and pulmonary arteriovenous (AV) shunts are possible pathogenic factors. The possibility of circulating vasodilators has been entertained. The kallikrein-bradykinin system cannot be implicated.[32] Plasma kallikreinogen is depressed in cirrhosis, whereas kallikrein in-

Table 10.3. Altered immunologic status in alcoholic liver disease.

Alcoholic cirrhosis	Mechanism
↑ IgG, IgA, and IgM, especially IgA	? stimulation of peripheral lymphoid tissue by gut derived antigens bypassing the damaged liver
↑ viral and bacterial antibodies	Same as above
↓ leukocyte chemotaxis	Serum inhibitor of chemotaxis
↓ granulocyte adherence (chemotaxis and leukocytic killing remain intact)	Mechanism unknown
↓ skin reactivity to DNCB candida	↓ cellular immunity; mechanism unknown

Alcoholic hepatitis	Mechanism
↑ lymphocyte transformation (LT) to autologous liver and Mallory bodies	↓ cellular immunity
↑ MIF production to both antigens	↓ cellular immunity
↓ LT to PHA	↓ T-cells

hibitor, Hageman factor, and bradykinin levels are normal or moderately depressed. It appears that impairment of liver function decreases plasma kallikreinogen production. Renal dysfunction in these cirrhotics is not associated with elevated bradykinin concentration. Other evidence of circulatory abnormalities include:

1. Vascular spiders: These are not AV anastomoses but vascular anomalies, although they may pulsate.
2. Clubbing: This is found in 5% of patients with alcoholic cirrhosis. Severe clubbing is more frequent in biliary cirrhosis.
3. Oxygen unsaturation: This is attributed to intrapulmonary, portapulmonary, and systemic pulmonary shunting, but apparently it is not due to displacement of the hemoglobin dissociation curve for oxygen. A shift of the oxygen dissociation curve to the right is not observed in cirrhosis. The 2,3-diphosphoglycerate concentration in erythrocytes is, however, elevated.

Mineral deficits: Storage of both zinc and magnesium is affected in cirrhosis.[33,34] Plasma zinc levels, which correlate with albumin concentrations, appear depressed in both fasting and postcibal states. The increased urinary excretion of zinc, among other factors, accounts for the

Table 10.4. Hematological disorders in chronic alcoholic disease.[30,31]

Disorder	Mechanism
Macrocytic anemia	Folate deficient diet Malabsorption of folate
Vacuolated forms and ring sideroblasts in bone marrow	Folate deficiency
Hypochromic anemia	Iron deficiency from blood loss
Hemolytic anemia, compensated or uncompensated	Shortened RBC life span due to damage to cells during passage through liver; sequestration by hyperactive spleen; rare auto-antibody
Hemolytic anemia with stomatocytes	? intrinsic RBC defect
Acanthocytes (10% incidence)	Membrane lipid change
Spur cells (rare)	LCAT deficiency
Transient hemolytic anemia, with jaundice, hyperlipemia and fatty liver (Zieve's syndrome)	Anemia not due to hyperlipemia; disease indistinguishable from alcoholic pancreatitis with fatty liver
Thrombocytopenia	Direct ethanol toxicity, or suppression of platelet production; hypersplenism; dietary folic acid deficiency
Leukopenia	Diminished granulocytic reserve due to folate deficiency and ethanol toxicity
↓ leucocyte mobilization with intact phagocytosis and intracellular killing during ethanol infusion	Unknown

low hepatic content of the metal. Skeletal magnesium is lowered in cirrhosis but concentrations in bone and erythrocyte are normal. The change in magnesium stores is ascribed to the secondary aldosteronism encountered in cirrhosis.

Pathology. Grossly, the liver is diffusely scarred, with normal lobules replaced by either macronodules or micronodules (< 1 cm), with a tough, leathery consistency, and yellowish-brown or green-tinged in color (Fig.

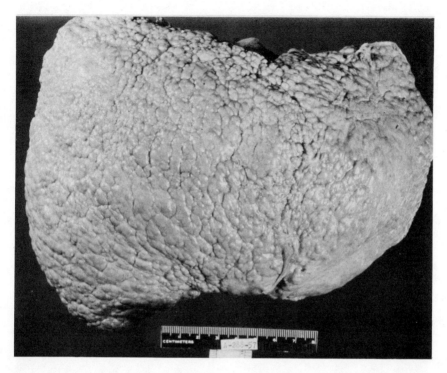

Fig. 10.7. The micronodular liver of alcoholic cirrhosis. The small uniform nodules average less than 1 cm in size.

10.7). The nodular size is determined by the stage of the disease.[35] The micronodular appearance represents a midpoint in the evolution of alcoholic cirrhosis, in which necrosis, inflammation, fibrosis, and nodular regeneration have occurred at more or less equal rates, and in all lobules. The progression of micronodular deformation produces the final common pathway lesion of macronodular, or a mixed micronodular-macronodular cirrhosis. In this continuum, uneven necrosis and inflammation damage some parts of the liver more severely than others. This occurs among alcoholics who drink in sprees interspersed by relatively alcohol-free periods.

The terms micronodular and macronodular are purely descriptive and noncommittal for etiologic purposes. They have replaced Laennec's or portal, and postnecrotic cirrhosis, respectively. Microscopically, the essential features consist of regenerative nodules replacing the lobular pattern, diffuse fibrosis, and varying degrees of inflammation and necrosis (Fig. 10.8). The degree of activity is judged by the extent of necrosis and inflammation at the periphery of the nodules.

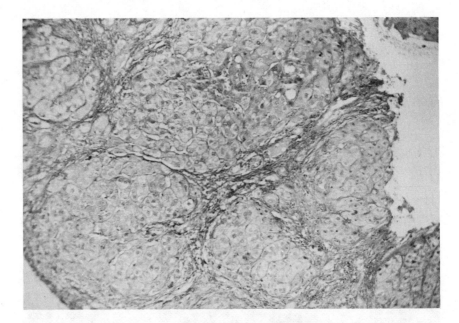

Fig. 10.8. Micronodular cirrhosis. Thin bands of portal fibrosis subdivide the lobules into small regenerative nodules. Mallory's trichrome, X100.

Diagnosis.   The clinical, physical, and laboratory findings are characteristic but not definitive. A liver biopsy is required for confirmation in most instances. Cirrhotic features are easily recognized by liver biopsy, although the disease is not excluded by the procedure. Sampling variation or subtle alterations, which are difficult to interpret, may provide a false impression. Subtle changes are not uncommon with biopsies obtained by Menghini needles, which tend to glance off hard fibrous tissue. In the specimens, often only the edges of regenerative nodules are obtained. The fragments do frequently reveal structural abnormalities: disturbance of afferent-efferent vessel relationships, variation in cell appearance, and evidence of double-cell plates and mitosis at the periphery. The lesions of cirrhosis are not specific for a disease entity. The histological appearances of all types of cirrhosis are similar, especially at the end stages. The presence of fat, especially in portal macrophages, and Mallory bodies favors the impression of alcoholic cirrhosis but is not diagnostic. Differentiation from other types of cirrhosis depends heavily on the history (Table 10.5).

Treatment.   Prevention of further damage by abstinence from alcohol is desirable. Abstention prolongs useful life, although the effect may not

Table 10.5. Contrast between alcoholic and nonalcoholic cirrhosis.

Features	Alcoholic cirrhosis	Nonalcoholic cirrhosis
Age	Generally above 40	Any
Sex	Male predominance	Variable
Antecedent history	Alcohol	Others
Malnutrition (sore tongue, peripheral neuritis)	Common	Uncommon
Parotid hypertrophy Dupuytren's contracture Gynecomastia Testicular atrophy	30–70%	Rare
Peptic ulcer	15%	Uncommon
Hepatoma development	< 5%	> 5% (higher, especially in hemochromatosis)

be seen in the milder forms of cirrhosis. Supportive therapy for the major sequalae, ascites, and portal hypertension should be employed. No beneficial effect with long-term steroids is noted in patients with cirrhosis. In fact, mortality of treated patients (44%) was greater than that in the control group (25%).[36] Drugs inhibiting fibrogenesis such as colchicine, penicillamine, and certain peptide compounds are currently undergoing investigation.

Prognosis. The causes of death are hepatic coma 50%, ruptured variceal hemorrhage 30%, infection 5%, renal shutdown 5%, others 10%. Prognosis has improved over the years, as the following comparison of two studies shows:

	Powell-Klatskin[37] series, 1968		Ratnoff-Patek series, 1942
		Five-year survival, %	
Cirrhotic Patients	*Drinkers*	*Abstainers*	
With jaundice	34	60	10
With ascites	34	53	7
With hematemesis	22	36	19

Overall five-year survival rate is in the range 40–70%.

REFERENCES

1. Isselbacher KJ, Greenberger NJ: Metabolic effects of alcohol on the liver. *New Eng J Med* 270:351–356, 402–410, 1964.
2. Lieber CS: Hepatic and metabolic effects of alcohol (1966–1973). *Gastroenterology* 65:821–846, 1973.
3. Bennion LJ, Li TK: Alcohol metabolism in American Indians and Whites: Lack of racial differences in metabolic rate and liver alcohol dehydrogenase. *New Eng J Med* 294:9–13, 1976.
4. Korsten MA, et al: High blood acetaldehyde levels after ethanol administration: Difference between alcoholic and nonalcoholic subjects. *New Eng J Med* 292:386–389, 1975.
5. Lieber CS: Effects of ethanol upon lipid metabolism. *Lipids* 9:103–116, 1974.
6. Johansson BG, Medhus A: Increase in plasma alpha-lipoproteins in chronic alcoholics after acute abuse. *Acta Med Scand* 195:273–277, 1974.
7. Kreisberg RA, Siegal AM, Owen WC: Glucose-lactate interrelationships: Effect of ethanol. *J Clin Invest* 50:175–185, 1971.
8. Mendelson JH: Biologic concomitants of alcoholism. *New Eng J Med* 283:24–32, 71–81, 1970.
9. Porta EA, Koch OR, Hartroft WS: Recent advances in molecular pathology; A review of the effects of alcohol on the liver. *Exp Molec Path* 12:104–132, 1970.
10. Schaffner F, Popper H: Alcoholic hepatitis in the spectrum of ethanol-induced liver injury. *Scand J Gastroent,* suppl 7, pp 69–78, 1970.
11. Terris M: Epidemiology of cirrhosis of the liver: National mortality data. *Amer J Pub Health* 57:2076–2088, 1967.
12. Rubin E, Lieber CS: Fatty liver, alcoholic hepatitis and cirrhosis produced by alcohol in primates. *New Eng J Med* 290:128–135, 1974.
13. Rubin E, Lieber CS: Alcohol-induced hepatic injury in nonalcoholic volunteers, *New Eng J Med* 278:869–876, 1968.
14. Zetterman RK, Luisada-Opper A, Leevy CM: Alcoholic hepatitis: Cell-mediated immunologic response to alcoholic hyalin. *Gastroenterology* 70:382–384, 1976.
15. Kanagasundaram N, Leevy CM: Transfer factor in alcoholic hepatitis: Its occurrence and significance. *Gastroenterology* 69:A-33/833, 1975.
16. Lischner MW, Alexander JF, Galambos JT: Natural history of alcoholic hepatitis: 1: The acute disease. *Amer J Dig Dis* 16:481–494, 1971.
17. Alexander JF, Lischner MW, Galambos JT: Natural history of alcoholic hepatitis. II: Long-term prognosis. *Amer J Gastroenter* 56:515–525, 1971.
18. Resnick RH, Iber FL: Treatment of acute alcoholic hepatitis. *Gut* 13:68–73, 1972.
19. Campra JL, et al: Prednisone therapy of acute alcoholic hepatitis: Report of a controlled trial. *Ann Intern Med* 79:625–631, 1973.
20. Peters RL, Gay T, Reynolds TB: Post-jejunoileal-bypass hepatic disease: Its similarity to alcoholic hepatic disease. *Amer J Clin Path* 63:318–331, 1975.
21. Partin JS, et al: Liver ultrastructure in abetalipoproteinemia: Evolution of micronodular cirrhosis. *Gastroenterology* 67:107–118, 1974.

22. Kuhn C, Kuo TT: Cytoplasmic hyalin in asbestosis: A reaction of injured alveolar epithelium. *Arch Path* 95:190–194, 1973.
23. Christoffersen P: Light microscopical features in liver biopsies with Mallory bodies. *Acta Path Microbiol Scand Sect A* 80:705–712, 1972.
24. Gerber MA, et al: Hepatocellular hyalin in cholestasis and cirrhosis: Its diagnostic significance. *Gastroenterology* 64:89–98, 1973.
25. Yokoo H, et al: Morphologic variants of alcoholic hyalin. *Amer J Path* 69:25–40, 1972.
26. Adlercreutz H: Hepatic metabolism of estrogens in health and disease. *New Eng J Med* 290:1081–1083, 1973.
27. Baker HWG, et al: A study of the endocrine manifestations of hepatic cirrhosis. *Quart J Med* 45:145–178, 1976.
28. Van Thiel DH, Lester R: Sex and alcohol. *New Eng J Med* 291:251–253, 1974.
29. Straus B, Berenyi MR: Infection and immunity in alcoholic cirrhosis. *Mt. Sinai J Med* 40:631–641, 1973.
30. Eichner ER, Hillman RS: The evolution of anemia in alcoholic patients. *Amer J Med* 50:218–232, 1971.
31. Eichner ER: Hematologic disorders of alcoholism. *Amer J Med* 54:621–630, 1973.
32. Wong P, et al: Kallikrein-bradykinin system in chronic alcoholic liver disease. *Ann Intern Med* 77:205–209, 1972.
33. Walker BE, et al: Plasma and urinary zinc in patients with malabsorption syndromes or hepatic cirrhosis. *Gut* 14:943–948, 1974.
34. Lim P, Jacob E: Magnesium deficiency in liver cirrhosis. *Quart J Med* 163:291–300, 1972.
35. Scheuer PJ: Liver biopsy in the diagnosis of cirrhosis. *Gut* 11:275–278, 1970.
36. Copenhagen Study Group for Liver Diseases: Sex, ascites and alcoholism in survival of patients with cirrhosis: Effect of prednisone. *New Eng J Med* 291:271–273, 1974.
37. Powell WJ Jr, Klatskin G: Duration of survival in patients with Laennec's cirrhosis: Influence of alcohol withdrawal, and possible effects of recent changes in general management of the disease. *Amer J Med* 44:406–420, 1968.
38. Wu A, et al: Reduced serum somatomedin activity in patients with chronic liver disease. *Clin Sci Molec Med* 47:359–366, 1974.
39. Lunzer MR, et al: Impaired cardiovascular responsiveness in liver disease. *Lancet* 2:382–385, 1975.

VIRAL HEPATITIS AND CHRONIC HEPATITIS

11

VIRAL HEPATITIS

Acute viral hepatitis (VH) refers to the two clinically similar but immunologically dissimilar diseases caused by hepatitis virus type A (infectious or epidemic hepatitis) and type B (serum hepatitis). A third hepatitis virus, non-A and non-B, has been implicated in a recent epidemic in Costa Rica.[1] The role of the third agent in the etiology of VH has not been clarified. Other viruses, such as yellow fever, Epstein-Barr virus (infectious mononucleosis), rubella, cytomegalovirus, herpes simplex, echo, and coxsackie, may produce clinical and pathological features similar to VH. However, the liver is not the primary target organ in these viral infections.

Acute VH remains a major infectious disease, accounting for about 30,000 overt cases a year in the United States. In addition, there are 3–5 times more anicteric cases. VH is responsible for 1500–3000 deaths in the United States each year. The virus type, mode of spread, host susceptibility, and environmental factors determine the clinical variants of VH (Table 11.1).

Hepatitis A and B Virus

A and B virus have not been propagated under laboratory conditions. Hepatitis A virus (HAV) has been recently identified in the stools of patients with hepatitis A. The agent is 27 nm in size, and appears to be either a parvovirus or an enterovirus (Fig. 11.1a).[2] The A virus is characterized as an RNA virus inactivated by ultraviolet light, heating to 100°C for five minutes, and dilute formalin.[3] Hepatitis B virus (HBV) has been extensively studied in serum, liver, and other tissue sources by electron microscopy, immunofluorescence, and immune electron microscopy techniques. Under the electron microscope the HBV appears in three distinctive particle forms (Fig. 11.1b). In two of these, the chief components are small 20-nm spherical and filamentous forms. The third form is a double-shelled 42-nm (Dane) particle with a 27-nm core. The inner core

Table 11.1.   Clinical types of viral hepatitis.

Acute viral hepatitis (VH)
  Icteric
  Anicteric
  Cholestatic
Acute sequelae
  Prolonged (unresolved) acute VH
  Relapsed acute VH
  Acute fulminant hepatitis
Hepatitis in high risk groups
  Neonatal viral hepatitis
  Chronic asymptomatic carrier
  Drug-abuse-associated hepatitis
  Acute VH in hemodialysis/transplant unit
  Posttransfusion hepatitis
Chronic sequelae
  Chronic hepatitis: chronic persistent hepatitis
    and chronic active hepatitis
  Postviral hepatitis cirrhosis

structure resembles that of a picornavirus. The Dane particle is probably the infectious viron of type B hepatitis. The core is thought to proliferate in the nucleus of the hepatocyte, whereas the surface double-shelled material is added on in the cytoplasm. The purified HBV particle has an MW of 3×10^6, 5% of which is RNA.[4] This amounts to about 450 nucleotides that could code 150 amino acids, which is unusually small for a virus.

All three particle forms show a surface antigenic determinant, HB$_s$Ag. The corresponding antibody in type B hepatitis infection is HB$_s$Ab. HB$_s$Ag resists heating to 60°C for 10 minutes, or to 100°C for brief periods. It is not extracted by ether, nor is it digested by the usual proteolytic enzymes. The 27-nm core of the Dane particle contains DNA polymerase and carries an antigenic determinant, known as HB$_c$Ag. The corresponding antibody is HB$_c$Ab. The presence of HB$_c$Ab reflects continuing virus multiplication, while DNA polymerase correlates with peak virus replication.[5] Analysis of HB$_s$Ag reveals it is not a homogeneous antigen but rather is composed of several distinct antigenic specificities.[6] A common group determinant, a, is present, as well as two sets of mutually exclusive subtype determinants y and d, and r and w. Three subdeterminants of the group type, a, designated a_1, a_2, a_3, are described but their significance is unknown at the present time. The common group and subtype determinants give rise to four possible phenotypes: ayr, ayw, adr, adw. Other subtype determinants are also reported (see below).

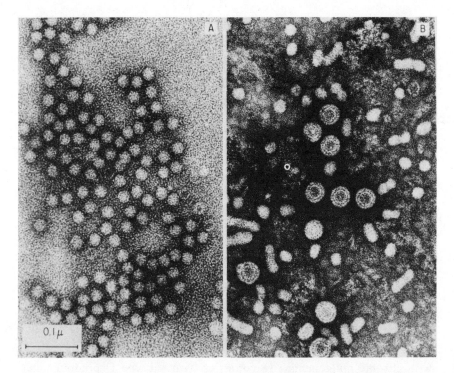

Fig. 11.1. A. Purified CR326 strain human hepatitis A virus prepared by CsCl density gradient separation from infected marmoset serum. B. Purified Australia antigen, filamentous and Dane particles prepared from sera from a human hepatitis B carrier. Courtesy of Dr. M. H. Hilleman (Merck Institute for Therapeutic Research).

Epidemiology. Hepatitis A virus is usually associated with childhood hepatitis or rural epidemics. It is transmitted preferentially by the oral-fecal route, although parenteral and urinal spread is possible. It accounts for hepatitis occurring under crowded, poor sanitary conditions, after pollution of the drinking water, or by milk contaminated by polluted water used to wash dairy equipment, or by eating raw clams or oysters from polluted waters.

A common source for the epidemics can often be identified or suspected. Sporadic, urban hepatitis is associated with HBV. Infection spreads parenterally by contaminated syringe needles, blood, and blood products. Other modes of transmission for HBV are oral, airborne, and sexual. There is some evidence that the incubation period (60–100 days) is shorter by parenteral transmission than by oral spread. The virus has been identified in practically all body fluids and excreta, including stool, urine, saliva, sweat, semen, and menstrual blood.

The infectious dose is as minute as 1 ml $\times$ 10^{-7} dilution of HB_sAg-positive blood.[7] The role of blood-sucking mosquitoes and other arthropods as vectors of transmission in the tropics has been raised.[8] HBV does not replicate in the mosquitoes; it is carried passively. Infection can be effected by mechanical means, whereby the infected meal of the mosquito penetrates the skin. This method may account for the high prevalence of chronic HB_sAg-carrier state in the tropics (10-20 times the temperate zone). The epidemic also depends on the high rate of exposure during the early years of life mediated in part by the mechanical transmission due to infected blood-sucking arthropods. The spread of HBV in the United States is also largely conditioned by socioeconomic status. In low-socioeconomic populations the virus appears endemic, and the exposure occurs early. The frequency of HB_sAb in the adolescent age group is increased compared to the similar age group in high-socioeconomic status.[9]

HB_sAg subtypes serve as useful markers of the infection in different settings. Of the four possible subtype variants described, one (ayr) is very rarely isolated.[10] The other subtypes vary in their epidemiological characteristics (Table 11.2). In countries with subtype Y predominance, such as Greece, Y is found in association with acute and chronic hepatitis and with chronic antigenemia. In countries with subtype D predominance, such as the United States, D is found more often among healthy chronic carriers and patients with chronic active hepatitis or cirrhosis. Subtype Y occurs more frequently in patients with drug abuse and in hemodialysis units. Posttransfusion hepatitis may belong to either Y or D subtype. It appears that the D strain virus greatly outnumbered the Y-type virus at one time. The dominance is diminished by a resurgence of the Y strain, which is closely identified with drug addiction. The clinical features of the subtype disease reflect epidemiological factors rather than biological differences. The association of Y or D with a disease does not mean that the disease will be more severe than were Y or D absent.

Another antigen complex, e, has been recently described.[11] Closely associated but not identical with the HB_sAg system, e-antigen is found only in HB_sAg-positive patients; e-antigen occurs more commonly in cases of chronic active hepatitis (60% positivity) and cirrhosis (30%) than in those with acute hepatitis (10%). Thus e-antigen may serve as a useful prognostic marker in acute viral hepatitis since over 50% of positive reacting cases progressed to chronic liver disease. Patients with acute viral hepatitis and serologically positive HB_sAg and e-antigen differ from e-negative (but HB_sAg-positive) cases. The former group shows lower serum concentrations of bilirubin and aminotransferase activity. Liver

Table 11.2. HB$_S$Ag subtypes: Their geographical distribution and disease association.[10]

Subtypes	Geographical predominance	Disease association
adw (D)	North America, Europe, multifocal, among remote groups of S. Africa, S. America (ancient subtype)	Chronic carriers, chronic active hepatitis, cirrhosis
adr (R)	Restricted to Far East, Oceania, where D is also common but not Y	
ayw (Y)	Middle East, Mediterranean, where D is also common	Strong association with drug abusers, hemodialysis patients
ayr	Very rare	

histology reveals more frequent piecemeal necrosis of the periportal limiting plate and more severe Kupffer cell proliferation. The nature of e-antigen is obscure but a relationship with the Dane particle (core antigen) is proposed. Other antigenic subtypes—f, and (l)—have been identified. Their relationship to liver disease is not clarified at the present time.

Experimental models. Both HAV and HBV are transmissible to animals.[12] Rhesus monkeys and chimpanzees are susceptible to HVB infections. In infected animals, Kupffer cell proliferation and a lymphocytic triaditis are found in the early stages (six months or so) after inoculation. Subsequently, HB$_s$Ag and HB$_c$Ag particles become evident in both hepatocellular and cytoplasm nuclei by electron microscopy and immunofluorescence. Serological and biochemical changes mimic the human disease. HAV has been transmitted to marmoset monkeys. Cross-challenge experiments indicate that there are at least two different antigenic strains of HAV.

Liver histology shows focal and diffuse hepatic necrosis with periportal and centrolobular lymphocytic inflammation. It is not known if phagocytosis of human hepatitis virus by Kupffer cells is required before the virus enters into hepatocytes. Other hepatotropic viruses such as those of yellow fever and canine hepatitis apparently first infect Kupffer cells before involving the hepatocytes. Humans who are experimentally infected with viral hepatitis reveal extensive ultrastructural changes in the liver. The rough endoplasmic reticulum is dilated with detachment of polysomal particles. Mitochondria swell. Autophagic vacuoles are prominent and surround foci of cytoplasmic degeneration. The nucleus shows nucleolar enlargement and inclusions derived from the cytoplasm. No ultrastructural distinction can be made between type A and type B hepatitis unless viral particles are present. HB$_s$Ag particles may be found in both the cytoplasm and nuclei of liver cells. The pattern and degree of viral particle deposition varies with the severity of the lesion and the development of other sequelae. It is not clear if hepatitis virus damages the liver and other organs by a direct cytopathic effect or by an immunologically mediated mechanism. The evidence so far favors the latter hypothesis, or a combination of both.

HB$_s$Ag in liver disease. The incidence of HB$_s$Ag in the normal population, acute VH, and other liver diseases varies by geographical distribution, the phase of the disease, and the sensitivity of the methods of determination (Table 11.3). In general, the titer of HB$_s$Ag bears no relation to the severity of liver disease.[13] In fact, the reverse appears to be true. Serum HB$_s$Ag titer and hepatic content of antigen are highest in chronic carriers who have little or no biochemical evidence of hepatic injury, less in chronic persistent hepatitis, and least in chronic active hepatitis. Circulating titers are also low in fulminant hepatitis and primary liver carcinoma. HB$_s$Ag appears to exert little cytopathic effect. The immunologic evidence suggests that the cell-mediated response evoked by HB$_s$Ag is the pathogenic mechanism for liver injury (Table 11.4). Liver cell necrosis is initiated by an immune response controlled by T-cells to

Table 11.3. Incidence of HB$_s$Ag in the normal population and in liver diseases.

	Incidence (% positive)
Normal population:	
USA	0.1
Taiwan	5
Peruvian Indians	20
Type B hepatitis	40–80
Type A hepatitis	0
Chronic active hepatitis	25
Chronic persistent hepatitis	30–50
Hepatoma:	
USA	5
Uganda	40
Taiwan	80
Halothane hepatitis	Same as normal population
Primary biliary cirrhosis	Same as normal population

Table 11.4. Immunological abnormalities in viral hepatitis.

	HB$_S$Ag positive	HB$_S$Ag negative
Immunoglobulins	↑ IgG, ↑ IgA, smaller ↑ IgM	Similar early ↑ IgM
Smooth muscle antibody	Slightly higher titers; correlates with serum bilirubin	↑ in 75% of cases
Lymphocyte transformation	↓ PHA reactivity, ? due to lymphocyte defect	Similar ↓
	↑ response to HB$_S$Ag after acute attack	
MIF	↑ with HB$_S$Ag during acute stage	

the infective agent. This may also account for the predominant lympho-cytic, rather than polymorphonuclear cell, infiltrates in viral hepatitis. Suppression of this response, either by corticosteroids or immune paralysis due to high-antigen load or defective T-cell function, results in little or no liver damage, but the virus continues to proliferate. This constitutes the carrier state. Infections of the newborn and those during early childhood are likely to be followed by persistence of HB$_S$Ag an-tigenemia, perhaps due to a quantitative defect of T-cells at these early ages.

Acute Icteric Viral Hepatitis

Both type A (infectious) and type B (serum) hepatitis produce identical clinical features. The two diseases can be differentiated only on epidemiologic grounds and serologic studies (Table 11.5). Type A hepatitis has a short incubation period, spreads mainly by the fecal-oral route, and gives a positive test for HAAb. A long incubation period, predilection for the parenteral mode of transmission, and HB$_S$Ag positiv-ity distinguish type B hepatitis. For both forms of VH, there is a preicteric phase lasting one week or less preceding the onset of jaundice. The phase is marked by a flu-like syndrome with malaise, weakness, loss of appetite, and nausea, which occurs in over 90% of the patients. Less common but also frequent (75% of cases) are mild fever, headache, vomiting, and abdominal discomfort. The preicteric illness may be recog-nized by the patient when the urine turns brown due to the bilirubinuria. With the onset of jaundice the symptoms may abate or progress in

Table 11.5. Contrast between type A and type B viral hepatitis.

Synonyms	Type A infectious hepatitis	Type B serum hepatitis
Serologic test	HAAb	HB_sAg
Incubation period	2–6 weeks	8–15 weeks
Seasonal incidence	Autumn, winter	All year
Age preference	< 20 years	Any age
Epidemiology	Epidemic, rural	Sporadic, urban
Transmission:		
Parental	+	+ +
Oral-fecal	+ +	+
Sexual	?	+
Contagiousness	+ + +	+ +
Socioeconomic status	Any	Low
Severity	Mild	Severe
Prophylaxis	Gamma globulin effective	Passive-active immunity with HBV immune globulin
Immunity:		
Homologous	Yes	Yes
Cross	No	No

severity, especially the malaise and GI manifestations. The liver is slightly enlarged, often tender. Splenomegaly occurs in 10% of the cases.

Liver function tests characteristically show hyperbilirubinemia (usually below 20 mg/dl), marked aminotransferase elevations (> 500 IU/l; in 75% of the cases AlAT exceeds AsAT), and the presence of HB_sAg if caused by HBV. Serological tests for HAAg and HAAb have been recently introduced. For the HAAb test, the antigenic material is derived from infected marmoset liver.[14] The procedures and their modifications are under current evaluation. They will undoubtedly become standard routine tests. High titers of HAAb are detected during the course of HAV infection, which may persist for years unrelated to the symptoms. The rise in bilirubin peaks at the same time as the increase of aminotransferase. The enzyme levels do not correlate with the severity or the prognosis of the disease. The pattern of appearance for positive hepatic tests and antigenemia is depicted in Fig. 11.2. HB_sAg, HB_sAb, and HB_cAb may become positive in various combinations with different significance (Table 11.6).

The symptoms and biochemical abnormalities subside in the ensuing 4-6 weeks after the appearance of icterus. Children usually recover more

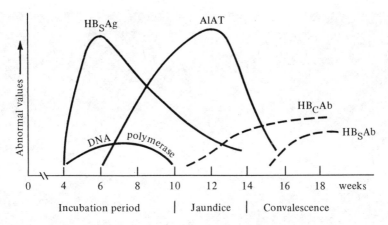

Fig. 11.2. Sequence of enzyme and serological changes in acute type B hepatitis.

rapidly than adults. Liver histology shows diffuse spotty necrosis with lymphocytes, variations in hepatocellular staining and cell size, Kupffer cell hyperplasia, and portal tract lymphocytic infiltration (Fig. 11.3). The changes are characteristic but not diagnostic of VH. Infectious mononucleosis in particular reveals a similar hepatic histology (see Chapter 16).

Table 11.6. Patterns of reactivity for HB$_S$Ag, HB$_S$Ab, and HB$_C$Ab.

HB$_S$Ag	HB$_S$Ab	HB$_C$Ab	Possible interpretations
+	−	−	Early course of HBV disease
+	−	+	1. Late in course of HBV infection 2. Chronic HB$_S$Ag carrier
−	+	+	Convalescent stage
−	+	−	1. Late convalescence 2. Recovery from acute infection
−	−	+	1. Early convalescence 2. Chronic carrier with subdetectable levels of HB$_S$Ag 3. Rising titer indicates immunity, not primary infection

From J. H. Hoofnagle, R. J. Gerety, and L. F. Barker, *Lancet* 2:869–873, 1973.

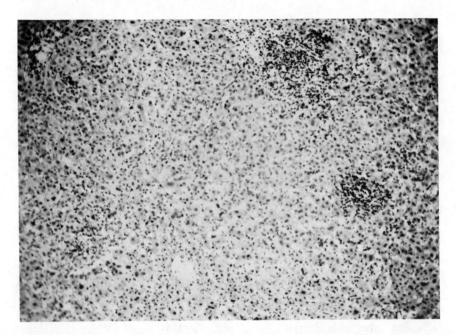

Fig. 11.3. Acute viral hepatitis. Two portal triads are inflamed. Liver cells in the centrolobular area (lower middle) appear in disarray, while Kupffer cells proliferate in the sinusoids. H and E, X100.

The morbidity for acute VH increases with age. Children fare better than older adults. Ninety-five percent of childhood cases recover completely; less than 5% develops chronic sequelae such as chronic active hepatitis or cirrhosis, and less than 1% progresses into acute fulminant hepatitis (Fig. 11.4).

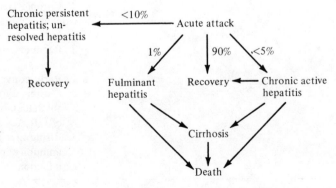

Fig. 11.4. Sequelae of acute viral hepatitis.

Prophylaxis and management. Gamma globulin modifies infection due to type A virus. The usual dose is a single injection of 0.02-0.04 ml/kg body weight. The injection is recommended for those in close contact with victims, and also to immunize residents in endemic areas and to control epidemics. The resultant passive-active immunity exceeds the half-life of gamma globulin (about three weeks). Protection apparently lasts for about six months. Prophylaxis of type B hepatitis has been clarified only recently, in contrast to the experience with type A hepatitis. Hepatitis B immune globulin (HBIG) containing significant HB$_s$Ab titers modifies or prevents type B infection or the carrier state in an endemic setting.[15,16] Standard immune serum globulin (ISG) with little or no HB$_s$Ab can also reduce the incidence of type B hepatitis after low-level exposure to HBV. It is not clear if ISG can substitute for HBIG when the exposure to HBV is intense. ISG has two advantages over HBIG: it is a currently licensed product that is available, and it may be more effective than HBIG in inducing passive-active immunity to HBV. Active immunity against type B hepatitis can be induced by heat-treated HBV serum. The experimental vaccine consists of 22-nm HB$_s$Ag units without Dane particles. This means of prevention is still under study.

Treatment of symptoms consists of supportive measures. Absolute or prolonged bed rest does not facilitate recovery. The usual isolation procedures and techniques for control of infectious disease should be practiced. Corticosteroids which cause a rapid decline of bilirubin and elevations in aminotransferase in VH are contraindicated because these drugs suppress immune response and are likely to prolong HB$_s$Ag antigenemia.

Extrahepatic manifestations.[17] Urticaria and arthritis may occur in the preicteric phase of HB$_s$Ag-positive hepatitis in 5-20% of the cases, disappearing by the onset of jaundice. HB$_s$Ag-HB$_s$Ab immune complexes are deposited in the skin and joints, with consumption and fall in serum complement. The finding suggests a pathogenic phenomenon akin to serum sickness (see also Chapter 4). A similar mechanism is invoked in the rare association between glomerulonephritis and acute VH. A direct virus effect on synovial tissue has also been implicated in the production of arthritis associated with hepatitis.[18]

A curious association between aplastic anemia and VH has been reported (less than 200 cases so far).[19,20] The patient is usually a young male, under 20 years of age, who develops profound pancytopenia 1-7 months after complete resolution of the hepatitis. The prognosis is grave, and death commonly results from septicemia. The pathogenesis is unexplained. Exposure to drugs or chemicals is usually excluded. It is hypothesized that the virus directly damages the stem cells or induces chromosome abnormalities in the hemopoietic cells, resulting in bone-marrow failure. A further possibility is that hepatocellular injury impairs the liver's detoxifying mechanism to handle a metabolite which in turn damages the marrow cells.

Acute anicteric viral hepatitis.   The symptoms and course in adults are similar to the icteric infection, except for lack of jaundice. For this reason the disease is often not recognized clinically. In children the symptoms are mild and are not specific. The disease may progress to chronic active hepatitis or cirrhosis. The chronic carrier state is also more likely to develop from this subclinical state.

Acute cholestatic viral hepatitis.   This form accounts for up to 20% of all acute VH; the figure may be much higher in some epidemics. In its severest manifestations it mimics extrahepatic cholestasis. The bilirubin level and alkaline phosphatase concentration are higher than those encountered in icteric VH. Liver biopsy serves to differentiate the lesion from other more serious conditions.

Prolonged acute viral hepatitis.   Prolonged or unresolved VH may persist longer than the usual six weeks for periods up to 1-2 years (less than 5% of cases). Patients complain of variable malaise, fatigue, and weakness. Jaundice is mild. Liver function tests do not reveal progressive deterioration but fluctuate with a gradual return to normality. Recovery is the invariable rule. Liver biopsy shows a mild hepatitis with prominence of Kupffer cells loaded with lipofuscin. Replacement of the lobular pattern by a cobblestone appearance of liver cells, focal hepatocytolysis, and portal lymphoid hyperplasia are other histological features. Prolonged VH is difficult to distinguish from chronic persistent hepatitis (see below).

Relapsed acute viral hepatitis.   A relapse complicates 5-10% of the cases of the acute disease. The second attack duplicates the first. Serious sequelae are unlikely and recovery is complete.

Acute fulminant viral hepatitis.   Fortunately, this dreaded complication occurs in less than 1% of the patients with acute viral hepatitis. The clinical and biochemical features are identical to other disorders which cause massive hepatitis necrosis. Chapter 8 discusses this more fully.

Hepatitis in High-Risk Groups

Neonatal viral hepatitis.[21]   HB$_s$Ag may be transmitted from mother to infant by transplacental crossing in utero, contamination during delivery, postpartum fecal-oral transmission, or transcolostral spread. The first two routes are documented; the latter two are likely but not proved. The frequency of HBV maternal to infant transmission is 40–75% when acute hepatitis occurs in the third trimester as compared to 10% if acute infection develops in the first two trimesters, and 5% if the mother is an asymptomatic chronic carrier. Antibody to HB_sAg (HB_sAb) is rarely detected in mothers, or in their infants during the first six months of life. In comparison, the antibody to core antigen (HB_cAb) appears regularly in carrier mothers and in umbilical cord blood, but disappears soon from the sera of newborns shortly after birth. The finding suggests that HB_cAb crosses the placental barrier readily in carrier mothers whereas HB_sAb does not. Only 10% of the infected infants become symptomatic; 80% develop chronic, sustained antigenemia. Liver histology in the latter group shows "unresolved" hepatitis.

The most common response of the infant to HBV infection is prolonged antigenemia. The important determinant of neonatal infection is the developmental period of exposure to the virus. The presence of antibody to e-antigen in asymptomatic mothers with HB_sAg affects the likelihood of transmitting HBV to their infants.[22] Infants born to mothers who have both HB_sAg, and the antibody to e do not develop HB_sAg antigenemia. When mothers are positive for the e-antigen and HB_sAg, then not only do the newborns become HB_sAg carriers but the elder siblings are also likely to be infected. The protective effect of anti-e against the vertical transmission of HB_sAg may be due to the fact that anti-e agglutinates the Dane particle.

Chronic asymptomatic carrier. Acquisition of the carrier state (defined as the presence of circulating HB_sAg detected for at least six months) is determined by the age of exposure (more likely during childhood), dose of infectious agent, modifying influence such as immunosuppressive therapy, immune status of the host (failure of T-cells to eliminate the virus), and perhaps genetic predisposition. The latter is suggested by the association of HL-A type, Sabell antigen, with the carrier state. About 900,000 persons in the United States are said to harbor HB_sAg without clinical symptoms. The carrier rate for health-care personnel, including physicians and dentists, is estimated to be as high as 3%. Health-care workers who are chronic HB_sAg carriers may present little risk to their patients.[23] The issue is, however, not fully resolved. It is not clear how carriers in sensitive occupations should be managed.[7]

Persistent HB_sAg antigenemia is also observed in other diseases and select groups (Table 11.7). The increased incidence is due either to a high exposure rate or presumably decreased host resistance in some disease states. The identification of the core antibody HB_cAb has extended the group of HB_sAg-positive asymptomatic carriers, since HB_sAg-negative

Table 11.7. Groups and diseases with increased incidence of HB_SAg.

Groups:
    Residents of prisons, mental institutions, communes
    Prostitutes
    ? Alcoholics
    Hospital personnel, especially those in hemodialysis/
        transplant and cancer chemotherapy units
    Recipients of blood transfusion, eg, hemophiliacs
    Drug abusers

Association with diseases:
    Down's syndrome
    Lymphocytic leukemia
    Hodgkin's disease
    Lepromatous leprosy
    Hemodialysis patients
    ? Polyarteritis nodosa
    ? Primary liver cell carcinoma

blood can still induce hepatitis. HB_sAg-negative donors are positive for HB_cAb, indicating continued virus multiplication. The carrier state should include not only HB_sAg-positive persons but also those who are both HB_sAg-negative and HB_cAb-positive. Recovery from the carrier stage is heralded by the disappearance of HB_cAb. HB_cAb is found in 100% of chronic HB_sAg carriers, in 98% of HB_sAg-positive blood donors and normal recipients of viral vaccines, and in 1% of volunteer HB_sAg-negative blood donors. Tests for HB_cAb are, however, not readily available in most laboratories.

Drug-abuse-associated hepatitis. Drug abuse is accompanied by an increased incidence of HB_sAb-positive hepatitis. Transmission occurs by means of contaminated needles used for drug injections. The ensuing liver disease covers a wide spectrum: chronic antigenemia, aminotransferase elevations, overt acute hepatitis, chronic persistent and active hepatitis, and cirrhosis. Opiates or chronic methadone therapy in themselves do not cause hepatic dysfunction, although the vehicular medium in which drugs are diluted, eg, talcum powder, may produce liver changes. The hepatitis usually involves the subtype Y. There are several other epidemiological characteristics. Infection is endemic in low-socioeconomic areas. It is more frequent among younger addicts. White addicts are more liable to develop signs and symptoms than are black addicts.[24] The tendency for hepatitis to reoccur is high and so is the likelihood of its progression to chronic liver disease.

Hepatitis in hemodialysis/transplant units.[25,26] Most hepatitis cases reported in dialysis/transplant units in the United States belong to subtype Y, whereas subtype D hepatitis predominates among other hospital residents and personnel. The primary source for perpetuating the infection appears to be within the unit involving lateral transmission between patients and staff personnel. The duration and frequency of dialysis therapy are important determinants of infection prevalence among patients. Hepatitis in staff members correlates with the degree, intensity, and length of exposure to the equipment and material used in dialysis procedure. Symptomatic infection in patients is generally mild, well-tolerated, and often presenting as a chronic antigenemia. Acute hepatitis among staff personnel tends to be more severe than the average case in the general public. HB_sAg can be detected in about 15–20%, and HB_sAb in 30–40% of patients undergoing dialysis.[6] The incidence of Hb_sAg is about 3% in staff members but the incidence for HB_sAb is similar to that in patients. Family members of patients and medical personnel also share a five to eightfold increased risk of contracting hepatitis compared to control groups.

Patients who become HB_sAg-positive while on immunosuppressive therapy may develop an acute hepatitis once the drugs are withdrawn. The recovery of host immune function is thought to initiate the clinical attack.

Posttransfusion hepatitis (PTH). In only 25% of PTH cases is HB_sAg detected and type B hepatitis implicated.[27,28] Other viruses, cytomegalovirus and EB virus, are known to account for a relatively small percentage of PTH cases. The major proportion is of unknown etiology. It is not certain if HAV is blameless in most cases of PTH. Recently, a third hepatitis virus, non-A and non-B, has been proposed as a causative agent for PTH, particularly in those cases with a long incubation period.[29] The third virus may be related to the virus recently described in an epidemic in Costa Rica.[1]

The incidence of HBV-associated PTH depends on the incidence of HB_sAg in donor blood, proportion of commercial blood products, transfusion volume, and the nature of the blood product (Table 11.8). The proportion of subtypes D and Y in the donor varies according to the source. Estimates of the incidence rate vary widely, depending on the donor, recipient population, and case follow-up. In the United States 65% of the patients who have had multiple transfusions and who received at least one unit of HB_sAg-positive blood develop PTH.[27] The figure is about 4½ times the incidence following transfusion of HB_sAg-negative blood. In another study the incidence of hepatitis after receipt of whole blood or blood products (average risk category) is 2.8% with a 0.1%

Table 11.8. Risks of hepatitis from blood and blood products.[48]

Average risk:
 Whole blood, packed red blood cells, single donor plasma, platelet-rich plasma
High risk:
 Pooled plasma stored at room temperature or at 31.6°C for six months,
  irradiated pooled plasma, fibrinogen, antihemophilic globulin
"Safe" products:
 Serum albumin, thrombin, immune and hyperimmune globulin

---

mortality rate.[30] In contrast, PTH develops in 9% of recipients of pooled plasma and in 19% of those receiving fibrinogen (high-risk category). The mortality in the latter group averages 4%. The incidence of hepatitis following very large numbers (> 10 units) of blood transfusions is three times greater than that occurring with fewer volumes. The incubation period for PTH is approximated to be 16–180 days. Hepatitis with a short incubation period (less than 16 days) would suggest other unrelated causes: halogenated anesthesia and postperfusion syndrome, both of which occur much less frequently than PTH. The transfusion of blood containing HB_sAb does not increase the risk of PTH.[31] Donors who are incubating hepatitis form a more dangerous source of infection than chronic long-term carriers without signs of liver disease. Donors who are healthy chronic carriers of HB_sAg, especially those with antibodies against e-antigen, present little risk of transmitting hepatitis to possible recipients.[32] Pretransfusion prophylaxis with high titer HB_sAb immune globulin or normal gamma globulin reduces the incidence and severity of PTH due to hepatitis B.

The introduction of screening methods for the detection of HB_sAg in donor blood has reduced the incidence of PTH significantly. However, cases of serum hepatitis continue to occur in patients who received blood negative for HB_sAg screened by the most sensitive methods. Apparently HBV can replicate even when subdetectable HB_sAg circulates. The supposition is borne out by the finding of HB_cAb in 1% of volunteer HB_sAg-negative blood donors. The small group is responsible for PTH following receipt of HB_sAg-negative blood.

Chronic Sequelae of Viral Hepatitis

Chronic hepatitis with its two subtypes, chronic persistent and chronic active hepatitis, and postviral hepatitis cirrhosis all represent the late effects of the hepatitis virus, although the virus is but one of the causes for chronic active hepatitis. All three sequelae reflect the range of hepatic damage in humans, chronic persistent hepatitis being the mildest form, chronic active hepatitis the intermediate form, and postviral hepatitis cirrhosis the severest form. Accordingly, prognosis is excellent for chronic persistent hepatitis, variable for chronic active hepatitis, and poor for postviral hepatitis cirrhosis.

The clinical, biochemical, and morphological features of postviral hepatitis cirrhosis are identical to those of cryptogenic cirrhosis, except for the serological finding of HB_sAg (see also Chapter 9). In cases of hepatitis-associated cirrhosis, the evidence for infection in the late stage is often not present. Adverse factors predisposing toward development of chronic liver disease include:[33] presence of both HB_sAg and e-antigen,[34] drug addiction, severe hypergammaglobulinemia, positive antinuclear and smooth muscle antibodies in high titers, and on liver histology, destruction of portal limiting plates and increased plasma cell infiltration.

CHRONIC HEPATITIS

Chronic hepatitis may be defined as a continuing inflammation of the liver lasting more than six months. Of the two subtypes, chronic persistent hepatitis is a benign, self-limited condition. In contrast, chronic active hepatitis often has a virulent course and may progress to cirrhosis. Chronic active hepatitis is not a homogeneous entity in terms of etiology (Table 11.9).

Table 11.9. Classification of chronic active hepatitis.

---

1. Cryptogenic (idiopathic, autoimmune, HB_sAg-negative)
2. Virus-induced, HB_sAg-related
3. Drug-induced:
   a. Frequent offenders:
      Isoniazid, oxyphenisatin, methyldopa
   b. Infrequent offenders:
      Methotrexate, chlorpromazine,[49]
      salicylates, sulfonamides, phenyl-
      butazone, hydralazine
4. Association with:
   a. Wilson's disease
   b. Primary biliary cirrhosis, early phase
   c. Alpha-1-antitrypsin deficiency
   d. Cryptogenic cirrhosis
5. Rarely with:[41]
   a. Fibrosing alveolitis
   b. Cryoglobulinemia
   c. Periarteritis nodosa
   d. Eosinophilia with Coomb's positive hemolytic anemia

Chronic Persistent Hepatitis[35]

Less than 10% of the cases with acute viral A or B hepatitis develop this condition. Other causes have not been identified. Sequelae of viral hepatitis such as unresolved hepatitis and chronic HB_sAg-carrier state represent variants of the same condition as chronic persistent hepatitis. The symptoms are vague, including malaise, weakness, loss of appetite, right-upper-quadrant discomfort, and occasionally mild icterus. In about 50% of the cases, patients remain asymptomatic. Abnormal physical signs are sparse and include slight liver tenderness and enlargement. Among the mildly perturbed hepatic tests, serum aminotransferase rarely exceeds 100 IU/l. Serum bilirubin above 5 mg/dl is unusual. Both IgA and IgM may be moderately elevated. Circulating autoantibodies are absent or found in low titers. Histological examination of the liver reveals a portal mononuclear cell inflammation with preservation of the limiting plates, and slight, if any, fibrosis (Fig. 11.5). Intralobular necrosis and inflammation are generally mild or even absent. Prognosis is excellent. Most patients recover but a few cases may convert to chronic active hepatitis.

Chronic Active Hepatitis (CAH)[36,37]

In contrast to chronic persistent hepatitis, liver destruction and severe inflammation are characteristic of CAH. Activity is recognized by the elevated aminotransferase level, hyperglobulinemia, and circulating autoantibodies. There are several causes of CAH: the cryptogenic and viral types comprise the majority of cases (90%); the incidence of drug-induced CAH seems to be on the rise (Table 11.9). The biochemical and liver biopsy features are similar for the various types of CAH. The difference depends on the antecedent history, clinical features, other disease associations, serological tests, remission after withdrawal of the offending drug, and response to steroid treatment.

Cryptogenic Type. About 60-70% of all patients with CAH belong to this group. Striking hypergammaglobulinemia, the florid presence of nonorgan and nonspecies specific autoantibodies, and response to immunosuppressive drugs characterize cryptogenic CAH. A subvariety with detectable LE (lupus erythematosus) cells has been known as lupoid hepatitis. It is likely that lupoid hepatitis does not exist as a separate entity but represents part of the continuum encountered in CAH. The etiology is unknown. A viral infection during the early stage of pathogenesis has not been excluded. Patients with acute HB_sAg-positive hepatitis can develop antigen-negative CAH.[38]

Two other differences distinguish the cryptogenic variety from other types of CAH (Table 11.10). First, a serum autoantibody directed against

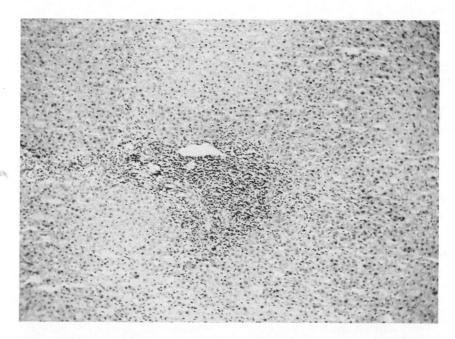

Fig. 11.5. Chronic persistent hepatitis. The mononuclear inflammatory infiltrate is confined to the portal triad without erosion of the limiting plate. Mild Kupffer cell hyperplasia and focal hepatocellular injury are present. H and E, X100.

liver-specific lipoprotein membrane is found only in cryptogenic CAH.[39] The IgG antibody can be detected fixed in a linear pattern to the membrane of isolated hepatocytes. In contrast, in HB_sAg-related CAH and other liver conditions, IgG, presumably a different autoantibody or immune complex, is deposited in a granular fashion on the hepatocellular membrane. The restricted presence of liver-membrane autoantibody in the cryptogenic group suggests that different pathogenic mechanisms underlie the subtypes of CAH.

Second, there is a genetic predisposition which is absent in HB_sAg-related and other types of CAH. The cryptogenic group is strongly associated with histocompatibility antigens, HL-A1 and A8. In addition, an association exists with other autoimmune disease complexes such as Hashimoto's thyroiditis, rheumatoid arthritis, Sjögren's syndrome, ulcerative colitis, periarteritis nodosa, idiopathic thrombocytopenic purpura, and hemolytic anemia. The early phase of some cases of cryptogenic CAH share a common clinical and functional background as primary biliary cirrhosis, a stage which has been termed "autoallergic" hepatitis.

Table 11.10. Contrast between cryptogenic and HB$_S$Ag-related CAH.

	Cryptogenic CAH	HB$_S$Ag-related CAH
Age and sex preference	Adolescent, young female	Middle-aged male
Genetic predisposition	Strong association with HL-A1 and A8, and other autoimmune diseases	Absent, or weak association
Pathogenic factor	Liver-membrane autoantibody	HB$_S$Ag
Liver histology:		
Features of acute VH	Absent, or mild	Present
Plasma cell infiltration	Prominent	Mild or absent
Incidence of nonspecific autoantibodies	High, with high titers	Low or absent
Hypergamma-globulinemia	Marked elevation	Slightly raised or normal
Response to immunosuppression	Good	?
Prognosis	Early mortality	Slow progression

The clinical presentation contrasts with that of alcoholic liver disease (Tables 11.11, 10.5). Patients often do not appear malnourished or particularly ill. Poorly defined complaints of weakness, fatigue, and anorexia are offered. Jaundice is not usually observed until late, with evidence of fairly severe disease. Pruritus is common. In adolescent girls, disturbed endocrine functions such as amenorrhea, acne, hirsutism, and cushingoid features are manifested.

Laboratory findings depend largely on the stage of the disease. Serum bilirubin rarely exceeds 10 mg/dl. Aminotransferase does not rise above 300 IU/l, although occasionally values reach 1000 IU/l. Hypergammaglobulinemia averages 5.5 g/dl or about 2-3 times normal level. The rise is predominantly in the IgG fraction. Alkaline phosphatase is elevated in about 10% of the cases. The autoantibodies, particularly smooth muscle antibodies, are characteristically detected in high titers. Other serologic findings include agglutination titers to salmonella and other gram-negative bacteria, positive CEA test, and cryoglobulinemia. Liver histology reveals widespread but not necessarily diffuse inflammation, piecemeal necrosis, and varying degrees of parenchymal hepatocellular injury. The biopsy lesions evolve through a spectrum that correlates with the clinical and biochemical findings (Table 11.12).[40]

Table 11.11. Clinical and laboratory features of cryptogenic CAH.[41]

Clinical features:	Incidence, %
Female sex	75
Age 10–30	30
Acute onset	60
Associated with auto-immune disease	20
Symptoms:	
Jaundice	90
Weakness and anorexia	40
Fever	20
Abdominal pain	50
Amenorrhea	50
Arthralgia	30
Physical findings:	
Hepatomegaly	75
Splenomegaly	50
Ascites	25
Laboratory features:	
Positive LE cell	20
Immunoglobulin IgG	80
IgA	60
IgM	20
Autoantibodies SMA	70
AMA	30
ANA	70–80

Table 11.12. Histological features of chronic active hepatitis (CAH).[40,41]

Features	Mild CAH	Subacute hepatitis With bridging	With multi-lobular necrosis
Inflammation	Periportal	Bandlike triad to triad or to central veins	Panlobular
Limiting plate	Destroyed	Eroded	Destroyed
Necrosis	Perilobular	Bridging	Panlobular
Viral hepatitis stigmata	Not infrequent	Not infrequent	Not distinguish-able
Balloon cells	Many, periportal	Few	Few
Kupffer cells	Prominent	Prominent	Prominent
Cholestasis	Less frequent	Frequent	Frequent
Abnormal bile ducts	Florid	Less florid	Less florid
Fibrosis	Periportal	Bridging	Thick, diffuse

In the mild, and presumably early form of the disease (25% of cases), CAH resembles the changes in CPH except that the piecemeal necrosis becomes prominent (Fig. 11.6). The mononuclear inflammation is most apparent in the perilobular area. Plasma cells are commonly seen. Hepatocytes in the perilobular zone are swollen, sometimes multinucleated, and often arranged in a rosette formation.

In a second, more severe stage of the disease (25% of cases), necrosis, collapse, and inflammation are found in neighboring portal triads, or between triads and central veins (Fig. 11.7). This pattern of bridging necrosis is known as subacute hepatitis with bridging (also termed subacute hepatic necrosis). Subacute in this context does not have a temporal meaning.

Progression of the destructive process leads to the third stage of the disease (Fig. 11.8), subacute hepatitis with multilobular necrosis (25% of cases). Necrosis of contiguous hepatic lobules, as well as severe chronic inflammation, is observed.

In the fourth and final stage, fibrosis and regenerative nodules predominate among the biopsy findings. Macronodular cirrhosis accounts for 25% of all the cases with CAH. Differential diagnosis includes CAH due to virus, drugs, and other disease associations. PBC, systemic lupus

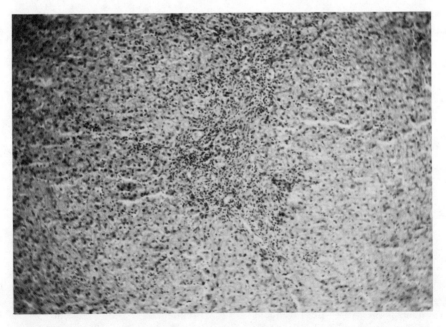

Fig. 11.6. Chronic active hepatitis. Lymphocytes and plasma cells break through the portal confines into the perilobular zones (piecemeal necrosis). H and E, X100.

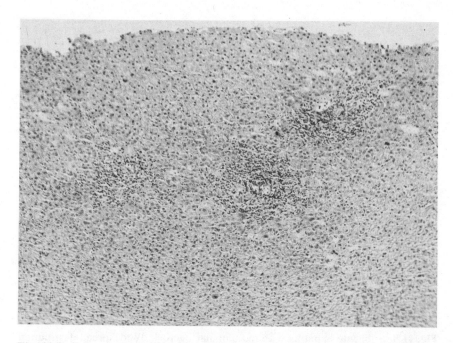

Fig. 11.7. Subacute hepatitis with bridging. Two portal triads (left side) approximate each other with collapse and necrosis of intervening parenchyma. H and E, X100.

erythematosus (liver involvement in this disorder is not common), and ulcerative colitis with pericholangitis are among other diseases which may simulate CAH. Diagnosis is based on clinical presentation, laboratory findings, and above all liver histology; morphological confirmation is necessary not only for diagnosis but also for management.

Treatment is based mainly on immunosuppressive drugs, that is, prednisone with or without azathioprine. The treatment schedule and experience with these drugs vary from institution to institution, depending on the type of patient selected for therapy. Success of corticosteroid treatment is less likely in the advanced stage of the disease. Unfavorable factors include cirrhosis and HB_sAg antigenemia. No general standard has been established.

One set of guidelines which proved effective in a well-controlled and studied group of patients is that proposed by the Mayo group. Steroid therapy is started according to the Mayo Clinic[40,41] criteria when there is (1) clinical and biochemical evidence of serious liver dysfunction, (2) histological findings of subacute hepatitis, and (3) CAH and continued 10-week elevation of AsAT (10 × normal), or AsAT (5×) and gamma globu-

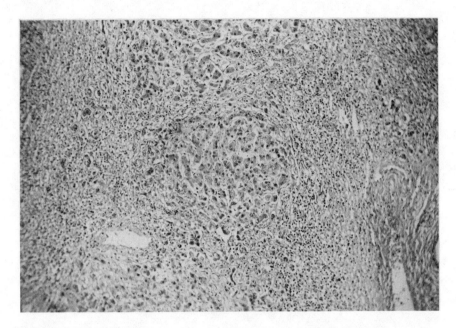

Fig. 11.8. Subacute hepatitis with multilobular necrosis. Widespread destruction and inflammation delimit remaining cirrhotic nodules. H and E, X100.

lin (2×). Prednisone is given initially in a loading schedule with 60 mg/day for one week, then 40 mg/day for one week, and finally 30 mg/day for two weeks. The maintenance schedule follows, with 20 mg prednisone per day, or 10 mg prednisone and 50 mg azathioprine per day. After treatment for two years or longer, 67% of the patients became symptom-free in six months; in 75% of the cases abnormal biochemical or immunological findings disappeared. Most remissions occurred within one year. At the end of the second year 90% were well clinically and biochemically; in 70% liver histology returned to normal or inactive hepatitis. Relapse followed cessation of therapy in 50% of the cases within six months. Treatment failure is said to occur in 20% of cases.

Prognosis for CAH is not especially good: approximately 40% of the patients die without steroid treatment, whereas 20% spontaneously improve. The remaining 40% progress to cirrhosis. The propensity of mild CAH to develop cirrhosis is 10%; for subacute hepatitis with bridging, 30%; and for subacute hepatitis with multilobular necrosis, 40%.

Virus-induced, HB_sAg-related type. CAH associated with positive HB_sAg titer accounts for 20% of all patients in most series. Other viruses—hepatitis A virus, Epstein-Barr, and cytomegalovirus—may also cause chronic hepatitis but their incidence is unknown. Approximately

5% of acute viral hepatitis cases develop HB_sAg antigenemia lasting more than three months.[42] Ninety percent of this high-risk group progresses into CAH. The probability of contracting the chronic sequelae is not dependent on the height of the virus titer or virus numbers in liver tissue. In fact, the opposite may be true. Host-cell-mediated reactions to HB_sAg are the primary determinant of hepatocellular injury. HB_sAg-related CAH differs from the cryptogenic type in several respects (Table 11.10). This group is not easily distinguished from the cryptogenic type on the basis of symptoms or liver histology alone. The use of steroid therapy for this group is not definitely established.

Drug-induced type. Isoniazid, oxyphenisatin, and alpha-methyldopa produce disease that simulates CAH in every respect.[43,44,45] Other drugs, such as methotrexate, chlorpromazine, and salicylates may rarely cause a similar picture. Isoniazid is probably the most frequent offender among the group of drugs. Chapter 15 contains a fuller discussion of isoniazid-induced toxicity. Laxatives containing oxyphenisatin usually require a latent period of at least several months before symptoms and laboratory findings appear. Positive LE-cell test, raised autoantibodies, and other evidence of hepatocellular injury have all been reported. Liver histology reveals piecemeal necrosis, diffuse inflammation, hepatocellular collapse, and fibrosis. Improvement follows withdrawal of the drug in all cases. Challenge with oxyphenisatin causes an abrupt rise in serum amino-transferase. It is not clear whether hepatic damage is dose-related or results from a hypersensitivity reaction. Laxatives containing oxyphenisatin are no longer on the market in the United States.

Methyldopa produces hepatic injury, usually after several weeks, in dosages ranging from 250 mg to 1 g daily. The features resemble acute viral hepatitis. With prolonged exposure to methyldopa, the disease becomes chronic, accompanied by histologic lesions and abnormal serum immunologic reactions typical of CAH. In rare instances, the course is fulminant and terminates in hepatic coma. The lesions regress with cessation of drug use. Methyldopa-induced liver injury probably occurs on a hypersensitivity basis. Five percent of patients on regular methyldopa therapy develop mild aminotransferase increases. In general, drug-induced CAH does not progress spontaneously unless drugs are taken continuously. The hepatic lesions regress on withdrawal of the medication. Steroid therapy is not indicated.

CAH-associated Diseases

Wilson's disease.[46] CAH may be the first manifestation of Wilson's disease, usually in patients under age 30. This group probably accounts for less than 5% of all cases of CAH. Jaundice, splenomegaly, other signs

of portal hypertension, and laboratory evidence of hepatic dysfunction
may all antedate the neurologic manifestations characteristic of Wilson's
disease. Not infrequently the illness begins like viral hepatitis, or infectious mononucleosis that does not resolve. Diagnosis is established by the
finding of Kayser-Fleischer rings, low-serum ceruloplasmin ($<$ 20 mg/dl),
and increased hepatic content of copper ($>$ 250 μg/g dry liver); see also
Chapter 13.

Primary biliary cirrhosis. The identity of CAH and the early stage of
primary biliary cirrhosis in some cases is discussed above and in Chapter 4.

Alpha-1-antitrypsin deficiency. The syndrome of neonatal hepatitis,
CAH, and alpha-1-antitrypsin deficiency is described in Chapter 9.

Cryptogenic cirrhosis. The entity probably represents the end phase
of cryptogenic CAH. In Europe, CAH is recognized as a subgroup of
cryptogenic cirrhosis. The disease occurs in premenopausal middle-aged
women who manifest multisystemic symptoms. These may include
amenorrhea, arthralgia, thyroiditis, and chronic renal disease. Hyperglobulinemia and other immune markers such as antinuclear, smooth
muscle, and mitochondrial antibodies are prominent. Liver histology is
indistinguishable from other types of CAH. Cirrhotic features in the late
phase provide no clue as to the prior cause. Steroids both improve
symptoms and retard the fatal outcome.

Immunosuppressive Therapy

Corticosteroids and azathioprine are used in the treatment of chronic
hepatitis.

Corticosteroids. Corticosteroids exert a wide range of metabolic and
tissue effects. Metabolically, they are antianabolic, increase gluconeogenesis, promote salt and water retention, and stimulate erythropoiesis.
The tissue effects of corticosteroids include: anti-inflammatory properties, lysis of lymphocytes and eosinophiles, decreased vascular permeability, inhibition of cellular DNA synthesis, and decrease of MIF production. In humans, steroids do not affect antibody synthesis. The induced
lymphopenia is attributed to a redistribution of T-lymphocytes to the
bone marrow. Prednisone and prednisolone are both effective in the
treatment of CAH. Theoretically, prednisone may be relatively less effective since it is activated by hepatic dehydrogenase to prednisolone, the
active steroid.

In practice, no therapeutic difference is observed between the two corticosteroids. The incomplete conversion of prednisone to prednisolone is balanced by the impairment of prednisolone degradation. This, plus the low plasma binding of unbound prednisolone, the active moiety, accounts for the higher level of circulating unbound prednisolone in patients with liver disease.[47] The concentration of active steroids is higher than that obtained with equivalent doses of prednisone and prednisolone in subjects without liver disease. This finding explains the efficacy of relatively low doses of prednisone (15–20 mg/day) in the treatment of chronic hepatitis. At these doses the serious complications of long-term steroid administration are minimized, although side effects such as diabetes mellitus, osteoporosis, peptic ulceration with gastrointestinal bleeding, and psychological disturbances may still occur.

Azathioprine. Azathioprine is a purine analogue of 6-mercaptopurine, which inhibits the synthesis of adenosine monophosphate from inosinic monophosphate. The altered purine biosynthesis suppresses DNA production. Azathioprine must also undergo hepatic biotransformation to active metabolites. In liver disease impaired conversion does not interfere with the therapeutic action of the antipurine agent. In the treatment of CAH, azathioprine is used in low doses (50–100 mg/day) in combination with corticosteroids. The regimen permits patients who may not tolerate corticosteroids to use small doses of steroids. It also avoids the toxic effect of azathioprine-induced bone-marrow depression. Azathioprine does not affect the binding of prednisolone by normal plasma. The additive effect with corticosteroids is not due to any alteration of unbound circulating steroid.

REFERENCES

1. Villarejos VM, et al: Evidence for viral hepatitis other than type A or type B among persons in Costa Rica. *New Eng J Med* 293:1350–1352, 1975.
2. Maynard JE: Hepatitis A: Perspectives and recent advances. *Amer J Path* 81:683–694, 1975.
3. Editorial: Virus hepatitis updated. *Lancet* 1:1365–1366, 1975.
4. Blumberg BS: The nature of Australia antigen: Infections and genetic characteristics, in Gen Ref No. 9, pp 367–379.
5. Krugman S, et al: Viral hepatitis, type B: DNA polymerase activity and antibody to hepatitis B core antigen. *New Eng J Med* 290:1331–1335, 1974.
6. Melnick JL, Dreesman GR, Hollinger FB: Approaching the control of viral hepatitis type B. *J Infect Dis* 132:210–229, 1976.
7. Chalmers TC, Alter HJ: Management of the asymptomatic carrier of the hepatitis-associated (Australia) antigen: Tentative considerations of the clinical and public-health aspects. *New Eng J Med* 285:613–617, 1971.

8. Prince AM, et al: Hepatitis B antigen in wild-caught mosquitoes in Africa. *Lancet* 2:247–250, 1972.
9. Cherubin CE: The emerging epidemiology of hepatitis B antigen. *Ann Intern Med* 79:745–746, 1973.
10. LeBouvier GL: Subtypes of hepatitis B antigen: Clinical relevance. *Ann Intern Med* 79:894–896, 1974.
11. Nielsen JO, Dietrichson O, Juhl E: Incidence and meaning of the "e" determinant among hepatitis-B-antigen positive patients with acute and chronic liver diseases. *Lancet* 2:913–915, 1974.
12. Sabesin SM, Koff RS: Pathogenesis of experimental viral hepatitis. *New Eng J. Med* 290:944–950, 996–1002, 1974.
13. Dudley FJ, Fox RA, Sherlock S: Cellular immunity and hepatitis-associated, Australia antigen liver disease. *Lancet* 1:723–726, 1972.
14. Krugman S, Friedman H, Lattimer C: Viral hepatitis, type A: Identification by specific complement fixation and immune adherence tests. *New Eng J Med* 292:1141–1143, 1975.
15. Alter, HG, Barker LF, Holland PV: Hepatitis B immune globulin: Evaluation of clinical trials and rationale for usage. *New Eng J Med* 293:1093–1094, 1975.
16. Editorial: Specific immunoglobulin in prevention of hepatitis B. *Lancet* 2:1132–1134, 1975.
17. Editorial: Extrahepatic manifestations of serum hepatitis. *Lancet* 2:805–806, 1971.
18. Schumacher HP, Gall EP: Arthritis in acute hepatitis and chronic active hepatitis: Pathology of the synovial membrane with evidence for the presence of Australia antigen in synovial membranes. *Amer J Med* 57:655–664, 1974.
19. Ajlouni K, Doeblin TD: The syndrome of hepatitis and aplastic anemias. *Brit J Hematol* 27:345–355, 1974.
20. Hagler L, Pastore RA, Bergin JJ: Aplastic anemia following viral hepatitis: Report of two fatal cases and literature review. *Medicine* 54:139–164, 1975.
21. Schweitzer IL, et al: Viral hepatitis B in neonates and infants. *Amer J Med* 55:762–771, 1973.
22. Okada K, et al: e-Antigen and anti-e in the serum of asymptomatic carrier mothers as indicators of positive and negative transmission of hepatitis B virus to their infants. *New Eng J Med* 294:746–749, 1976.
23. Alter HJ, et al: Health-care workers positive for hepatitis B surface antigen: Are their contacts at risk? *New Eng J Med* 292:545–547, 1975.
24. Whaley WH, Galambos JT: Race and risk of hepatitis in narcotic addicts. *Amer J Dig Dis* 18:460–466, 1973.
25. Pattison CP: Hepatitis as a hemodialysis hazard. *Amer Heart J* 88:386–387, 1974.
26. Hamilton JD, Hatch MH, Gutman RA: Serological evidence of cross infection in a dialysis unit hepatitis-B epidemic. *Kidney Internat* 6:118–122, 1974.
27. Alter HJ, et al: Clinical and serological analysis of transfusion-associated hepatitis. *Lancet* 2:838–841, 1975.
28. Feinstone SM, et al: Transfusion-associated hepatitis not due to viral hepatitis type A or B. *New Eng J Med* 292:767–770, 1975.

29. Prince AM, et al: Long-incubation post-transfusion hepatitis without serological evidence of exposure to hepatitis-B virus. *Lancet* 2:241–246, 1974.
30. Grady GF, et al: Risk of posttransfusion hepatitis in the United States: A prospective cooperative study. *JAMA* 220:692–701, 1972.
31. Aach RD, et al: Risk of transfusing blood containing antibody to hepatitis-B surface antigen. *Lancet* 2:190–193, 1974.
32. Magnius LO, et al: A new antigen-antibody system: Clinical significance in long-term carriers of hepatitis B surface antigen. *JAMA* 231:356–359, 1975.
33. Dietrichson O, et al: Acute viral hepatitis: Factors possibly predicting chronic liver disease. *Acta Path Microbiol Scand* 83A:183–188, 1975.
34. El Sheikh N, et al: e-Antigen-antibody system as an indicator of liver damage in patients with hepatitis B antigen. *Brit Med J.* 4:252–253, 1975.
35. Javitt NB, Hand R, Finlayson NDC: Persistent viral hepatitis. *Amer J Med* 55:799–810, 1973.
36. Sherlock S: Active chronic hepatitis, in Gen Ref No. 6, pp 342–360.
37. Sherlock S: Chronic hepatitis. *Gut* 15:581–597, 1974.
38. Galbraith RM, et al: Chronic liver disease developing after outbreak of HB$_s$Ag-negative hepatitis in haemodialysis unit. *Lancet* 2:886–890, 1975.
39. Hopf U, Meyer zum Büschenfelde K-M, Arnold W: Detection of a liver-membrane autoantibody in HB$_s$Ag-negative chronic active hepatitis. *New Eng J Med* 294:578–582, 1976.
40. Summerskill WHJ, Ammon HV, Baggenstoss AH: Treatment of chronic hepatitis, in Gen Ref No. 12, pp 216–226.
41. Summerskill WHJ: Chronic active liver disease reexamined: Prognosis hopeful. *Gastroenterology* 66:450–464, 1974.
42. Nielsen JO, et al: Incidence and meaning of persistence of Australia antigen in patients with acute viral hepatitis: Development of chronic hepatitis. *New Eng J Med* 285:1157–1160, 1971.
43. Gjone E, et al: Laxative-induced chronic liver disease. *Scand J Gastroenterol:* 7:395–402, 1972.
44. Schweitzer IL, Peters RL: Acute submassive hepatic necrosis due to methyldopa: A case demonstrating possible initiation of chronic liver disease. *Gastroenterology* 66:1208–1211, 1974.
45. Toghill PJ, et al: Methyldopa liver damage. *Brit Med J* 3:545–548, 1974.
46. Sternlieb I, Scheinberg IH: Chronic hepatitis as a first manifestation of Wilson's disease. *Ann Intern Med* 76:59–64, 1972.
47. Powell LW, Axelsen E: Corticosteroids in liver disease: Studies on the biological conversion of prednisone to prednisolone and plasma protein binding. *Gut* 13:690–696, 1972.
48. Mosley JW, Galambos JT: Viral hepatitis, in Gen Ref No. 14, p 529.
49. Goldstein GB, Lam KC, Mistilis SP: Drug induced active chronic hepatitis after chlorpromazine ingestion. *Amer J Dig Dis* 18:177–184, 1973.

DRUG-INDUCED AND TOXIC LIVER INJURY

12

DRUG-INDUCED LIVER INJURY

Drug-liver interaction has two distinguishable but related aspects: hepatic modification of drug action and hepatic reaction to drugs.[1] The metabolism of drugs in the liver proceeds in a two-step reaction. The first step consists of reactions classified as oxidation, reduction, and hydrolysis. Groups such as OH, COOH, NH_2, and SH are introduced into the drug molecule so that in the second stage conjugation can occur.[1]

$$\text{Drug} \xrightarrow[\text{enzymes}]{\text{Stage I}} \begin{array}{c}\text{Oxidation,}\\ \text{reduction,}\\ \text{hydrolysis}\\ \text{intermediates}\end{array} \xrightarrow[\text{enzymes}]{\text{Stage II}} \begin{array}{c}\text{Conjugation}\\ \text{products}\end{array}$$

Not all drugs undergo a two-step metabolism. Drugs possessing appropriate groups, such as OH, may be directly conjugated. Some drugs need only undergo step I reactions. The majority of drugs, however, are detoxified by the two-step reaction. For example, phenobarbital (active compound) is hydroxylated to hydroxyphenobarbital (inactive) before being conjugated as bound hydroxyphenobarbital (inactive). The net result is that lipid-soluble drugs are converted to water-soluble polar drugs, which are readily excreted by the kidney. The active hepatic site of drug metabolism consists of the microsomal fraction plus cytosol. The microsome contains the drug-metabolizing enzymes and cytosol, the cofactors for enzyme activity, mainly NADPH. There are two catalysts in the microsome: NADPH-cytochrome-c reductase (oxidizing flavoprotein) and cytochrome P-450 (a carbon monoxide-binding hemeprotein). Oxidation of a drug by the hepatic microsomal system can be represented as follows:

$$\text{NADPH} + \text{Cytochrome P-450} + \text{H}^+ \rightarrow (\text{cytochrome P-450})\text{H}_2 + \text{NADP}$$
$$(\text{cytochrome P-450})\text{H}_2 + \text{O}_2 \rightarrow \text{active O}_2$$

$$\text{Drug} + \text{active O}_2 \rightarrow \text{Cytochrome P-450} + \text{Oxidized drug} + \text{H}_2\text{O}$$

Hepatic Modification of Drug Action[2]

The process has several different aspects. First, altered disposal of drugs by impaired hepatic function: Acute and chronic liver diseases increase the plasma half-life disappearance of phenylbutazone, chloramphenicol, isoniazid, and rifampin, but not salicylic acid, aminopyrine, dicumarol, and antipyrine. Second, increase of the microsomal drug metabolizing enzyme system: Nonspecific inducers of the microsomal enzyme system, such as phenobarbital, diphenylhydantoin, alcohol, and many other chemicals affect drug interactions. With drugs that are themselves toxic, and not the metabolites, enzyme induction will protect against damage. Toxicity that is due to metabolites but not the parent drugs will be enhanced by enzyme induction. A clinical example is the concurrent administration of phenobarbital and coumarin derivatives. Severe hemorrhage may appear with discontinuation of the sedative. Experimentally, pretreatment with phenobarbital protects the liver against aflatoxin, toluene, and benzene, but potentiates the toxicity of CCl_4, halothane, and methoxyflurane. Third, drug-induced inhibition of hepatic metabolism of other agents: Allopurinol and chloramphenicol are examples. Allopurinol inhibits the metabolism of bishydroxycoumarin and antipyrine, and chloramphenicol inhibits the metabolism of tolbutamide and diphenylhydantoin.

Hepatic Reaction to Drugs[3,4,5]

Two types of hepatic reactions to drugs are recognized (Table 12.1): (1) idiosyncrasy, caused by drug hypersensitivity or accumulation of an abnormal toxic metabolite; and (2) direct hepatotoxicity. Factors modifying such reactions are sex, age, nutrition, dose, route and frequency of drug administration, concurrent disease, other drugs or foreign compounds, and genetic factors.

Idiosyncratic Drugs

These agents, in contrast to direct hepatotoxins, cause hepatic damage by hypersensitive reactions, the mechanism of which in most cases is obscure, or by some abnormality in drug metabolism (Tables 12.1 and 2). Drug sensitization is manifested by distinctive clinical features: (1) a relatively fixed and long latent period of 1–4 weeks; (2) high incidence of drug fever, rash, urticaria, and arthralgia which appear abruptly; (3) prompt recurrence of symptoms and hepatic dysfunction on challenge with small doses of the drug; (4) concurrent blood dyscrasia depending on the nature of the injury; (5) eosinophilia, although this is not invariably found; (6) a previous history of atopic or other allergies. Evidence of a

Table 12.1. Characteristics of idiosyncratic and hepatotoxic drugs.

	Incidence	Animal model	Dose dependence	Latent period	Mechanism	Mortality	Examples
Idiosyncrasy:							
Hypersensitivity	Low (1:50 to 1:10,000)	No	No	Consistently long (1–4 weeks)	Drug allergy	Variable	Chloropromazine, PAS
Metabolic abnormality	Low	No	Maybe	Variable	Toxic metabolite	High	Cinchophen, ? halothane
Hepatotoxins:							
Direct	High	Yes	Yes	Minutes to hours	Membrane injury	Generally high	CCl$_4$, phosphorus
Cytotoxic	High	Yes	Yes	Days	Interference with metabolic pathways	Variable	Tetracycline
Cholestatic	High	Yes	Yes	Days	Interference with bile secretion	Low	Synthetic androgens

From H. J. Zimmerman, *Perspect Biol Med* 12:135–161, 1968; used with permission of author and The University of Chicago Press.

Table 12.2.   Hepatotoxic drugs.

Drug class	Mechanism	Frequency	Cholestasis	Hepatitis	Massive necrosis	Cirrhosis
Analgesics						
Acetaminophen (Tylenol, paracetamol)	T	++			X	
Papaverine	T	+		X		
Salicylate	T	++		X		
Anesthetics						
Chloroform	T	++			X	X
Halothane	H	+		X	X	
Methoxyflurane	H	+		X	X	
Antiarthritics						
Cinchophen	H	+			X	X
Gold compounds	H	+		X	X	
Indomethacin	H	+	X	X	X	
Phenylbutazone	H	++	X	X	X	X
Antibiotics						
Erythromycin estolate	H	+	X			
Novobiocin	H	+	X	X	X	
Penicillin	H	+	X	X		
Rifampin	H	+		X		
Tetracycline	T	+		X		
Anticonvulsants						
Diphenylhydantoin	H	+	X		X	
Antihypertensives						
Methyldopa	H	+		X	X	
Chemotherapeutic agents						
Arsenicals	T	++				X
Isoniazid	T	++		X	X	X
Sulfonamides	H	+		X	X	
PAS	H	+	X	X	X	
Hormonal and metabolic agents						
Synthetic androgens	T	+ to ++	X		X	
Oral contraceptives	? H or T	+	X			
Antithyroid drugs	H	++	X	X	X	
Tolbutamide	H	+	X		X	
Immunosuppressive agents						
Methotrexate	T	++		X		X
Urethane	T	+			X	X

Table 12.2 Hepatotoxic drugs—*continued.*

Drug class	Mechanism	Frequency	Chole-stasis	Hepa-titis	Massive necrosis	Cir-rhosis
Psychopharmacologic agents						
Monamine oxidase inhibitors	H	+ +		X	X	
Phenothiazines	H	+ +	X		X	X
Sedatives						
Phenobarbital	H	+	X	X		
Others						
Iopanoic acid (Telepaque)	H	+	X			
Oxyphenisatin	? H or T	+ +	X	X		X
Nicotinic acid	T	+	X			

Mechanism: T = toxic; H = hypersensitivity. Frequency: + + = frequent (incidence 1% or greater); + = infrequent. From G. Klatskin, in F. Schaffner, S. Sherlock, and C. M. Leevy (eds.), *The Liver and Its Diseases,* 1974, pp 164–166; used with permission of author and Stratton Intercontinental Medical Book Corp.

particular drug allergy is usually inferred by the presence of the above clinical features and the absence of direct toxic effects. Direct proof is usually not available, as the pathogenic mechanism is not understood.

In animals, a drug of low-molecular weight acts as a hapten, which once bound to protein serves as an antigen. The ensuing hypersensitivity is usually of the humoral variety, with antibodies directed against the hapten-protein complex. In humans, skin sensitizing and circulating antibodies reactive to drug antigens are not often demonstrable. Some agents do evoke immunologic abnormalities, which provide secondary evidence that immune phenomena are involved. For instance, procainamide toxicity is associated with the appearance of LE cell, antinuclear, and mitochondrial antibodies. Cell-mediated hypersensitivity is documented for halothane, penicillin, sulfonamides, and chlorpromazine by laboratory tests (lymphocyte transformation or macrophage migration inhibition factor). The laboratory tests can detect the susceptible individual, although they are not routine or practical procedures.

Liver histology reveals two different tissue patterns, hepatitis and cholestasis. They are not invariably separate. Some drugs evoke a mixed morphology. Hepatitic lesions faithfully mimic viral hepatitis with spotty necrosis and diffuse lymphocytic infiltration. The presence of more than the usual eosinophiles or other features atypical of viral hepatitis, such as fat and granuloma, suggests drug-induced hepatitis. Drugs that produce the hepatitis morphology are more dangerous than drugs that result in cholestasis, and carry a high mortality (10–50%). Fortunately, hepatitic reactions are less frequent than the cholestatic types.

The cholestatic form of liver injury resembles that of intrahepatic cholestasis due to other causes. Initially, the bile stasis appears centrolobularly, within canaliculi and hepatocytes. A mild chronic inflammatory infiltrate, sometimes rich in eosinophiles, distends the portal spaces. Hepatocellular necrosis is not a feature unless the damage is severe. The changes resolve without residual effects in most cases, although biliary cirrhosis may develop in rare instances. Biochemically, drug-induced hepatitis is accompanied by striking aminotransferase elevations, the levels correlating with the extent of the injury. High transient levels of alkaline phosphatase are not uncommon. Reduction of prothrombin activity or serum albumin signifies the onset of massive necrosis. In cholestasis related to drugs, the picture simulates that of extrahepatic biliary obstruction. The serum alkaline phosphatase rises earlier than that seen in obstruction, usually accompanied by a similar peaking of aminotransferase. The abnormal values subside quickly and do not persist unless complications occur. Diagnosis for either form of drug-induced liver damage rests heavily on liver histology, which must differentiate these conditions from viral hepatitis and extrahepatic biliary obstruction.

Direct Hepatotoxins

The effects in this group are reproducible, often constant, and dose-related (Tables 12.1 and 2). The hepatic lesions may consist of necrosis, fatty change, and cholestasis. Five mechanisms of injury are involved: (1) cell membrane injury, (2) interference with metabolic pathways, (3) interference with bile secretion, (4) interference with bilirubin metabolism, and (5) covalent binding with hepatic macromolecules.

Cell membrane injury. The prototype toxin, extensively studied in animals, is carbon tetrachloride (CCl_4). The toxic action of CCl_4 is due to its metabolites, such as CCl_3 free radicals, after undergoing breakdown in the endoplasmic reticulum. Enzyme inducers, such as phenobarbital, enhance the toxicity of CCl_4 whereas protein deficiency diminishes it, presumably because of decreased endoplasmic reticulum. CCl_4 produces zonal necrosis and steatosis in a regular and predictable manner (Table 12.3). CCl_4 poisoning is not limited to the liver but, like other cellular toxins, affects a variety of host organs, particularly the kidneys. The injurious effect is due to lipid perioxidation of unsaturated lipids in cell membranes by free radicals. Attack of mitochondrial and endoplasmic reticulum membranes produces the necrosis and steatosis characteristic

Table 12.3.   Sequence of CCl_4-induced cell injury.

Time	Mechanism	Effect
1 hour	↓ ER synthesis of protein	↑ fat content
3 hours	↓ ER synthesis of protein	Visible fat
5 hours	Lysosomal destruction	Focal necrosis
10 hours	Mitochondrial injury	Zonal necrosis

From H. J. Zimmerman, *Perspect Biol Med* 12:135–161, 1968; used with permission of author and The University of Chicago Press.

of the agent. Whether other halogenated aromatic hydrocarbons, such as halothane, produce liver damage on the basis of lipid peroxidation is not clear.

Lipid peroxidation would tie together several known features of halothane damage. The anesthetic is dechlorinated by microsomal activity. A toxic metabolite, presumably free radicals, could explain the increased risk noted after phenobarbital and previous halothane exposure. Both drugs are known microsomal enzyme inducers. Other direct hepatocellular toxins include yellow phosphorus, tannic acid, and heavy metals. Therapeutic drugs do not belong in this category.

Interference with metabolic pathways. The prime example is ethionine, a metabolic antagonist which competes with methionine for ATP. The resultant deficiency in messenger-RNA synthesis leads to decreased lipoprotein synthesis and fat accumulation histologically. Tetracycline, urethane, methotrexate, and other antimetabolites are among the known inhibitors of cellular metabolic pathways.

Interference with bile secretion.[2]   Drugs in this category produce intrahepatic cholestasis. They include 17-alpha-alkyl substituted estrogens and other steroids, particularly the 19-norsteroids, components of oral contraceptives, and chlorpromazine. The mechanisms for decreased bile secretion have been attributed to increased permeability of the bile ducts to water; inhibition of Na^+K^+ ATPase-dependent transport system of biliary cell membrane, with consequent decrease of bile salt independent fraction of bile flow; inhibition of hepatic bile salt metabolism; secretion of poorly soluble monohydroxy bile acids secondary to hypoactive hypertrophic smooth endoplasmic reticulum (the hypoactivity refers to in.-

paired ring hydroxylation of the cholesterol molecule); and direct interference with micelle formation. The precise point of interference with bile secretion for the aforementioned drugs has not been identified.

Interference with bilirubin metabolism. Some drugs produce a moderate unconjugated hyperbilirubinemia, which has little serious effect in humans. Novobiocin, rifampin, male-fern extracts, and bunamiodyl all interfere with bilirubin uptake by liver cells. Novobiocin may also inhibit glucuronyl transferase activity necessary for bilirubin conjugation.

Covalent binding with hepatic macromolecules.[6] Drugs causing hepatic necrosis such as acetaminophen (paracetamol), phenacetin, and furosemide are converted in the liver to reactive arylating agents which bind tissue macromolecules. The extent of hepatic covalent binding correlates with the degree of hepatic necrosis. A threshold dosage for toxicity exists for some drugs. For example, acetaminophen is safe in therapeutic doses, although large amounts of 10–20 g cause massive hepatic destruction. Under normal conditions, acetaminophen is detoxified by preferential conjugation with hepatic glutathione. When large doses of the drug deplete the available glutathione, excess metabolite arylates nucleophilic macromolecules in liver cells, resulting in hepatic necrosis. Glutathione appears essential for protecting the body against toxic drug metabolites. Administration of cysteamine, a glutathione-like nucleophile, prevents arylation of cellular macromolecules and hepatic necrosis due to acetaminophen in humans and animals. Reactive metabolites, hepatic content of glutathione, and covalent binding of hepatic macromolecules are interrelated processes in the pathogenesis of drug-induced liver necrosis.

Commonly Used Drugs with Hepatotoxicity

Chlorpromazine. The incidence of cholestasis with this phenothiazine derivative is about 1%. It usually occurs 1–4 weeks after drug exposure and is not dose-related. The incidence of hepatic dysfunction as gauged by serum aminotransferase activity is much higher, involving up to 50% of the patients. This has cast some doubt on whether or not chlorpromazine injures by an allergic mechanism. The cholestasis may result from its direct inhibition of micellar formation of bile salt.

Halothane.[7,8] Liver necrosis secondary to exposure to the anesthetic (estimated at 1–7 per 10,000 administrations) is among the leading causes of fulminant hepatic necrosis in the United States. Halothane hepatitis is much more common in patients who are exposed to halothane repeatedly rather than only once. Toxicity is thought to reflect a hypersensitivity state, but the pathogenesis is not clear. Fever, the first symptom, appears 8–14 days postoperatively. The latent period becomes abbreviated to 1–11 days on multiple exposures. Characteristically, the jaundice follows fever in about a week. The asynchrony between fever and jaundice aids in the differential diagnosis of the causes of postoperative jaundice. Hepatomegaly is not a common physical finding. The white cell count is usually not remarkable, except for eosinophilia in about 50% of the cases. In 15% of the patients serum bilirubin is not elevated. Levels above 10 mg/dl are rare. Rises in serum aminotransferase are in the same range as those of viral hepatitis; in 50% of instances values exceed 500 IU/l. Circulating antibodies to mitochondria and cell nuclei are usually low or transiently elevated. Halothane-induced lymphocyte stimulation in sensitized patients is recorded, but the phenomenon is questioned by some authors.[8]

Liver histology is indistinguishable from that of viral hepatitis, with spotty necrosis, acidophilic body formation, and diffuse inflammation. In addition, steatosis and granulomas are not uncommon, both of which are atypical for viral hepatitis. Cholestasis is inconspicuous. In severe cases, submassive hepatocellular necrosis is observed. During the healing stage, residual hepatocytes regenerate to form a pseudoductular arrangement. Extensive collagen deposition may also occur as part of the regenerative process.

Electron microscopy reveals some differences from acute viral hepatitis. The striking abnormality involves the mitochrondrial membranes which show segmented loss of the outer membrane and infolding of the inner layer. In viral hepatitis, the mitochrondrial changes consist mainly of swelling and pallor of the matrix. The rough endoplasmic reticulum is often fragmented and lysosomes are increased in numbers. Both structures are essentially unchanged in halothane hepatitis. The severity of halothane injury varies widely, rendering prognosis difficult in individual cases. About 30% of cases have a fulminant course, with a fatality rate of 80–90%. Unfavorable factors are obesity, early onset of jaundice after anesthesia, and abnormal coagulation tests. Repeated exposures to halothane may result in significant elevation of aminotransferase levels after the postoperative period.[9] The differential diagnosis between halothane injury and viral hepatitis and other forms of drug-induced liver injury is usually not difficult.

Oral contraceptives.[10] These drugs contain a mixture of synthetic progestin and synthetic estrogen, commonly in the ratio 10:1. Both components belong to the class of 19-norsteroids substituted on Cl7 alpha position by alkyl groups. Contraceptive drug-induced cholestasis is distinctively less frequent than hepatic dysfunction with mild BSP retention which can be detected in 40% of the patients. Synthetic androgens, estrogens, and progestins interfere with BSP uptake by hepatocytes. In high doses the steroids produce hepatic damage and cholestasis. About 40% of the patients who develop postcontraceptive jaundice give a history of recurrent cholestasis of pregnancy. Both conditions are said to occur on a genetic basis. Epidemiologically, susceptible patients have a higher incidence of previous hepatitis, gallstone symptoms, and cholecystectomy than matched pair controls.[11] Sisters and mothers of afflicted women experience pruritus during pregnancy and oral contraceptive treatment, and have cholecystitis and cholecystectomies more frequently than comparable controls. The findings support the thesis that genetic factors play a part. Additional factors probably exist in predisposed women. Pruritus, malaise, anorexia, and nausea may occur after the first few cycles of usage. Such symptoms suggest hepatic dysfunction and further tests should be performed. Mild BSP retention alone is not an indication to stop the drugs. If jaundice appears or other evidence of abnormal hepatic tests exists, the drugs should be avoided. In the presence of viral hepatitis or other liver disease, oral contraceptives should be discontinued.

Other rare hepatic complications of the contraceptive pill are fatal thrombosis of hepatic veins (Budd-Chiari syndrome) in young women, and development of hepatic adenoma (see Chapter 17). More recently, a few cases of hepatocellular carcinoma have appeared in women on cyclic hormones.[12] Those on birth control pills also have a 2-2.5 times greater risk of developing gallstones than normal persons. Gallbladder bile supersaturated with cholesterol has been observed during contraceptive therapy.[13]

Isoniazid.[14,15] The incidence of isoniazid hepatotoxicity approaches 2-3% in patients over age 50. The clinical syndrome simulates viral hepatitis, usually occurring within three months of treatment. A prodromal period of fatigue, weakness, anorexia, and malaise heralds the onset of jaundice.

The histological picture is that of viral hepatitis with necrosis and inflammation. Severe hepatic necrosis and fibrosis are not uncommon. Fulminant hepatic failure is reported in 10-20% of cases. The mechanism of liver injury is not settled. Both hypersensitivity reaction or direct drug toxicity have been considered. Genetic factors are involved in the metabolism of isoniazid. The rate of acetylation of the drug is related to pseudocholinesterase polymorphism. Slow acetylators maintain a higher blood level of isoniazid than is maintained by those who acetylate more rapidly. Rapid acetylators, however, hydrolyze more isoniazid to isonicotinic acid and acetylhydrazine than slow acetylators.[16] Acetylhydrazine acts as a potent acylating agent which covalently binds to tissue macromolecules, thus producing hepatic necrosis.

Other variables influence the outcome of isoniazid-induced hepatic reaction. A fatal course is likely if liver disease appears after the first two months of therapy and if hyperbilirubinemia exceeds 20 mg/dl. The fatality rate is higher in black females than in black males or whites of either sex. Isoniazid should be withdrawn when symptoms of malaise, fatigue, nausea, and weight loss appear, or when there is evidence of liver dysfunction (two to threefold elevations of aminotransferases and alkaline phosphatases). Monitoring of patients for symptoms is a more sensitive index of drug toxicity than periodic determinations of serum aminotransferase levels. The enzyme may be elevated in 10% of patients without overt hepatitis.

Methotrexate. Two groups of patients on methotrexate therapy show a high incidence of liver damage: those treated for psoriasis and children receiving the drug as cancer chemotherapy. Relatively few are spared the ill effects. In one study, only 10% were free from hepatic injury. About 50% of the cases developed fatty livers, another 20% showed hepatic fibrosis, and 20% had cirrhosis.[17] Hepatoxicity is more severe with a continuous, low-dose schedule than with intermittent therapy.

Paracetamol.[18] Ordinarily paracetamol (acetaminophen) is a safe and effective analgesic medication, and in the usual therapeutic range causes no liver damage. Drug overdose is, however, a popular means of suicide in England. It is estimated that at least 13 g are required to produce liver injury, and that 25 g causes death. Paracetamol has been extensively studied in animals, serving as a predictable direct hepatotoxin in large doses. In humans, fulminant liver failure is similar to that due to viral hepatitis. Liver morphology during the recovering period shows centrolobular necrosis. Mortality is high, about 20% in one series.

Salicylates.[19] Chronic serum salicylate levels exceeding 25 mg/dl produce hepatic dysfunction, evidenced primarily by raised aminotransferase activity and serum alkaline phosphatase value. Eosinophilia is common. Mild triaditis and focal hepatocellular necrosis are present in liver biopsies in approximately 20-30% of the cases.

Rifampin.[20] Usually given in conjunction with other antituberculosis drugs, it is difficult to pinpoint rifampin toxicity in clinical situations. Evidence for the existence of rifampin hepatotoxicity is usually indirect. About 20% of the cases develop modest rises of serum aminotransferase; 10% of the patients show clinical hepatitis. Symptoms of malaise, nausea, vomiting, and jaundice appear rather early, usually within three weeks. Aside from AsAT elevations, serum bilirubin is increased up to 15 mg/dl, with other biochemical changes resembling viral hepatitis. Liver morphology reveals diffuse liver-cell damage with acidophilic bodies, but the inflammatory response is sparse, a feature which differentiates rifampin hepatitis from viral hepatitis. The course is mild, although massive hepatic necrosis may occur.

TOXIC LIVER INJURY

Mushroom Poisoning[4]

The *Amanita* genus of mushroom is responsible for almost all cases of mushroom poisoning in the United States. The species *A. phalloides* accounts for over 90% of the fatalities. Occasionally, *A. muscaria* may cause a rapid form of death. The symptoms are due to the muscarine effect, appearing within minutes to two hours of ingestion: marked lacrimation, salivation, dyspnea, abdominal pains, and shock. In fatal cases, death occurs within hours. Atropine is the specific antidote. The delayed form of mushroom poisoning due to *A. phalloides* is more common than the rapid type. *A. phalloides* contains two toxins: phallin, thermolabile and easily destroyed by cooking; and amanitatoxin, the active toxic polypeptide. Symptoms occur 6–15 hours after ingestion, with severe abdominal pains, hematemesis, and bloody diarrhea. Jaundice develops in 2–3 days. The poison causes a characteristically fatty change and necrosis of the liver, kidney, and myocardium. The central nervous system lesions are found later, accounting for coma in fatal cases. Mortality is at least 50%. In patients who recover, liver histology is marked by striking centrolobular necrosis without significant inflammation or fatty change.[21] The damaged areas are surrounded by macrophages filled with iron-positive ceroid.

Heatstroke

Liver damage occurs in heatstroke as part of a generalized tissue injury. In 10% of the cases severe hepatic injury may contribute to the fatal outcome.[22] Jaundice and hepatomegaly appear in severely ill patients, accompanied by serum bilirubin levels above 20 mg/dl and mild increases of alkaline phosphatase and aminotransferase activities exceeding 1000 IU/l. The elevated enzymes are also derived from the damaged heart, kidney, and muscle. Either hepatic failure or a hepatorenal syndrome supervenes in fatal cases. In 90% of the patients, the hepatocellular damage is either mild or moderate. In general, the incidence of severe liver injury correlates with that of acute renal failure in heatstroke. The liver biopsy typically shows severe centrolobular necrosis, congestion, hydropic degeneration of cells, and triaditis.[23] In fatal cases, cholestasis is marked and portal venules appear dilated. The liver injury has been attributed to anoxia due to circulatory collapse, increased oxygen requirement resulting from the hyperpyrexial state, direct thermal injury, and disseminated intravascular coagulation. Complete restitution of normal histology follows clinical recovery.

Radiation Hepatitis

The human liver tolerates radiation up to 3500 rads without ill effects.[24] Radiation exceeding this level and sometimes dosages as low as 1400 rads may produce acute radiation hepatitis. Clinically, the course resembles Budd-Chiari syndrome, with ascites, hepatomegaly, abdominal pains, and jaundice. Pathologically, the liver shows marked subintimal sclerosis of the central and sublobular hepatic veins, with panlobular sinusoidal congestion and secondary liver cell atrophy. The morphological changes usually resolve without sequelae within three months or may leave some centrolobular fibrosis. An undetermined but sizable number of cases develop chronic radiation hepatitis. The liver becomes atrophic, with severe vascular alteration, lobular collapse and distortion, and portal fibrosis. Bile duct epithelial damage and extramedullary hematopoiesis may also be observed. Nodular regeneration is rarely seen, probably because of the impaired regenerative capacity of the liver following radiation. Severe right heart failure and other causes of the Budd-Chiari syndrome must be distinguished from this condition. The severity of the clinical features does not correlate well with the extent of the morphologic alterations. Patients may be asymptomatic in the presence of an abnormal liver biopsy, or the reverse can occur.

REFERENCES

1. Williams RT: Hepatic metabolism of drugs. *Gut* 13:579-585, 1972.
2. Berthelot P: Mechanisms and prediction of drug-induced liver disease. *Gut* 14:332-339, 1973.
3. Zimmerman HJ: The spectrum of hepatotoxicity. *Perspect Biol Med* 12:135-161, 1968.
4. Klatskin G: Toxic and drug-induced hepatitis, in Gen Ref No. 14, pp 604-710.
5. Klatskin G: Drug-induced hepatic injury, in Gen Ref No. 12, pp 163-178.
6. Mitchell JR: Drugs and the liver. *Viewpoints Dig Dis* 6:5, 1974.

7. Moult PJA, Sherlock S: Halothane-related hepatitis: A clinical study of twenty-six cases. *Quart J Med* 44:99-114, 1975.
8. Walton B, et al: Lymphocyte transformation: Absence of increased responses in alleged halothane jaundice. *JAMA* 225:494-498, 1973.
9. Wright R, et al: Controlled prospective study of the effect on liver function of multiple exposures to halothane. *Lancet* 1:817-820, 1975.
10. Ockner RK, Davidson CS: Hepatic effects of oral contraceptives. *New Eng J Med* 276:331-334, 1967.
11. Dalen E, Westerholm B: Occurrence of hepatic impairment in women jaundiced by oral contraceptives and in their mothers and sisters. *Acta Med Scand* 49:459-463, 1974.
12. Davis M, et al: Histological evidence of carcinoma in a hepatic tumor associated with oral contraceptives. *Brit Med J* 4:496-498, 1975.
13. Bennion LJ, et al: Effects of oral contraceptives on the gallbladder bile of normal women. *New Eng J Med* 294:189-192, 1976.
14. Israel HL: Isoniazid-associated hepatitis: Reconsideration of the indications for administration of isoniazid. *Gastroenterology* 69:539-542, 1975.
15. Black M, et al: Isoniazid-associated hepatitis in 114 patients. *Gastroenterology* 69:289-302, 1975.
16. Mitchell JR, et al: Isoniazid liver injury: Clinical spectrum, pathology, and probable pathogenesis. *Ann Intern Med* 84:181-192, 1976.
17. Dahl MGC, Gregory MM, Scheuer PJ: Liver damage due to methotrexate in patients with psoriasis. *Brit Med J* 1:625-630, 1971.
18. Clark R, et al: Hepatic damage and death from overdosage from paracetamol. *Lancet* 1:66-70, 1973.
19. Editorial: Does aspirin harm the liver? *Lancet* 1:667, 1974.
20. Scheuer PJ, et al: Rifampin hepatitis: A clinical and histological study. *Lancet* 1:421-425, 1974.
21. Wepler W, Opitz K: Histologic changes in the liver biopsy in Amanita phalloides intoxication. *Human Path* 3:249-254, 1972.
22. Kew M, et al: Liver damage in heatstroke. *Amer J Med* 49:192-202, 1970.
23. Bianchi L, et al: Liver damage in heatstroke and its regression: A biopsy study. *Human Path* 3:237-248, 1972.
24. Lewin K, Millis RR: Human radiation hepatitis: A morphologic study with emphasis on the late changes. *Arch Path* 96:21-26, 1973.

IRON AND COPPER OVERLOAD

13

IRON METABOLISM

The average Western diet provides 10-15 mg of iron daily, of which 5-10% is absorbed. Iron absorption takes place mainly in the upper jejunum. Dietary iron is mostly in the ferric form and must be reduced to the ferrous form before it can be absorbed. Reduction is facilitated by ascorbic acid and the SH groups in sulfur-containing amino acids, which form soluble macromolecular complexes with iron. Achlorhydria, phosphates, carbonates, and phytic acid in cereals retard its absorption. Iron crosses the intestine via the brush-border layer by two discrete steps: (1) uptake of iron from the intestinal lumen, and (2) mucosal transfer of iron to plasma. Both processes act as a regulatory mechanism which governs the entry of iron. Most of the iron is combined with the mucosal protein apoferritin to form ferritin, and is deposited in intestinal cells. The intracellular ferritin is lost when mucosal cells are regularly shed as part of their life cycle. A small portion of the iron combines with beta-globulin to form transferrin and is dispersed to storage sites or bone marrow.

In the adult male, total iron approximates 50 mg iron/kg body weight (about 2-5 g, varying also with the hemoglobin level), and in the female adult, about 35 mg iron/kg body weight. Two-thirds of this amount is in the form of hemoglobin, and about one-third is storage iron (about 1 g in males; 200-400 mg in females). Three mg circulates in plasma as transferrin. Myoglobin and heme enzymes account for 0.15 g iron. About 6 g of hemoglobin, containing 20 mg of iron, is turned over each day. Loss of iron from the body is kept to 1 mg/day in men, and 2.5 mg/day in menstruating women. Most of the lost iron is derived from shed mucosal cells, the skin, and menstrual blood.

The normal serum iron level varies 75-150 μg/dl. The iron-binding capacity of serum exceeds this concentration by a factor of three. A minute amount of circulating iron exists as serum ferritin.[1,2] Ferritin concentration is a good index of iron deficiency and iron excess. It becomes abnormal before the iron stores are exhausted and before the onset of anemia. The information ferritin provides is similar to that obtained from bone marrow stained for iron. Levels below 10 ng/ml indicate iron deficiency anemia and above 200 ng/ml signify conditions with increased iron stores, such as thalassemia major. Serum ferritin concentrations are also increased in inflammation, liver disease, and several types of cancer. The iron of ferritin apparently comes from the reticuloendothelial system, where it derives from senescent red cells. Ferritin transfers the iron to hepatocytes. Transferrin represents iron carriage from the liver parenchyma and the intestine to bone marrow.

The hyperferritinemia encountered in acute and chronic liver diseases depends on the degree of hepatocellular injury and liver iron store.[3] Serum ferritin varies with serum aminotransferase and liver iron concentration together, but not with serum iron or total iron-binding capacity. Serum ferritin correlates with liver iron store when the ferritinemia is expressed as a ratio to the aminotransferase value. Ferritin-aminotransferase ratio provides a useful index of liver iron excess, and as a monitor of progress for patients with primary hemochromatosis during treatment. Serum ferritin underestimates iron stores in the precirrhotic stage of familial hemochromatosis. Serum levels are normal in this condition, and do not identify those patients who require phlebotomies.[4]

Iron Overload in the Liver[5,6]

Iron excess in the liver occurs under the following situations:

1. Transfusional iron overload, and iron-loading anemias
2. Excess dietary intake of iron
3. Siderosis after portacaval shunt
4. Congenital transferrin deficiency
5. Iron overload in cirrhosis
6. Idiopathic (primary) hemochromatosis

The first five conditions are also grouped under the heading of secondary hemosiderosis or hemochromatosis. Hemosiderosis refers to tissue accumulation of iron; hemochromatosis implies the additional element of tissue damage and clinical symptoms. Both terms are often used interchangeably. Iron excess after transfusions (usually after 100 units of blood or more) is well recognized. In disorders marked by erythroid hyperplasia and by ineffective erythropoiesis, such as thalassemia, sideroblastic anemias, and hereditary spherocytosis, increased iron absorption leads to hepatic iron increase. Excess oral iron ingestion is seen in hypochondriacs taking medicinal iron, in South African Bantus who drink native beer brewed in iron pots, and in alcoholics who imbibe wine (2-6 mg iron/l) or alcohol with high-iron content. Liver iron excess may complicate portacaval shunt surgery but is rarely of any clinical significance. Iron in cirrhosis and primary hemochromatosis are discussed below.

Liver iron[7,8]

Normal liver iron concentration does not exceed 0.25% dry weight. The mean concentration varies about 0.1% dry weight, depending on the population group surveyed. At low-storage levels, iron is held predominantly as water-soluble but nonstainable ferritin. With increasing storage more of the iron is deposited as insoluble and histologically stainable hemosiderin. The liver with adequate iron stores shows a faint iron stain. With mild to moderate siderosis there is poor correlation with the chemical determination of hepatic iron concentration. Histological evidence of severe siderosis invariably signifies heavy iron excess. The absence of staining iron may be regarded as indicating suboptimal iron reserves. It is estimated that for every gram increase of total body iron storage, the liver iron concentration increases by about 170 μg/100 mg. Measurement of hepatic iron concentration is closely correlated with total chelatable body iron as determined by the differential ferrioxamine test, and indirectly provides a reliable estimate of total body iron.[9] In experimental conditions, iron is not fibrogenic or hepatotoxic unless superimposed on a previously injured liver such as choline deficiency. In humans the clinical picture suggests that iron acts as a low-grade fibrogenic agent when the liver is damaged over a long period of time.

Congenital Transferrin Deficiency[6]

In this rare disorder, blood-borne iron is not transported in the normal manner because of the lack of transferrin. As a result, the bone marrow characteristically becomes devoid of iron particles. Iron, however, does diffuse into other organs, notably the liver, pancreas, kidneys, and heart. Patients present with iron deficiency anemia in the presence of systemic hemosiderosis. Hepatic fibrosis and rarely cirrhosis may be found. The disease is probably inherited as an autosomal recessive trait.

Iron Overload in Cirrhosis[6,10]

A slight degree of hepatic hemosiderosis is observed in 80% of cases with alcoholic cirrhosis. The amount is usually not in the range that would be confused with primary hemochromatosis. In about 10% of the cases, the overload is great enough to mimic primary hemochromatosis. The clinical presentation of alcoholic pancreatitis, diabetes mellitus, testicular atrophy, and skin pigmentation in cirrhosis further adds to the diagnostic difficulty. A minority opinion holds that primary hemochromatosis does not exist as an inheritable error of iron metabolism but represents a variant of cirrhosis caused by either alcoholism or nutritional deficiency, with iron excess derived from diet, occurring coincidentally.[11] Siderosis in cirrhosis may be derived by several mechanisms: (1) the elevated iron content of alcohol; (2) increased iron absorption of chronic liver disease; (3) direct alcohol stimulation of iron absorption; and (4) portal systemic shunting. Hepatic siderosis develops in patients after portacaval shunt procedures and after the appearance of spontaneous collateral circulation. The siderosis may develop rather rapidly. The cause is not established, although increased absorption of iron is thought likely.

Liver biopsy usually distinguishes iron overload in cirrhosis from iron excess due to anemias or dietary ingestion. The latter conditions do not show the degree of fibrosis that is seen in cirrhosis. The presence of iron only in reticuloendothelial cells of the liver may indicate previous transfusions, hemolysis, or viral hepatitis. If iron appears in both RE cells and parenchyma in roughly equal proportions, then hemosiderosis associated with hematological disorders is likely. If the diffuse siderosis is accompanied by cirrhosis, the condition may be either primary hemochromatosis or cirrhosis with iron overload. In short, liver biopsy does not differentiate between siderotic cirrhosis and hemochromatosis.[12] Diagnosis rests on prior history, other clinical features, and the subsequent course.

Iron overload cirrhosis differs from primary hemochromatosis in several respects:[13] (1) Abnormalities of iron metabolism occur in relatives of patients with primary hemochromatosis but not in relatives of patients with other forms of cirrhosis. (2) Carbohydrate intolerance is more severe and insulin response to glucose load less marked in hemochromatotics as compared to cirrhotics. (3) The unusual and specific arthropathy of hemochromatosis with chondrocalcinosis affecting the metacarpophalangeal joints does not occur in cirrhotics. (4) Prognosis in hemochromatosis is better than in that of alcoholic cirrhosis. Furthermore, venesection prolongs life and reverses most of the pathological effects in hemochromatosis but not in cirrhosis.

Primary Hemochromatosis[13]

The disease is recognized as an inborn error of iron metabolism. There is an overwhelming male preponderance, with 10 males afflicted for every female, and a peak age incidence range of 40–60 years. The rarity of the disorder is indicated by an incidence of 1 in 20,000 hospital admissions. The way it is inherited is uncertain, although an autosomal dominance is likely. The underlying biochemical defect is disputed, but increased mucosal absorption of iron is considered the primary factor. The suggestion that gastric or pancreatic factors are involved has not been confirmed. Total iron increases from the normal 2-5 g to 10-20 g. Liver iron concentration increases from 0.25% to 2-4% dry weight.

A second, as yet not fully explored, abnormality involves the molecular configuration of tissue ferritin, the isoferritins.[14] In normal subjects, each organ shows a characteristic isoferritin profile which appears maintained in secondary iron overload associated with alcoholic cirrhosis and transfusional siderosis. By contrast, patients with primary hemochromatosis demonstrate an isoferritin pattern that is the same for all tissues, each resembling that of normal liver ferritin. The genetic abnormality in primary hemochromatosis may involve tissue ferritins rather than iron absorption.

A third hypothesis, not incompatible with the first two, proposes a defect in the internal distribution of iron. The increased iron absorption of hemochromatosis may be due to a failure to deposit iron in storage sites which would normally regulate iron absorption. Some studies show a preferential hepatic deposition of excess hemosiderin during the early stage of disease.[15] In contrast, the bone-marrow iron store is relatively low. The disassociation of iron accumulation in liver and bone marrow is important, since it is the bone-marrow iron store which controls the level of intestinal absorption of iron.

Widespread deposits of iron correlate with the major clinical manifestations: skin pigmentation, diabetes mellitus, liver and cardiac disturbances. Liver disease is said to be a constant feature of hemochromatosis. Hepatomegaly, jaundice, portal hypertension, and ascites are common results of liver involvement. Half of the cases show no hepatic dysfunction until late in the course of the disease. Serum iron concentration exceeds 150 μg/dl; the iron-binding capacity is fully saturated. The transferrin level is normal (250 μg/dl) or slightly depressed. Serum ferritin value is raised. Hepatoma develops in up to 15% of the cases.

Liver biopsy does not distinguish this disease from cirrhosis with siderosis (Fig. 13.1).[12] Skin biopsy shows an increase of iron and melanin. The latter pigment is also increased in patients with Wilson's disease. The other systemic features of hemochromatosis occur with high frequency and provide some diagnostic hints: skin pigmentation in 90% of the cases, diabetes mellitus in 80%, and cardiac failure in 30%. Testicular atrophy, arthropathy, and other endocrinopathy are also common. The endocrine signs are attributed to pituitary hypofunction. Prognosis is variable and long-term survival after diagnosis is not rare. The method of choice for iron removal is repeated venesection; generally two 500-ml phlebotomies are performed weekly until the iron stores are depleted.

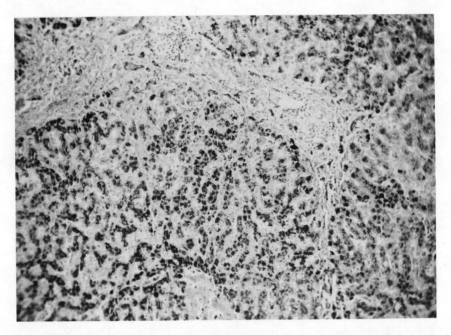

Fig. 13.1. Hemochromatosis. The iron granules are extensively deposited in all liver cells. Perl's iron, X100.

COPPER METABOLISM

The normal diet contains about 5 mg copper, of which 25% is absorbed in the stomach and upper jejunum. At least two mechanisms, active transport and passive diffusion, are involved but further details are lacking. Ceruloplasmin, copper-bound to alpha-2-globulin (MW 150,000 daltons), does not play a regulatory role in absorption. It does, however, represent 95% of the circulating serum copper. Normal ceruloplasmin concentration varies 27–37 mg/dl. Normal serum copper is 155 μg/dl $\pm$ 15 μg 1SD. Body copper content is maintained within a fairly narrow range of 100–150 mg, irrespective of age. The liver synthesizes ceruloplasmin which contains 0.5 mg copper of the body store. Bone, muscle, and liver account for 90% of the total copper store. The major pathway of disposal is through the bile. A small fraction is lost in the urine, and a negligible amount is excreted in feces, sweat, and menstrual blood.

Copper Overload

In humans copper overload occurs in Wilson's disease.

Wilson's disease.[16]   Wilson's disease (or hepatolenticular degeneration) is a rare derangement of copper homeostasis, resulting in copper accumulation in the liver, brain, kidney, cornea, and other organs. The disorder is very uncommon, appearing worldwide in 1 out of 200,000 persons. It is inherited as an autosomal recessive trait. The underlying biochemical lesion leading to metal retention is not fully elucidated, although a hepatic defect in biliary excretion of copper is considered likely. Possible mechanisms may include: (1) increased intestinal absorption of dietary copper; (2) increase of hepatic metal-binding protein with an abnormally high affinity for copper; (3) diminished ceruloplasmin synthesis with decreased excretion of ceruloplasmin-bound copper; and (4) decreased biliary disposal of copper.

Radioactive copper kinetic studies exclude the first possible mechanism (Table 13.1).[17,18,19] Intestinal absorption of copper is not different in patients with Wilson's disease. Recent evidence suggests that copperthioneine, a hepatic binding protein, in Wilson's disease has a copperbinding constant four times greater than that of the protein from control subjects.[20] This observation would not conflict with the fourth mechanism, that of decreased biliary excretion of copper, which has been documented by kinetic studies. The third hypothesis, lack of ceruloplasmin synthesis, could not be the major cause of copper retention since hypoceruloplasminemia or its complete absence in 10% of heterozygotes is not associated with the accumulation of the metal in tissue. Furthermore, 5% of patients with Wilson's disease have normal ceruloplasmin levels. The most intriguing evidence to date is the data analyzing the subcellular pools of ^{64}Cu after its administration to a patient with hepatolenticular disease who underwent surgery for gallstones.[21] The low specificity of ^{64}Cu in lysosomes resembles that of the common duct bile

Table 13.1.   Radioactive copper kinetics in Wilson's disease.[16,17,18,19]

Labeled copper half-time:	5 times normal
Calculated half-life of liver copper:	> 1800 days; control 20–30 days; in PBC 600–700 days
Plasma ^{64}Cu disappearance curve:	Prolonged, twice normal (in minutes to reach 10% of initial counts)
Incorporation into ceruloplasmin:	⅓ less than normal patient
Uptake by liver:	Slower but more persistent rise than controls; initial rate of uptake lower by 20% at 6 hours
Fecal excretion:	Decreased to about ¼ of normal
Urinary excretion:	Not different from control
Transfer into bile:	Almost absent

and differs from all the other subcellular pools of radioactive copper. The finding suggests that a defect in the lysosomal handling of copper is the basis for the reduction of biliary copper excretion. The mean biliary copper excretion rate in Wilson's disease is 8.6 ± 0.8 $\mu g/20$ minutes, as determined by duodenal perfusion studies.[22] The calculated rate of bile copper excretion is about 600 $\mu g/day$ in Wilson's disease as compared to the normal biliary excretion of 1250 $\mu g/day$. The net body accumulation of 650 $\mu g/day$ is much higher than the 50 $\mu g/day$ positive balance required to account for the copper retention in Wilson's disease. Urinary copper excretion increases during the course of the disease and may reduce the net positive copper balance.

The natural history of the disease is divisible into five stages (Table 13.2).[23] In general, during the first 20 years of life, the copper which initially accumulates in the liver redistributes to other organ sites. During this period there are usually no symptoms, but in some patients acute hepatic necrosis or hepatitis may occur when the intracellular copper shifts from hepatic cytoplasm to lysosomal sites. The sudden entrance of the metal into erythrocytes may lead to acute hemolysis, the other complication during this stage. For another 10 years or so, the brain accumulates copper without development of neurologic symptoms. After age 40, the full-blown syndrome of Wilson's disease is recognized by the classical Kayser-Fleischer corneal rings, liver cirrhosis and dysfunction, and basal ganglia disease. Neurologic manifestations consist mainly of extrapyramidal symptoms, Parkinsonian movements, and cerebellar ataxia. The renal deposition of copper produces tubular defects evidenced by aminoaciduria, uricosuria, and impairment of urinary acidification, dilution, and concentration capacities. Biochemical abnormalities include hypocupremia, hypoceruloplasminemia, and hypercupriuria (Table 13.3). Diagnosis is strengthened if the copper content of hepatic tissue exceeds 250 $\mu g/g$ dry weight. Only in prolonged extrahepatic biliary obstruction and primary biliary cirrhosis does hepatic copper reach similar concentrations. However, the clinical features would distinguish the two conditions from Wilson's disease.

Liver histology discloses a wide spectrum of lesions: acute hepatitis, fulminant hepatitis, chronic active hepatitis, fatty change, and macronodular cirrhosis. The morphological alterations alone are insufficient to establish the diagnosis.

Treatment consists of lifelong reduction of copper with chelating agents, primarily D-penicillamine. Potassium sulfide is added for a limited period to bind intragastrointestinal copper by the formation of insoluble copper sulfide. Pyridoxine prophylaxis prevents vitamin B_6 deficiency due to chelation. Liver transplants have been employed on a limited basis when there is severe decompensation.[24] In a healthy liver, the body

Table 13.2. The natural history of Wilson's disease.

Stage	Duration (in age)	Site of copper deposition	Kayser-Fleischer rings	Hepatic failure	Neurologic symptom	Serum copper	Ceruloplasmin	Urine copper
I.	0–5 yr	Liver	0	0	0	↓	↓	N↑
II.	5–20 yr	Slow redistribution, 60% asymptomatic, 30% hepatic failure,	±	+	0	N↑	↓N↑	N↑
		10% hemolytic crisis	±	0	0	N↑	↓	N↑
III.	30–40 yr	Brain	±	0	0	↓	↓	↑↑
IV.	40 yr	Brain, neurologic disease	+	0	+	↓↓	↓↓	↑↑
V.		Copper balance on therapy	0	0	0	↓	↓	↑

N = normal; ↑ = increase; ↓ = decrease. From A. Deiss et al, *Ann Intern Med* 75:57–65, 1971.

Table 13.3 Biochemical features of Wilson's disease.

	Wilson's disease	Normal person
Total body copper (mg)	1000–1500	100–150
Liver copper (μg/g dry weight)	> 250	35
Brain copper (μg/g fresh tissue)	4	58
Serum copper (μg/dl)	< 110	115
Ceruloplasmin (mg/dl)	< 20	35
Biliary copper (μg/20 min)	9	16
Urine copper (μg/24 hr)	> 100	15

copper stores are decreased without copper reaccumulating in the transplanted organ. This provides indirect evidence that Wilson's disease is primarily a liver disorder. The heterozygous state in which copper accumulates without clinical effects can be recognized by the prolonged biologic half-time of radiocopper, hypercupriuresis after penicillamine loading, increased hepatic and muscle copper concentration, aminoaciduria, and impaired urinary acidifying and diluting capacities.[25]

REFERENCES

1. Editorial: Serum-ferritin. *Lancet* 1:1263–1265, 1974.
2. Lipschitz DA, Cook JD, Finch CA: A clinical evaluation of serum ferritin as an index of iron stores. *New Eng J Med* 290:1213–1216, 1974.
3. Prieto J, Barry M, Sherlock S: Serum ferritin in patients with iron overload and with acute and chronic liver diseases. *Gastroenterology* 68:525–533, 1975.
4. Wands JR, et al: Normal serum ferritin concentrations in precirrhotic hemochromatosis. *New Eng J Med* 294:302–305, 1976.
5. Barry M: Iron and the liver. *Gut* 15:324–334, 1974.
6. Grace ND, Powell LW: Iron storage disorders of the liver. *Gastroenterology* 64:1257–1283, 1974.
7. Barry M, Sherlock S: Measurement of liver-iron concentration in needle-biopsy specimens. *Lancet* 1:100–103, 1971.
8. Barry M: Liver iron concentration, stainable iron, and total body storage iron. *Gut* 15:411–415, 1974.

9. Walker RJ, et al: Relationship of hepatic iron concentration to histochemical grading and to total chelatable body iron in conditions associated with iron overload. *Gut* 12:1011–1014, 1971.

10. Williams R, et al: Iron absorption and siderosis in chronic liver disease. *Quart J Med* 36:151–166, 1967.

11. MacDonald RA: Hemochromatosis and Wilson's disease, in Gen Ref No. 6, pp 466–479.

12. Kent G, Popper H: Liver biopsy in diagnosis of hemochromatosis. *Amer J Med* 44:837–841, 1968.

13. Powell LW: Hemochromatosis, in Gen Ref No. 1, pt A, pp 129–161.

14. Powell LW, et al: Abnormality in tissue isoferritin distribution in idiopathic haemochromatosis. *Nature* 250:333–335, 1974.

15. Valberg LS, et al: Distribution of storage iron as body iron stores expand in patients with hemochromatosis. *J Lab Clin Med* 86:479–489, 1975.

16. Sternlieb I, Scheinberg IH: Wilson's disease, in Gen Ref No. 12, pp 328–336.

17. Smallwood RA, et al: Copper kinetics in liver disease. *Gut* 12:139–144, 1971.

18. Gibbs K, Walshe JM: Studies with radioactive copper (^{64}Cu and ^{67}Cu): The incorporation of radioactive copper into ceruloplasmin in Wilson's disease and in primary biliary cirrhosis. *Clin Sci* 41:189–202, 1971.

19. Strickland GT, Beckner WM, Leu M-L: Absorption of copper in homozygotes and heterozygotes for Wilson's disease and controls: Isotope tracer studies with ^{67}Cu and ^{64}Cu. *Clin Sci* 43:617–625, 1972.

20. Evans GW, Dubois RS, Hambridge KM: Wilson's disease: Identification of an abnormal copper-binding protein. *Science* 181:1175–1176, 1973.

21. Sternlieb I, et al: Lysosomal defect of hepatic copper excretion in Wilson's disease (hepatolenticular degeneration). *Gastroenterology* 64:99–105, 1973.

22. Frommer DJ: Defective biliary excretion of copper in Wilson's disease. *Gut* 15:125–129, 1974.

23. Deiss A, et al: Long-term therapy of Wilson's disease. *Ann Intern Med* 75:57–65, 1971.

24. DuBois RS, et al: Orthotopic liver transplantation for Wilson's disease. *Lancet* 1:505–508, 1971.

25. Leu M-L, Strickland GT: Renal function in heterozygotes for Wilson's disease. *Amer J Med Sci* 263:19–24, 1971.

METABOLIC DISORDERS AND FATTY LIVERS

14

METABOLIC DISORDERS

Amyloidosis[1,2]

Amyloidosis refers to the deposition of glassy, amorphous, eosinophilic extracellular material in various organs, characterized histochemically by green birefringence after Congo-red staining; by fine, nonbranching fibrillar structure on electron microscopy; and biochemically, by the identity of one type of amyloid protein with the light polypeptide chain of immunoglobulins. The clinical classification of amyloidosis divides the disease into the following forms: (1) Primary type, with no known antecedent cause or disease. This may occur on a familial basis, such as Andrade's disease and familial Mediterranean fever, or appear sporadically. (2) Secondary type, associated with such chronic diseases as tuberculosis, leprosy (50% are complicated by amyloidosis in the United States), osteomyelitis, and bronchiectasis; and nonsuppurative illnesses such as rheumatoid arthritis, ankylosing arthritis, and ulcerative colitis. (3) Amyloidosis accompanying multiple myeloma. (4) Age-related amyloid deposition. Forty percent of autopsies of patients over age 60 reveals amyloid deposits in the pancreas, heart, and intracranial vessels. The liver is not normally involved in the aging process.

Pathologically, amyloid is deposited in two ways, perireticular or pericollagen. In the first type, amyloid may be laid down in reticulum tissue, starting in the basement-membrane area and spreading to the tunica media of a vessel. Secondary amyloidosis, familial Mediterranean fever, and some groups of idiopathic amyloidosis belong to the reticular group of amyloid deposition. In the second type, amyloid is laid down in the adventitial coat of a blood vessel and spreads inward toward the tunica media. Included in this group of pericollagen amyloid are the acquired amyloidosis of multiple myeloma, neuropathic or cardiopathic type, and certain cases of primary amyloidosis.

Chemically, several classes of amyloid substances exist, depending on the predominant type of amyloid protein. In secondary amyloidosis, familial Mediterranean fever, and certain experimental forms of amyloidosis, the fibrillar amyloid protein has an unusual amino acid composition unlike any other protein (type A amyloid protein, AA). In primary amyloidosis, and that associated with multiple myeloma, the fibrillar amyloid protein consists mainly of the variable portion of immunoglobulin light chains (type B). Mechanisms of amyloid formation are poorly understood but may involve macrophage degradation of antigen-antibody complexes producing fibril precursors, or circulating high concentration of free light chain immunoglobulin subunits synthesized in such diseases as multiple myeloma. Liver, kidney, and spleen are commonly involved in all three forms of amyloidosis. Renal disease and failure appear in 90% of the patients with secondary amyloidosis, 60% with primary amyloidosis, and 40% with amyloidosis associated with multiple myeloma.[3,4]

Clinical manifestations of hepatic deposits include right-upper-quadrant pain, jaundice (5% of all cases), ascites, and weight loss. Intrahepatic cholestasis, chronic liver disease, and death due to hepatic failure are rare complications.[5]

Among laboratory tests, increased BSP retention and elevated alkaline phosphatase concentration are the most reliable indicators of hepatic dysfunction in amyloidosis. Serum bilirubin and aminotransferase activity are either normal or slightly altered. A serum component related to amyloid protein AA (SAA) is usually present. A small quantity of SAA occurs in normal serum. It behaves as an acute-phase reactant, and is elevated in conditions other than amyloidosis such as pregnancy, chronic inflammatory disorders, and lymphoproliferative diseases.

Liver biopsy discloses either diffuse or spotty amyloid infiltration in sinusoids and vascular walls in portal spaces. The liver cells become secondarily compressed and atrophic in appearance. Inflammation and necrosis are unusual features. There is no known specific treatment. Prognosis correlates with the underlying cause and renal complications.

Diabetes Mellitus[6]

Pathologically, the liver in diabetes mellitus shows an excess of glycogen, nuclear glycogen, and fat.

Glycogen. Brittle diabetes in children tends to show increased liver glycogen with hepatomegaly and hypoglycemia. Intensive insulin therapy of diabetic acidosis may lead to temporary glycogen storage, manifesting as hepatomegaly, which usually disappears within a week. There is, in general, no correlation between fasting blood glucose, degree of ketosis, and hepatic glycogen or fat content.

Nuclear glycogen. This is observed in 80% of the patients with juvenile and maturity onset diabetes. The deposits are actively synthesized by cell nuclei, and chemically bear a similarity to skeletal muscle glycogen. The number of cells with nuclear glycogen but not the incidence increases with the rise of blood glucose. Nuclear glycogen is not specific for diabetes mellitus. It may be observed in healthy persons from the very young to the very old, and in such disorders as Wilson's disease, cirrhosis, chronic active hepatitis, tuberculosis, and leprosy.

Fat. The incidence of fatty liver in diabetes varies 20–80%, according to different reports. Although insulin deficiency causes fatty liver in animals, the condition is rarely found in human juvenile diabetes since most children are usually treated with insulin. Enhanced lipolysis is responsible for the increased hepatic fat. The fatty liver associated with maturity onset diabetes correlates with obesity. Accelerated lipogenesis accounts for the fatty change in the liver. Weight reduction usually results in mobilization of the fat from the liver in the adult diabetic. Oral antidiabetic drugs which stimulate insulin secretion are not effective since hepatic fat in this instance is not under insulin control. Mild to moderate liver dysfunction is frequent among patients with diabetes. BSP clearance is often abnormal and represents a useful test for detecting biochemical abnormality. The development of fatty liver does not appreciably alter the prognosis in diabetes mellitus. Fatty change by itself does not predispose toward the increased incidence of cirrhosis (5–30%) in patients with diabetes.

Clinically, diabetes mellitus may be complicated by viral hepatitis and cirrhosis.

Viral hepatitis. Studies from Europe report an increased frequency of viral hepatitis in patients with diabetes mellitus. Decreased host resistance to infection is held to play a role. However, the hypothesis is not tenable. Diabetics are more susceptible to bacterial and fungal but not viral infections than nondiabetics. It is likely that the increased exposure to needles during insulin injection accounts for the high incidence of viral hepatitis.

Cirrhosis. The incidence of cirrhosis in diabetes mellitus depends to a great extent on the definition of diabetes. Postmortem examinations show an increased association between the two diseases. Clinical studies, in general, fail to confirm a positive correlation. This is partly due to the fact that most clinical statistics exclude latent diabetes and include only manifest diabetes with persistent hyperglycemia and glycosuria. The other relationship, the increased frequency of diabetes mellitus in cirrhosis, has been well documented. Diabetes in cirrhotic patients is about 4–5 times more common than in the general population. There is no epidemiological evidence that diabetes mellitus is the causative agent of cirrhosis. The situation is probably the reverse, namely, that cirrhosis is diabetogenic. Normal or elevated insulin secretion after glucose load, increased nonesterified fatty acid level, decreased sensitivity to insulin with inappropriate lack of glucose fall, abnormal plasma binding of insulin leading to loss in biological activity, and decreased muscle utilization occur in the cirrhotic patient and contribute to the diabetic state. Clinical manifestations of overt diabetes are usually absent in the cirrhotic who is also diabetic.

Hepatic Porphyria

Porphyria is divided into two groups (Table 14.1): erythropoietic and hepatic, depending on the predominant site of overproduction.[7] The erythropoietic group consists of three types: in erythropoietic uroporphyria (congenital), uroporphyrin accumulates; in erythropoietic protoporphyria, protoporphyrin accumulates; and in erythropoietic coproporphyria, coproporphyrin accumulates. All three types are characterized clinically by photosensitivity and skin lesions. Although the skin is a major site of pigment deposit, other organs, including the liver, are flooded by the porphyrin overload. Liver function is usually normal. Hepatic morphology reveals fluorescent or polarizing brown pigment intracellularly, particularly in erythropoietic protoporphyria. The protoporphyrin deposits appear as birefringent needle-shape crystals and Maltese crosses. Liver damage is generally absent or mild. Cholestasis, ductal proliferation, portal fibrosis, and rarely cirrhosis may develop in severe cases.

Hepatic porphyria.   Three of the four hepatic porphyrias are familial in occurrence and inherited in a dominant mode: acute intermittent, porphyria variegata, and hereditary coproporphyria. The fourth, porphyria cutanae tarda (symptomatica), is acquired and often iatrogenically induced. Acute intermittent porphyria (AIP) is an uncommon disorder.[8] The basic defect appears to be a deficiency of urosynthetase (Fig. 14.1), leading to decreased heme production and reversal of aminolevulinic acid (ALA) synthetase inhibition.[9] The secondary induction of hepatic ALA synthetase results in increased production of ALA and porphobilinogen (PBG), which characteristically overflow into the urine. Clinical features consist of recurrent abdominal colic, constipation, hypertension, psychoneurotic behavior, and neuromuscular symptoms. Photosensitivity is notably absent. Attacks are often precipitated by barbiturates,

Table 14.1 Characteristics of porphyrin diseases.

	Hepatic				Erythropoietic
	Acute intermittent porphyria	Porphyria variegata	Porphyria cutanea tarda	Hereditary coproporphyria	Three types
Inheritance	Dominant	Dominant	Acquired	Dominant	Recessive or dominant
Age	Puberty	Puberty	Any age	Any age	Infancy
Symptoms	Abdominal, psychic, neurologic	Photosensitivity, may be abdominal		May be both, or none	Photosensitivity and skin lesions, no abdominal pains
Liver	↑ ALA synthetase ↓ urosynthetase	?	↑ ALA synthetase	↑ ALA synthetase	?
Urine color	Red	N or red	Red	N or red	Red or N
ALA and PBG	↑↑	↑	N	↑	N
Uro and copro'gen	↑	↑	↑	↑	N or ↑
Fecal uro'gen, etc.	↑	↑	↑	↑	N or ↑
RBC uro'gen, etc.	N	N	N	N	↑↑

ALA = aminolevulinic acid; PBG = porphobilinogen; uro'gen, copro'gen = uroporphyrinogen, coproporphyrinogen; urosynthetase = uroporphyrinogen 1-synthetase; N = normal. From U. A. Meyer et al, *New Eng J Med* 286:1277-1282, 1972.

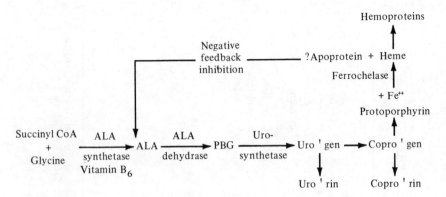

Fig. 14.1. Outline of porphyrin metabolism. ALA = aminolevulinic acid; PBG = porphobilinogen; Uro'gen, Copro'gen = uro and coproporphyrinogen; Uro'rin, Copro'rin = uro and coproporphyrin; Uro-synthetase = uroporphyrinogen 1-synthetase. (Adapted from U. A. Myers et al.[9])

alcohol, other drugs, and menstruation. The urine is an amber color initially but turns red on standing. The color change is explained by the fact that PBG (colorless) is excreted and not urobilinogen (red). ALA is also found in high concentration. Both ALA and PBG continue to be excreted during the latent stage. The liver fluoresces due to the accumulation of porphyrin compounds.

Histologically, it is either normal or may reveal nonspecific alterations. Hemosiderosis is prominent at times. Functionally, 90% of cases have abnormal BSP retention, often with values greater than 10%. In the latent, asymptomatic stage a large number of patients continue to have increased BSP retention. The defect is not in the uptake but rather in the conjugation and excretion of the dye. Other liver function tests are normal, except for hypercholesterolemia.

Porphyria variegata. This hereditary disease is characterized by skin lesions or abdominal pains and by the constant fecal excretion of coproporphyrin and protoporphyrin. Acute attacks may be accompanied by jaundice. It is believed that as long as the liver is capable of excreting porphyrin into the bile, the disease is latent. When this capacity is impaired or exceeded, symptoms appear. Hepatic derangements and lesions are similar to those described for acquired porphyria.

Hereditary coproporphyria. In this rare condition type III coproporphyrin is excreted in the urine and feces in large quantities. Protoporphyrin excretion is not increased. Clinical attacks simulate acute intermittent porphyria. Barbiturates and other drugs are inciting agents. Like other hepatic porphyrias, the liver contains excessive ALA synthetase.

Porphyria cutanea tarda (symptomatica). The causes of this condition are exogenous. Clinically, skin lesions and hypertrichosis predominate. Abdominal symptoms are conspicuously absent. Uroporphyrin and coproporphyrin are excreted in the urine in large amounts. Liver dysfunction with coexistence of liver disease is frequent. This disorder can occur in conjunction with other conditions, eg, cirrhosis in Bantu patients in South Africa, alcoholic cirrhosis, rare cases of hepatoma, and certain drug-induced illnesses. Estrogen therapy (for prostatic carcinoma) and hexochlorobenzene may induce the disease.

Liver histology shows fatty change, diffuse nonspecific hepatitis, or cirrhosis, depending on the underlying condition. Hemosiderosis, needle crystalline structures in hepatocytes, and fluorescent pigments are additional features.[10,11] Mild to moderate iron overload is common in this disease, but the cause is not fully understood. Experimentally, iron induces synthesis of ALA synthetase. Repeated venesection is the established treatment. Both tissue iron and hepatic ALA synthetase levels are reduced by blood letting. Porphyrin excretion, on the other hand, is raised.

Hyperthyroidism

The older studies, based mainly on autopsy examinations, related hepatic damage to increased morbidity in thyrotoxic patients. Jaundice and impaired drug and protein metabolism were among the abnormal features. In addition, a specific form of cirrhosis was thought pathognomonic of hyperthyroidism. More recent studies indicate that hepatic dysfunction in the disease is mild and inconstant, and histologic alterations of the liver are scanty.[12] Hepatic changes include mild to moderate steatosis, focal necrosis and inflammation, and mononuclear triaditis. Biochemically, serum alkaline phosphatase is mildly elevated. Other liver function tests are not abnormal. Congestive heart failure which complicates hyperthyroidism is associated with centrolobular congestion and necrosis.

Hypothyroidism[13]

The patient with myxedema may rarely develop ascites independent of cardiac failure. Liver biopsy reveals centrolobular congestion and fibrosis without an inflammatory response. The lesion resembles chronic hypervitaminosis A. The pathogenesis of the hepatic change in myxedema ascites is unknown.

Glycogenoses

At least 10 types of glycogen storage disease are recognized, involving enzyme defects in the anaerobic glycolytic cycle (Fig. 14.2; Table 14.2).[14,15] The conditions vary considerably in severity and clinical presentation, depending on the underlying chemical defect. All except types V and VII exhibit hepatomegaly, with and without hypoglycemia, metabolic acidosis, or hyperlipidemia. Histologically the enlarged liver cells show an empty cytoplasm, sometimes containing faintly eosinophilic material. Discrete small lipid vacuoles are usually also evident. Type IV glycogen storage disorder is the only one of the group that is regularly associated with cirrhosis. Diagnosis rests on biochemical demonstration of the enzyme deficiency in liver, muscle, and other tissues. Portacaval anastomosis has been advocated for treatment of types I and III, and possibly type IV disease. There is improvement of the hypoglycemia, metabolic acidosis, and survival time. Among other beneficial effects are accelerated body growth, increased bone mineralization, and decrease in liver size.

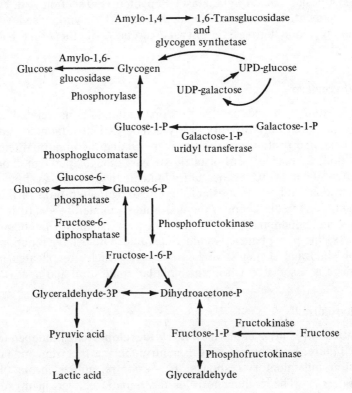

Fig. 14.2. Embden-Meyerhof pathway of anaerobic glycolysis.[14]

Table 14.2. Classification of glycogenosis. [14,15]

Type	Synonym	Enzyme defect	Liver morphology			
			Lobular pattern	Nuclear glycogen	Lipid	Septa formation
I.	Von Gierke's disease	Glucose-6 phosphatase	Mosaic	+	Large and small droplets	–
II.	Pompe's disease	Lysosomal acid alphaglucosidase	Nonmosaic; cytoplasmic microvesicular	–	–	–
III.	Cori's syndrome	Amylo-1, 6-glucosidase, "debrancher enzyme"	Mosaic	+	+	+
IV.	Amylopectinosis; Anderson's disease	Amylo 1,4→1,6-transglucosidase "brancher enzyme"	Peripheral amylopectin deposits	–	Large droplets	Cirrhosis
V.	McArdle's syndrome	Muscle phosphorylase	Normal	–	–	–
VI.	—	Liver phosphorylase	Mosaic	–	Small droplets	+
VII.	—	Phosphofructokinase	?	?	?	?
VIII.	—	Enzyme deficiency not yet demonstrated	Mosaic	–	–	–
IX.	—	Liver phosphorylase kinase	Mosaic	–	Small droplets	+
X.	—	Cyclic AMP dependent kinase	Mosaic	–	Small droplets	+

+ = present; − = absent. Reprinted with permission from G. Hug, Nonbilirubin Genetic Disorders of the Liver, monog no 13, *Internat Acad Path*, Williams and Wilkins Co, 1973, pp 28–31.

Other Storage Diseases

Many of these disorders represent lysosomal enzyme defects with secondary accumulation of metabolites (Tables 14.3 and 4).[14] Hepatic dysfunction and lesions form a relatively inconspicuous part of the generalized derangement, and are usually overshadowed by other clinical manifestations. Foamy macrophages and vacuolated hepatocytes are recognized on liver histology in the histiocytosis X complex (Letter-Siwe disease and Hand-Schüller-Christian disease, but usually not in eosinophilic

Table 14.3.   Lysosomal diseases.

Name	Enzyme affected	Material stored	Hepatic lesion
Pompe's disease	Acid 1,4 and 1,6-gluco-sidase	Glycogen	Abnormal lysosomes
Mucopoly-saccharidoses (at least 6 types)	Acid beta-ga-lactosidase	Mucopoly-saccharides	Cytoplasmic vacuoles, seen in Hurler's disease (zebra-like lyso-somes in brain)
Metachromatic leukodystrophy	Arylsulfa-tase A	Cerebroside sulfate	Abnormal lysosomes
Gaucher's disease	Acid beta-glucosidase	Glucocere-broside	Foamy macro-phages
Krabbe's disease	Galacto-cerebroside beta-galacto-sidase	Galactocere-broside	Abnormal lysosomes
Tay-Sachs disease	N-acetyl-beta-hexosaminidase component A	Ganglioside GM_2	Residual bodies with lamellar organization
Sandhoff's disease	Same, but com-ponent A and B involved	Ganglioside GM_2	Residual bodies with lamellar organization
Chediak-Higashi disease	?	?	Abnormal inclusions in Kupffer cells
Aspartylglu-cosaminuria	B-aspartyl-glucosylamide hydrolase	? and fat	Vacuoles in hepatocytes and Kupffer cells

Reprinted with permission from G. Hug, Nonbilirubin Genetic Disorders of the Liver, monogr no 13, *Internat Acad Path,* Williams and Wilkins Co, 1973, p 48.

Table 14.4. Other disorders of carbohydrate metabolism without glycogen storage.

Type	Enzyme defect	Clinical presentation	Liver lesions
Aglycogenosis	Glycogen synthetase	Fasting hypogly-cemia; mental retardation	?
Galactosemia	Galactose-1-phosphate uri-dyl transferase	Jaundice, cata-racts, hepato-splenomegaly, mental re-tardation	Cirrhosis
	Galactokinase	Cataracts, no hepatospleno-megaly or mental changes	No hepa-toxicity
Benign fruc-tosuria	Fructokinase	None	None
Hereditary fructose intolerance	1-phospho-fructaldolase	Vomiting and hypoglycemia after fructose ingestion, hepatomegaly	Cirrhosis
Fructose diphosphatase deficiency	Fructose-1-6 diphosphatase	Hepatomegaly, frequent metabolic acidosis	Severe fatty change

Reprinted with permission from G. Hug, Nonbilirubin Genetic Disorders of the Liver, monogr no 13, *Internat Acad Path,* Williams and Wilkins Co, 1973, p 24.

granuloma), Gaucher's disease, Niemann-Pick disease, Hurler's disease, cholesterol ester storage disease, Wolman's disease, abetalipo-proteinemia, Tangier disease (alpha-lipoprotein deficiency), Fabry's disease, and types I and V hyperlipoproteinemia. Because of the similarity of hepatic changes, one cannot distinguish the various storage diseases by histology alone.

Inherited Disorders with Hyperammonemia

The clinical manifestations are primarily neurological and similar in this group of ammonia toxicity (Table 14.5).[16] The syndromes vary according to the severity and nature of the biochemical defect (see also Fig. 1.9). Hyperammonemia is often fatal in the newborn, severe in infancy, and

Table 14.5. Inherited disorders with hyperammonemia.

Enzyme deficiency/ disorder	Mode of inheritance	Clinical severity	Protein intolerance	Biochemical features
I. Inborn errors of urea cycle enzymes				
1. Carbamyl phosphate synthetase (3 variants)	? recessive	Generally fatal in M; vari-able in F	Severe to moderate	None; ke-totic hyper-glycemia; ortic acid-uria
2. Ornithine transcarbamy-lase (4 variants)	X-linked dominant	Generally fatal in M; vari-able in F	Severe to moderate	Ortic acid-uria
3. Arginino-succinate synthetase	? autosomal recessive	Severe to fatal	Moderate	↑ citrul-line in blood, CSF, and urine
4. Argininosuc-cinase	Autosomal recessive	Moderate, severe, or chronic	Mild to moderate	↑ arginino-succinate and citrulline in blood, CSF, urine
5. Arginase (? 1 variant)	?	Moderate	Moderate	↑ arginine in blood, CSF, urine
II. Other inborn errors associated with hyperammonemia				
1. Ornithine (3 variants)	? autosomal recessive	Moderate	None to moderate	↑ blood ornithine
2. Hyperlysi-nemia, lysine dehydrogenase deficiency (3 variants)	?	Mild to moderate	None	↑ blood lysine
3. Hyperlysinuria with hyperammo-nemia (2 variants)	?	Mental re-tardation	Mild to none	↓ plasma lysine arginine with ↑ urine levels
4. Disorders of branched-chain metabolism (7 conditions)	? autosomal recessive	Mild or severe re-tardation	None to severe	Generally keto-acidosis and hyperglycemia

Y. E. Hsia, *Gastroenterology* 67:347–374, Williams and Wilkins Co, 1974.

chronic or intermittent in older children and adults. Diagnosis is established by identification of the liver enzyme defect, if present, and by analysis of blood, CSF, and urinary patterns of abnormal amino acids. Survival to adulthood without treatment or recognition of the hyperammonemia is possible in three of the conditions: female heterozygotes with ornithine transcarbamylase deficiency, argininosuccinic aciduria, and familial protein intolerance.

FATTY LIVERS

Fatty livers are diagnosed on the basis of liver histology. The normal liver contains 5% fat, which ordinarily is not visible on routine histological examination. Fat exceeding 7% of liver weight appears as vacuoles or droplets within the cytoplasm of hepatocytes (see also Fig. 10.2). Glycogen excess may also give a similar appearance. Fat and glycogen can be distinguished only on the basis of histochemical staining after proper fixation, or by biochemical tests. The causes of fatty liver are varied (Table 14.6). In many instances the exact block in the fat metabolism which leads to increased accumulation is not known. Fatty change by itself rarely indicates the etiologic process. In the common types of fatty liver, such as in alcoholism, kwashiorkor, obesity, jejunoileal bypass, and diabetes mellitus, the intracellular fat droplets are large and displace the nucleus of the hepatocyte (Table 14.7).[17] In acute fatty liver of pregnancy, tetracycline toxicity, Reye's syndrome, and cholesterol ester storage disease the vacuoles are small, microvesicular in appearance, and do not displace the nucleus. A centrolobular distribution of fat suggests acute fatty liver of pregnancy and CCl_4 poisoning but not tetracycline toxicity or Reye's syndrome. In general, however, lipid size and its lobular pattern are not reliable indicators of a specific disorder.

Lipid Composition of Fatty Livers

The distribution of the chief lipids does not vary with the type of disease. The lipid accumulation is chiefly due to the increase of triglycerides, exceeding phospholipids > free cholesterol > cholesterol ester level.[18,19] The triglyceride content varies inversely with the phospholipid fraction. The amount of cholesterol ester determines the surface area of the fat droplet. For similar triglyceride concentrations, fatty vacuoles tend to be smaller in cases with high cholesterol ester than those with low cholesterol ester. On a standard hospital diet, rich in long-chain triglycerides, the liver fatty acid composition from alcoholic patients does not differ in the presence or absence of cirrhosis.[20] Palmitic, stearic, oleic, and linoleic

Table 14.6.   Causes of fatty liver in humans.

Toxic
  Alcohol
  CCl_4, chloroform, other chlorinated hydrocarbons
  Yellow phosphorus

Drug-induced
  Tetracycline
  Halothane
  Corticosteroids

Nutritional
  Obesity
  Starvation
  Kwashiorkor
  Jejunoileal shunt
  Chronic hypervitaminosis A

Metabolic
  Diabetes mellitus
  Wilson's disease, early stage
  Cystic fibrosis (mucoviscidosis)
  Galactosemia
  Hyperthyroidism
  Refsun syndrome (phytanic oxidase deficiency)
  Hyperlipoproteinemia (types I, V)
  Abetalipoproteinemia
  Glycogen storage disease (types I, III, IV, VI,? VII, IX, X)
  Hepatic cholesterol ester storage disease (cholesterol ester hydrolase and
    triglyceride lipase deficiency)
  Hereditary fructose intolerance
  Tangier's disease (alpha-lipoprotein deficiency)
  Fabry's disease (alpha-galactosidase deficiency)
  Niemann-Pick's disease (phosphorylcholineceramidoses)
  Gaucher's disease (glycosylcerebrosidoses)
  Wolman's disease (cholesterol ester hydrolase and triglyceride lipase
    deficiency)
  Neonatal hepatic steatosis
  Lipoatrophic diabetes

Unknown
  Acute fatty liver pregnancy
  Reye's syndrome
  Ulcerative colitis
  Down's syndrome
  Intravenous hyperalimentation

Table 14.7. Histological features of fatty liver.

Disease	Lobular distribution of fat	Location of hepatocyte nucleus	Mechanism of fat accumulation
Alcoholic	Random	Eccentric	Impaired fatty oxidation; increased esterification
Kwashiorkor	Periportal when mild	Eccentric	Decreased apoprotein synthesis
Obesity	Centrolobular when mild	Eccentric	Increased fat stores
Jejunoileal bypass	Diffuse	Eccentric	?
Diabetes mellitus	Diffuse	Eccentric	Increased lipogenesis (adult onset); increased lipolysis (juvenile)
Acute fatty liver of pregnancy	Centrolobular	Central	?
Tetracycline toxicity	Diffuse	Central	Impaired release of lipoprotein
Reye's syndrome	Diffuse, most prominent in periportal area	Central	Impaired lipoprotein synthesis; increased fatty acid influx
Corticosteroids	Random	Eccentric	? increased fatty acid influx
Carbon tetrachloride	Centrolobular; early stage	Central	Impaired apoprotein synthesis
Phosphorus	Periportal	Central	Impaired apoprotein synthesis
Abetalipoproteinemia	Diffuse	Eccentric	Lack of beta-lipoprotein
Tangier	Focal	Central	Deficiency of high-density lipoprotein
Wolman's	Foamy macrophages, especially in periportal area	Eccentric	? increased synthesis of cholesterol ester; ? decreased catabolism
Cholesterol ester storage	Diffuse	Central	?

From A. M. Hoyumpa, Jr, et al, *Amer J Dig Dis* 20:1142–1170, 1975.

acids account for 70% of the total hepatic fatty acids in fatty livers, irrespective of cirrhosis. Feeding of medium-chain triglycerides (MCT) alters the fatty acid composition of the cirrhotic but not the noncirrhotic liver. The relative high concentration of the long-chain oleic acid decreases, while the shorter-chain myristic and pentadecanoic acids are higher in cirrhotic patients after MCT feeding than in controls. No difference occurs for the noncirrhotic group. Oral administration of MCT to cirrhotics produces a higher and more persistent serum elevation of medium-chain fatty acids (MCFA) than in noncirrhotics. The increased serum MCFA may account for the shift from long-chain fatty acids to shorter-chain fatty acids in the cirrhotic liver. MCT may exert a protective effect on the liver during the cirrhogenic process. Animals develop cirrhosis less frequently when MCT is substituted for long-chain triglycerides in the choline-deficient diets. The mechanism for the effect is not known. MCT exerts no neurotoxicity in humans, and produces no clinical and EEG changes.[21] No alteration of arterial ammonia levels in patients with cirrhosis has been noted.

Fatty Liver Disorders

Obesity. Hepatic accumulation of lipid is invariable in obesity, though hepatic lipid mass does not correlate with the absolute degree of obesity. The fatty liver of an obese patient represents more than local organ excess in the presence of generalized lipid deposition.[22] The mechanism for the hepatic increase of lipid is not known.

Failure of dietary and medical measures to control the excessive weight has led to the development of surgical techniques. Jejunoileal bypass surgery is perhaps the most commonly employed operation to date. The results are impressive. Substantial and prolonged weight loss occurs in patients. Unfortunately, the complications are many and serious. Aside from the expected side effects of diarrhea, electrolyte loss, depletion of calcium and magnesium, and vitamin deficits, other complications include hyperuricemia, renal calculi, gallstones, and liver disease. Steatosis, cholestasis, parenchymal necrosis and inflammation, alcoholic hepatitis with Mallory bodies, and rarely cirrhosis have all been reported.[23,24,25] Fatty liver is the most common hepatic complication, developing within 2-3 months after the operation and accompanied by tender hepatomegaly and signs of malnutrition. In many ways the effects of jejunoileal shunt resemble the features of kwashiorkor, although the analogy is not completely accurate. The hepatic complications are more severe than those encountered in kwashiorkor. The cause of liver disease after bypass surgery is not known. Speculated mechanisms, aside from protein deficiency, include (1) lack of lipotrope absorption, possibly choline; (2)

alteration of gut flora with production of bacterial toxin; and (3) abnormal bile salt metabolism, resulting in increased serum levels of lithocholic and chenodeoxycholic acids.

It is not clear what role preexisting hepatic abnormalities may play since many obese patients show changes in the liver prior to the surgery. Fat, mild inflammation, periportal fibrosis, and cirrhosis in 2–3% of the cases are commonly noted on liver biopsy.[26] Following bypass surgery, weight loss is accompanied by a net increase of hepatic lipid three times the intraoperative values. Liver function tests become abnormal with elevated levels of serum aminotransferase and alkaline phosphatase. The BSP test, however, does not correlate with the degree of lipid increase in the liver. Of the essential amino acids, plasma valine, isoleucine, leucine, phenylalanine, threonine, and lysine decline. The levels of nonessential amino acids, alanine, citrulline, cystine, tyrosine, ornithine, and arginine, also fall. Glycine and serine are elevated. The pattern of amino acid alteration resembles protein-caloric malnutrition. Supplementation with amino acids partly corrects the abnormal profile and improves liver function.

Alcoholic fatty liver. This disorder is dicussed fully in Chapter 10.

Kwashiorkor.[27,28] Kwashiorkor forms one end of the spectrum of protein-caolric malnutrition, in which deficiency of protein but not caloric content leads to a characteristic syndrome, including a fatty liver. The other polar form of malnutrition, marasmus, is due to a low caloric diet in which all nutrients are deficient (Table 14.8). The starvation diet, frequently accentuated by repeated febrile illness, produces the general inanition of marasmus, but not a fatty liver. In kwashiorkor, the starchy diet, although not optimal, will sustain adults but not growing children. Typically, the onset is precipitated by a bout of dysentery or other infection, such as measles. The child becomes weak and irritable, although the general appearance may not be one of poor nutrition. Body fat remains well maintained. Skin and hair changes are frequent. The abdomen is distended with hepatomegaly, not ascites. Jaundice is usually mild or absent.

Liver function tests are minimally altered. Biochemically, there are low plasma values for albumin, beta-lipoprotein, glucose, and amino acids (especially the branched-chain amino acids), raised free fatty acids, and impaired glucose tolerance. The cause for the fatty liver is not known, but depressed hepatic lipoprotein synthesis and increased lipogenesis from fatty acid generation have been observed. The fatty liver of kwashiorkor does not progress to cirrhosis.

Table 14.8. Contrasts between kwashiorkor and marasmus.

	Kwashiorkor	Marasmus
Deficit	Proteins; caloric value normal or high	All nutrients; calories low
Age	> 2 yr	< 1 yr
Season	Anytime	Summer and autumn
Onset	Acute, precipitated by infections	Chronic, often gastroenteritis
Feeding	Breast	Bottle
Community	Rural	Urban
Biochemistry	Markedly altered	May be unremarkable
Fatty liver	Yes	No

From D. S. McLaren, *Lancet* 2:93–96, 1974.

Diabetes mellitus.   Diabetes mellitus is discussed in the first section of this chapter.

Acute fatty liver of pregnancy.[17,29]   This rare disorder occurs mostly in primiparas, and appears in the last trimester of pregnancy. Many of the previously reported cases were probably related to tetracycline toxicity. Diagnosis of the idiopathic condition must exclude drug administration. Clinically, acute fatty liver of pregnancy resembles fulminant viral hepatitis, with deep jaundice, hematemesis, and severe headaches. Signs of renal failure appear in about half of the patients: oliguria, uremia, and metabolic acidosis. Pancreatitis is another prominent feature. Neither the mother nor the infant usually survive. Laboratory findings confirm severe hepatic and renal dysfunction. A helpful point for diagnosis is the striking leukocytosis in the absence of fever. Both the liver and kidney show fat. Treatment is symptomatic.

Reye's syndrome.   For a discussion of Reye's syndrome see Chapter 15.

Corticosteroid-induced fatty liver.   This may occur endogenously, as in Cushing's disease, or exogenously. A small dose of prednisolone in rabbits produces hepatic fatty change with ultrastructural alterations such as glycogen accumulation, swelling of mitochondria, proliferation of smooth endoplasmic reticulum, and increased liposomes.[30] Humans who receive high doses of corticosteroid over prolonged periods develop symptomatic fatty livers with hepatomegaly, BSP retention, and abnormal hepatic microstructure, including focal necrosis and hemorrhage. Abrupt withdrawl of steroid therapy, among other complications, can produce fat embolism, presumably the result of sudden fat mobilization from the liver. The cause of steroid-induced fat deposition is not known. It is generally thought that increased fatty acid mobilization from peripheral depots plays a role.

Tetracycline-induced fatty liver.[29]   The microfatty droplets distinguish this fatty liver from other types. The fatty change is seen with ordinary doses of tetracycline, although clinical toxicity usually occurs with doses of 2 g or above administered intravenously. Most of the cases reported are described in pregnant women. The illness was diagnosed in the past as fatty liver of pregnancy but appears in the majority of the cases to be due to tetracycline toxicity. The clinical features often resemble viral hepatitis, with weakness, nausea, vomiting, and abdominal discomfort. Jaundice and hepatomegaly are usual presentations. The pregnancy is hastened with premature labor or curtailed with fetal death.

Laboratory findings disclose hepatic dysfunction, renal failure, and pancreatitis. Serum bilirubin rises to 10 mg/dl, and aminotransferase activity is high, up to 1000 IU/l. Striking leukocytosis and high serum BUN, creatinine, and amylase are also noted. The pathogenesis of the fatty liver is due to inhibition of protein synthesis. The accumulation of triglycerides probably results from impaired lipoprotein synthesis and fat release. It is not known if pregnancy increases tissue sensitivity to tetracycline toxicity. The metabolic disposal of the drug is not different from that in the nonpregnant state. Diminished glomerular filtration rate due to preexisting or acute renal disease and vomiting enhances the tetracycline effect, since blood clearance of the drug is delayed. Maternal prognosis is poor; the mortality rate is high.

Carbon tetrachloride (CCl$_4$).   Acute or chronic CCl$_4$ poisoning may result from inhalation or ingestion of this well-known hepatotoxin. Acute intoxication may follow transient exposure to the vapor (maximal safe atmospheric concentration is 25 ppm for eight hours of exposure), or from either suicidal or accidental ingestion of cleaning fluid or fire extinguisher fluid. The fatal oral dose is as little as 2–4 ml in susceptible persons. Chronic intoxication usually results from industrial exposure.

Clinically, inhalational CCl$_4$ poisoning produces mucous membrane irritation, dizziness, and headache. The course may progress to convulsion, coma, and death due to central nervous system depression or from ventricular fibrillation. If the patient survives the acute stage, severe neurologic derangements and hepatic manifestations of jaundice, hepatomegaly, and ascites then appear by the third day.

In poisoning by ingestion, gastrointestinal symptoms including abdominal pains and hematemesis predominate. The possibility of liver injury is greater when CCl_4 is taken orally. This contrasts with the prominent renal damage in inhalation intoxication, but the distinction is not invariable. Laboratory findings disclose a high aminotransferase level and normal serum alkaline phosphatase. Renal failure is signaled by the elevated serum BUN and creatinine. Liver histology reveals, as in animals, the characteristic centrolobular necrosis and fatty change.

Treatment should be supportive. An initial measure is lavaging the stomach for any remaining poison. Of all hepatotoxins, CCl_4 is perhaps the best studied. It is believed that free radicals liberated by the metabolism of CCl_4 act by lipid peroxidation to damage organelle membranes (see Chapter 12). The impaired endoplasmic reticulum with decreased lipoprotein synthesis and diminished secretion of triglycerides produces the fatty liver.

Phosphorus poisoning. Yellow phosphorus is hepatotoxic; the red form is not. Poisoning may be acute or chronic. The acute type usually results from ingestion of insecticides, rodent poisons, or firework powder. The clinical presentation is characterized by nausea, vomiting, abdominal pains, and bloody diarrhea, followed by jaundice and tender hepatomegaly. Aside from the liver, other target organs are the heart, kidney, muscles, and brain.

Liver histology shows extensive periportal fatty change and necrosis. Hepatic derangements may be profound with severe hypoprothrombinemia and hypoglycemia. The increase in hepatic triglycerides has been ascribed to impairment of the secretory mechanism, resulting from lipid peroxidation, an effect similar to CCl_4 toxicity, or from direct inhibition of lipoprotein synthesis. Death rapidly ensues. The fatal dose for humans is about 60 mg. Chronic poisoning follows protracted exposure to yellow phosphorus at lower doses, as in an industrial setting with volatile fumes. Necrosis of the facial bones and jaw, liver cirrhosis, and chronic renal disease are observed.

REFERENCES

1. Cohen AS: Amyloidosis. *New Eng J Med* 277:522–530, 1967.
2. Glenner GG, Ein D, Terry WD: The immunoglobulin origin of amyloid. *Amer J Med* 52:141–147, 1972.

3. Brandt K, Cathcart ES, Cohen AS: A clinical analysis of the course and prognosis of forty-two patients with amyloidosis. *Amer J Med* 44:955–969, 1968.

4. Barth WF, et al: Primary amyloidosis: Clinical, immunochemical and immunoglobulin metabolism studies in fifteen patients. *Amer J Med* 47:259–273, 1969.

5. Levy M, Fryd CH, Eliakim M: Intrahepatic obstructive jaundice due to amyloidosis of the liver: A case report and review of the literature. *Gastroenterology* 61:234–238, 1971.

6. Creutzfeldt W, Frerichs H, Sickinger K: Liver diseases and diabetes mellitus, in Popper H, Schaffner F (eds.): *Progress in Liver Disease.* New York, Grune and Stratton, 1970, pp 371–407.

7. Editorial: Enzymes in the hepatic porphyrias. *Lancet* 2:121, 1972.

8. Stein JA, Tschudy DP: Acute intermittent porphyria: A clinical and biochemical study of 46 patients. *Medicine* 49:1–16, 1970.

9. Meyer UA, et al: Intermittent acute porphyria—demonstration of a genetic defect in porphobilinogen metabolism. *New Eng J Med* 286:1277–1282, 1972.

10. Waldo ED, Tobias H: Needle-like cytoplasmic inclusions in the liver in porphyria cutanae tarda. *Arch Path* 96:368–371, 1973.

11. Klatskin G, Bloomer JR: Birefringence of hepatic pigment deposits in erythropoietic protoporphyria: Specificity and sensitivity of polarization microscopy in the identification of hepatic protoporphyrin deposits. *Gastroenterology* 67:294–302, 1974.

12. Klion FM, Segal R, Schaffner F: The effect of altered thyroid function on the ultrastructure of the human liver. *Amer J Med* 50:317–324, 1971.

13. Baker A, Kaplan M, Wolfe H: Central congestive fibrosis of the liver in myxedema ascites. *Ann Intern Med* 77:927–929, 1972.

14. Hug G: Nonbilirubin genetic disorders of the liver, in Gen Ref No. 6, pp 21–71.

15. McAdams AJ, Hug G, Bove KE: Glycogen storage disease, types I to X: Criteria for morphologic diagnosis. *Human Path* 5:463–488, 1974.

16. Hsia YE: Inherited hyperammonemic syndromes. *Gastroenterology* 67:347–374, 1974.

17. Hoyumpa AM Jr, et al: Fatty liver: Biochemical and clinical considerations. *Amer J Dig Dis* 20:1142–1170, 1975.

18. Permanen A, Miettinen TA, Nikkila EA: Qualitative lipid analysis of human liver needle biopsy specimens. *Acta Med Scand* 186:149–150, 1969.

19. Laurell S, Lundquist A: Lipid composition of human liver biopsy specimens. *Acta Med Scand* 189:65–68, 1971.

20. Malagelada JR, et al: Effect of medium-chain triglycerides on liver fatty acid composition in alcoholics with or without cirrhosis. *Amer J Clin Nutrition* 26:738–743, 1973.

21. Morgan MH, et al: Medium chain triglycerides and hepatic encephalopathy. *Gut* 15:180–184, 1974.

22. Holzbach RT, et al: Hepatic lipid in morbid obesity: Assessment at and subsequent to jejunoileal bypass. *New Eng J Med* 296:296–299, 1974.

23. Drenick EJ, Simmons F, Murphy JF: Effect on hepatic morphology of treatment of obesity by fasting, reducing diets and small-bowel bypass. *New Eng J Med* 282:829–834, 1970.
24. Buchwald H, Lober PH, Varco RL: Liver biopsy findings in seventy-seven consecutive patients undergoing jejunoileal bypass for morbid obesity. *Amer J Surg* 127:48–52, 1974.
25. Moxley RT III, Pozefsky T, Lockwood DH: Protein nutrition and liver disease after jejunoileal bypass for morbid obesity. *New Eng J Med* 290:921–926, 1974.
26. Kern WH, et al: Fatty metamorphosis of the liver in morbid obesity. *Arch Path* 96:342–346, 1973.
27. Davidson CS: Malnutrition and fatty liver: Kwashiorkor, in Gen Ref No. 3, pp 130–134.
28. McLaren DS: The great protein fiasco. *Lancet* 2:93–96, 1974.
29. Combes B, Whalley PJ, Adams RH: Tetracycline and the liver, in Gen Ref No. 9, pp 589–596.
30. Bhagwat AG, Ross RC: Prednisolone-induced hepatic injury: Ultrastructural and biochemical changes in rabbits. *Arch Path* 91:483–492, 1971.

LIVER DISEASES DURING INFANCY AND CHILDHOOD

15

The spectrum of liver disorders occurring during infancy and childhood resembles that in adulthood. The exception is the increased incidence of congenital conditions and infections in the pediatric age group. Hyperbilirubinemia and cholestasis are early manifestations, while portal hypertension and liver failure appear somewhat later. Liver disease in the early period of life may be classified on the basis of the age predilection (Table 15.1).[1,2]

Table 15.1. Classification of liver diseases based on age predilection.

I. Liver disease during the neonatal period (first four weeks of life).
  A. Unconjugated hyperbilirubinemia due to:
    1. Slow maturation of glucuronyl transferase enzyme, or Y and Z protein; "physiological jaundice" of newborn; hyperbilirubinemia of newborn
    2. Inhibition of conjugation: breast fed infants; transient familial neonatal hyperbilirubinemia (Lucey-Driscoll syndrome)
    3. Deficiency of red blood cell enzymes, eg, glucose-6-phosphate dehydrogenase deficiency, pyruvate kinase deficiency
    4. Sepsis
    5. Drugs, eg, vitamin K analogs (Synkayvite) primaquine, sulfamethoxypyridazine (Kynex), novobiocin
    6. Interruption of the enterohepatic circulation, eg, pyloric stenosis
    7. Hypothyroidism; infants of mothers with diabetes mellitus
    8. Hemolysis due to maternal-fetal blood group incompatibility: Rh, ABO, and other red cell antigen systems
  B. Conjugated hyperbilirubinemia due to:
    1. RH isoimmunization (inspissated bile syndrome)
    2. Idiopathic neonatal hemosiderosis
  C. Cholestasis
    1. Neonatal hepatitis
    2. Atresia of bile ducts, extrahepatic and intrahepatic
    3. Congenital infections: rubella, syphilis, cytomegalic virus, toxoplasmosis
    4. Other infections: herpes simplex, coxsackie B, varicella, listeria, viral hepatitis

Table 15.1. Classification of liver diseases based on age predilection. (*Cont.*)

    5. Sepsis

    6. Metabolic diseases: galactosemia, tyrosinemia

    7. Genetic disorders: Down's syndrome, trisomy 17-18 (E), familial intrahepatic cholestasis (Byler's disease)

    8. Neonatal, recurrent cholestasis with lymphedema (Norwegian-type hereditary cholestasis)

    9. Idiopathic

II. Liver disease in older infants and children

  A. Acute hepatitis

    1. Viral hepatitis, virus A and B

    2. Other viral infections

    3. Drug-induced

  B. Chronic hepatitis

    . Chronic active hepatitis

    Chronic hepatitis in Wilson's disease

  C. Hyperbilirubinemias

    1. Unconjugated: Gilbert's disease, Crigler-Najjar syndrome (types I and II)

    2. Conjugated: Dubin-Johnson syndrome, Rotor syndrome, recurrent intrahepatic cholestasis

  D. Reye's syndrome (fatty liver with encephalopathy)

  E. Cirrhosis

    1. Primary

      a. Galactosemia

      b. Hereditary fructose intolerance

      c. Wilson's disease

      d. Chronic active hepatitis

      e. Fanconi's disease

      f. Indian childhood cirrhosis

      g. Congenital hepatic fibrosis, with or without polycystic kidney disease

      h. Alpha-1-antitrypsin deficiency

      i. Cystic fibrosis

    2. Secondary

      a. Biliary atresia

      b. Neonatal hepatitis

      c. Congenital infections: see above

  F. Tumors

    1. Benign: cavernous hemangioma, hemangioendothelioma, hamartoma

    2. Malignant: hepatocellular carcinoma, hepatoblastoma

    3. Metastatic: metastatic neuroblastoma

    4. Choledochus cyst

  G. Metabolic diseases (other than in E)

    1. The glycogeneoses (10 variants)

Table 15.1. Classification of liver diseases based on age predilection. (*Cont.*)

2. Lysosomal diseases with storage
3. Inherited disorders with hyperammonemia
4. Cholestatic syndromes[3]
   a. Paucity of intrahepatic biliary ducts
   b. Bile salt disorders
5. Familial hepatosteatosis
6. Hereditary lymphedema
7. Zellweger's syndrome (biliary dysgenesis)

Hyperbilirubinemia: Jaundice in the Newborn

The depth of jaundice in the newborn bears no constant relationship to the degree of hyperbilirubinemia. Unconjugated bilirubinemia imparts a bright yellow or orange color to the skin, whereas conjugated bilirubinemia gives the skin a greenish or muddy-yellow color. The temporal appearance of jaundice in the newborn provides diagnostic clues (Table 15.2).

Bilirubin levels in neonates are not affected by the previous use of oral contraceptives, maternal smoking habits, methods of infant feeding, or epidural analgesia.[4] Hyperbilirubinemia is associated with artificial interruption of pregnancy, induced by amniotomy and either oxytocin or prostaglandin E_2. Maturation of liver enzymes in the fetus occurs around the time of the spontaneous onset of labor. They may not develop to a comparable level when labor is artificially hastened. The surge of fetal cortisol production which accompanies spontaneous labor contributes to the induction of liver enzyme systems. Some of these enzymes are also induced by corticosteroids under experimental conditions.

Table 15.2. Differential diagnosis of jaundice in the newborn.

Appearance of jaundice	Likely disease
First 24 hours	Hemolysis due to Rh incompatibility
48 hours	Physiological jaundice
After 72 hours	Septicemia; congenital infections (rubella, toxoplasmosis)
After first week	Septicemia, biliary atresia, neonatal hepatitis

Physiological Jaundice of the Newborn

Fifty percent of full-term and most premature newborns have a mild unconjugated hyperbilirubinemia during the first 3–8 days of life. The serum bilirubin does not exceed 10 mg/dl in full-term newborns, or 15 mg/dl in the premature newborn. The mechanism for the hyper-bilirubinemia is attributed to delayed maturation of the glucuronyl trans-ferase conjugating enzyme, and the Y and Z binding proteins in hepatic cells. Another factor is the increased enterohepatic circulation of biliru-bin. In newborn infants, bilirubin is not completely reduced to urobilino-gens because of the limited number of enteric bacteria. Intestinal beta-glucuronidase within mucosal cells continues to deconjugate bilirubin. Excessive unconjugated bilirubin accumulates in the intestine, resulting in increased reabsorption and presenting an increased load on the liver.

Unconjugated Hyperbilirubinemia of Prematurity

This condition represents an exaggeration of the process responsible for physiological jaundice. Serum bilirubin exceeds 15 mg/dl and persists longer than eight days. The defect is similar to that mentioned for physiological jaundice, except that the delayed maturation of the con-jugating enzyme lasts even longer. The incidence of the disorder among full-term infants is about 5%, higher in premature infants, and even higher among Orientals. The significance of unconjugated hyperbilirubinemia is in the increased risk of kernicterus (Table 15.3).

Causative Factors of Jaundice in Newborns:
Circulating Inhibitors

Breast-milk jaundice.[5] In about 1% of breast-fed infants jaundice develops during the second week of life, reaching the peak by one month of age and receding thereafter gradually. The steroid, pregnane-$3(\alpha),20(\beta)$-diol, has been identified in the milk of the mothers. It inhibits

Table 15.3.   Relation of serum bilirubin level to the incidence of kernicterus.

Serum bilirubin concentration (mg/dl)	Kernicterus
10–18	0%
19–24	7%
25–29	30%
30–40	70%

hepatic glucuronyl transferase in several mammalian species but not in the adult human liver. The cause of breast-milk jaundice is not known. The unconjugated hyperbilirubinemia does not exceed the levels associated with kernicterus. Breast-milk jaundice is not a contraindication to breast feeding. The benign condition must be distinguished from the more serious and rarer disorder, transient familial neonatal hyperbilirubinemia, in which a circulating inhibitor of conjugation is also implicated.

Transient familial neonatal hyperbilirubinemia. Also known as Lucey-Driscoll syndrome, all infants of a mother show severe unconjugated hyperbilirubinemia in the first four days of life. The jaundice resolves during the second to third week of life. The inheritance of the disorder is not clear, although it appears to be familial. Kernicterus may occur as a complication. The basic defect is an inhibitor of glucuronyl transferase activity present in both maternal and infant sera. The nature of the inhibitor has not been identified.

Drug-induced

Drugs administered to pregnant women near term such as long-acting sulfa compounds, chloramphenicol, and novobiocin increase the risk of kernicterus for newborns. Infants with glucose-6-phosphate dehydrogenase deficiency, prevalent in certain races, are particularly susceptible. Prenatal drugs aggravate neonatal jaundice by inhibiting the glucuronyl transferase conjugating enzyme or by competing with carrier-mediated mechanisms of bilirubin disposal.

Interruption of the Enterohepatic Circulation

In pyloric stenosis and duodenal atresia intestinal contents do not reach the lower gut, resulting in a limited intestinal bacterial flora. Under normal conditions the bacteria reduce the bilirubin to urobilinogens. Instead, the conjugated bilirubin is deconjugated by intestinal beta-glucuronidase to the unconjugated pigment, which is subsequently reabsorbed to produce the unconjugated hyperbilirubinemia. Antibiotics which suppress the intestinal flora achieve a similar effect.

Hemolysis from Rh and ABO Incompatibilities

About 15% of Caucasian persons are Rh negative. Rh-negative women develop antibodies to minute amounts of fetal blood (Rh-positive antigen)

which enter maternal circulation during pregnancy. Fortunately, sensitization rarely occurs during the first pregnancy but in subsequent ones the
maternal antibodies may reach a high level, cross the placenta, and react
with fetal erythrocytes to cause hemolysis. Only 5% of Rh-negative
mothers have infants with hemolytic disease. This figure is declining due
to prevention with anti-D-gamma-globulin immunization injected into
mothers 72 hours after delivery. The hemolysis leads to a striking elevation of unconjugated bilirubin appearing within the first 24 hours of life,
and declining by the end of a week. The risk of kernicterus increases
appreciably when serum bilirubin concentration exceeds 20 mg/dl. Occasionally in newborns with hemolytic disease due to Rh incompatibility,
the hyperbilirubinemia persists and is associated with elevated, conjugated as well as unconjugated bilirubin. The jaundice may last 2–3 months
but usually resolves on its own. The intrahepatic cholestatic syndrome,
also known as inspissated bile syndrome, is confused with extrahepatic
biliary atresia, although evidence of biliary obstruction is seldom complete. The increase in conjugated bilirubin probably reflects hepatocellular injury rather than "overloading" with bile pigment.

Treatment of Hyperbilirubinemia

There are three methods available which reduce the frequency and severity of hyperbilirubinemia and avoid the complication of kernicterus:
phenobarbital therapy, phototherapy, and exchange transfusion.
Phenobarbital given to the mother before delivery and/or to the neonate
lowers the bilirubin level of the newborn, presumably by stimulating the
glucuronyl transferase enzyme. Two to five days elapse before the drug
effect is seen. The indications for the use of phenobarbital in the newborn
period are not well defined. The slow onset of action and its depression of
vitamin-K-dependent factors are some of the drug's disadvantages.

Phototherapy is another frequently employed prophylactic technique.
Neonates are placed in a chamber exposed to blue light. Monochromatic
light at the wavelength of 450 nm causes oxidation of bilirubin to more
polar mono- and dipyrrole derivatives, which are water-soluble and
weakly albumin-bound. Phototherapy also enhances hepatic uptake,
biliary secretion of unconjugated bilirubin, and renal excretion of the
pigment. A potential danger is that phototherapy obscures the underlying
cause. Without the jaundice, early signs of the disease can be missed.
Phototherapy is effective in reducing the incidence of serious hyperbilirubinemia among premature infants. Both phenobarbital therapy and
phototherapy have reduced the severity of hyperbilirubinemia and the
need for exchange transfusion. The indications, risks, and technique of

exchange transfusion are well worked out. It remains the most useful method for rapid removal of bilirubin in cases of extreme and dangerous hyperbilirubinemia.

Cholestasis in Newborns: Neonatal Hepatitis

Neonatal hepatitis refers to the idiopathic syndrome of prolonged cholestasis in neonates which shows a definable set of histological changes on liver biopsy.[2] Specific causes which may bring about a similar syndrome such as rubella, herpes simplex, varicella, cytomegalovirus, listeria, syphilis, coxsackie B, toxoplasmosis, and viral hepatitis are not included. The possibility that neonatal hepatitis may be caused by an unrecognized virus infection acquired in utero has not been excluded. This disease and biliary atresia account for 85% of cholestasis in the newborn period. Both probably occur with equal frequency. A familial incidence has been suggested for neonatal hepatitis, with an autosomal recessive mode of inheritance. An association with alpha-1-antitrypsin deficiency (Z-Z phenotype) is noted in 25–40% of the patients, all of whom may display an acute hepatitis-like illness or cirrhosis.[6]

The symptoms of neonatal hepatitis are indistinguishable from those of biliary atresia. Jaundice develops within the first 2–4 weeks of life and increases in intensity. It is accompanied by acholic stools. The infant often appears surprisingly well, but in some cases develops weight loss and lethargy and expires within a few weeks. The liver and sometimes the spleen become enlarged.

Hepatic tests show high aminotransferase activity (> 500 IU/l), serum bilirubin levels above 10 mg/dl, and other evidence of biliary obstruction. Liver histology shows giant cell transformation of hepatocytes and disorganization of liver cell cords. The overall lobular architecture is, however, preserved. Variable extramedullary hemopoiesis is found. Neonatal hepatitis is not easily distinguished from biliary atresia. Diagnosis rests on subtle differences revealed by laboratory and liver biopsy findings (Tables 15.4 and 5).[2,7] The numerous available procedures suggest that no single test is adequate. Biliary excretion of radioactive material and bile acid profile are among the more popular and promising tests. [131]I rose bengal uptake, a test for major duct patency, suffers from false positives. Serum bile acid determinations, especially the pattern before and after cholestyramine administration, appear to be a reliable method of distinguishing intrahepatic from extrahepatic cholestasis (see below).[8] Further experience is required to evaluate the value of the tests.

Table 15.4. Laboratory tests in the differential diagnosis of cholestasis in the newborn.[2,5]

Tests	Comment
Peripheral blood smear	One-fourth of neonatal hepatitis cases show hemolytic anemia with burr cells
Maternal and cord blood for HB$_S$Ag	Positive in viral B hepatitis
Cord IgM > 60 mg/dl	Indicative of in utero infection
Liver function tests	Complete resolution of jaundice within 3 months points to neonatal hepatitis
Urine:	
1. Positive reducing substance	Absence excludes galactosemia
2. Amino acid profile	Detects tyrosinemia
Sweat chlorides > 60 meq/l	Suggests cystic fibrosis
Positive LP-X test	10% of neonatal hepatitis give false positive
Serum alpha-fetoprotein[21]	90% positivity in neonatal hepatitis, and 90% negativity in biliary atresia
Skull x-ray	50% of congenital toxoplasmosis reveal intracranial calcifications
Long-bone films	Abnormalities present in congenital rubella
Upper GI series	Locates choledochus cyst or other rare anomaly
Red-cell peroxide hemolysis	Dependent on bile salt, and presence and absorption of vitamin E; lack of vitamin E enhances red cell to hemolysis; hemolysis greater in atresia than in neonatal hepatitis
Vitamin E absorption	Serum level increases in neonatal hepatitis but not in atresia
^{131}I rose bengal excretion:	
1. After phenobarbital pretreatment	Increases in hepatocellular disease but not in biliary atresia; effect due to phenobarbital stimulation of bile flow
2. After cholestyramine	Increases in neonatal hepatitis but not in atresia; the resin binds bile acids, reduces body pool of bile salts, and decreases cholestasis

Table 15.4. Laboratory tests in the differential diagnosis of cholestasis in the newborn.[2,5]

Tests	Comment
Serum bile acid pattern:	
1. After cholestyramine pretreatment	Resin binds chenodeoxycholate in gut preferentially; raises serum cholate to chenodeoxycholate ratio in hepatitis but not in atresia
2. After phenobarbital	Enhances bile flow and thus lowers serum bile salts in neonatal hepatitis but not in biliary atresia

Table 15.5. Comparison of histological features in neonatal hepatitis and biliary atresia.[2,7]

Histological features	Neonatal hepatitis	Biliary atresia
Giant cell transformation of hepatocytes	+++	++
Lobular disarray	++	+
Inflammation	Parenchymal = portal	Portal > parenchymal
Extramedullary hemopoiesis	+	+
Cholestasis		
1. Intracellular, canalicular	++	++
2. Bile duct	+	++
Duct proliferation	+	+++
1. Distortion	±	+++
2. Absence	No	Rare
Fibrosis		
1. Periportal	+	++
2. Cirrhosis	Rare	Not unusual
Hepatic artery: medial wall hypertrophy	++	+++

Treatment is empirical. Steroids have no therapeutic efficacy. Phenobarbital may provide temporary relief by decreasing serum bile acid levels.[9] Prognosis is grave: 25% of the patients die, 50% have residual liver damage, and 25% recover completely.

Biliary Atresia

Biliary atresia, neonatal hepatitis, and choledochal cyst probably represent variants of the same process, neonatal obstructive cholangiopathy.[10] The basic abnormality may involve a disorder of bile acid metabolism.[11] High levels of monohydroxy bile acids, synthesized by the fetal liver, and relative hepatic deficiency of sulfate conjugation (an important mechanism for detoxifying bile acids) may be responsible for the destruction of the fetal hepatobiliary system. In some cases, biliary atresia is associated secondarily with infectious diseases such as congenital rubella and cytomegalovirus disease, and with chromosomal abnormalities such as trisomy 17,18 and Down's syndrome. Association with congenital anomalies is also common, particularly cardiac malformations and polysplenia. Extrahepatic biliary atresia (EBA) outnumbers the intrahepatic form by a ratio of 5 or 6 to 1. EBA is said to occur in 1:8000–10,000 live births. Females are affected more often than males, with a distinct predominance among whites. A genetic predisposition is not noted, as in neonatal hepatitis. Several anatomic variations are possible: complete atresia from porta hepatis to duodenum which is most common, occurring in over 50% of cases; partial or segmental atresia; extrahepatic atresia with intrahepatic atresia. Jaundice and hepatomegaly are striking signs but are delayed during the first 2–3 weeks of life. Acholic stools and splenomegaly appear somewhat later. Growth and health may be maintained for the first three months, until portal hypertension and malabsorption supervene.

Laboratory data show a moderate anemia, initial serum bilirubin below 10 mg/dl which steadily rises, raised aminotransferase activity (not above 300 IU/l), and a moderately elevated alkaline phosphatase. Among diagnostic procedures, the ^{131}I rose bengal test provides useful information. False positives are recorded in 5–20% of cases, especially in those with severe intrahepatic cholestasis, regardless of the cause. Analysis of serum bile acid before and after cholestyramine administration provides a new, apparently diagnostic method for distinguishing extrahepatic from intrahepatic cholestasis. Infants with biliary atresia show a predominant chenodeoxycholate elevation in plasma in contrast to those with intrahepatic cholestasis who have mainly cholic acid in plasma.[8,12] Cholestyramine, an insoluble quaternary ammonium anion exchange resin, binds bile acids (preferentially chenodeoxycholic acid) in the duodenum, interrupting the enterohepatic circulation and secondarily stimulating hepatic synthesis. Patients with intrahepatic cholestasis show a marked response to cholestyramine by an increase of the cholic acid to chenodeoxycholic acid ratio; patients with biliary atresia or extrahepatic cholestasis with primarily chenodeoxycholate in plasma show little or no response. Phenobarbital also diminishes serum bile acids and bilirubin in infants with intrahepatic but not extrahepatic cholestasis. A liver biopsy used in conjunction with other procedures (Tables 15.4 and 5) affords a correct diagnosis in 80–90% of the patients.

Treatment is primarily surgical. A laparotomy is usually undertaken for diagnostic purposes and to salvage the 5% that have long-term postsurgical success. Only 10–15% of cases have a patent extrahepatic biliary duct suitable for anastomosis. Hepatic portoenterostomy (the Kasai operation) promotes biliary drainage in 90% of selected patients with extrahepatic biliary atresia.[13] A successful result is achieved only in infants under 12 weeks of age, who demonstrate microscopic ductules in the excised scarred portion of the extrahepatic bile duct. Early surgery is indicated because of the irreversibility of cirrhosis after the age of 12 weeks. Despite postoperative bile drainage, long-term survival and cure of the disease process are obtained in very few patients. Ascending cholangitis is the chief complication.

Intrahepatic Biliary Atresia

This subgroup is associated with several diseases: congenital rubella syndrome, trisomy 17-18 (E) and 21, and Byler's disease. Some cases may even follow from unresolved neonatal hepatitis. Patients appear with three modes of presentation: (1) prolonged jaundice indistinguishable from extrahepatic biliary atresia or neonatal hepatitis; (2) xanthoma and pruritus at 2–5 years of age after earlier jaundice has disappeared; and (3) normal serum bilirubin but elevated serum bile acids. It is not known how bilirubin is excreted in the patients. The course in all three groups is variable, although eventually hepatic fibrosis and portal hypertension occur. For unknown reasons, patients with both extrahepatic and intrahepatic biliary atresia fare better and live longer than those with extrahepatic block alone. Survival into the teenage years is not uncommon for those with intrahepatic biliary atresia.

Diagnosis is made primarily on liver biopsy. Portal ducts are either entirely absent or diminished in number and are hypoplastic. There is variable cholestasis, inflammation, and fibrosis (Table 15.5). Other hepatic and laboratory tests show similar abnormalities as for extrahepatic biliary atresia (Table 15.4). Treatment consists of cholestyramine for control of pruritus, vitamins and medium-chain fatty acids for correction of the loss by steatorrhea, and phenobarbital to lower bile pigment and salt.

Congenital Disorders:
Rubella Syndrome

Fetal tissues are particularly susceptible to damage by rubella virus infection in utero. The risk of serious disturbance in embryogenesis for the fetus is 50% when the mother acquires the infection during the first trimester of pregnancy. The resultant congenital syndrome consists of low birth weight, cataracts, microcephaly, congenital heart disease, thrombocytopenia, and evidence of organ infection such as hepatitis, pneumonitis and, and osteomyelitis. Jaundice appears within the first two days of life. Hepatosplenomegaly is usual. Hepatic tests show serum bilirubin and aminotransferase elevations. In the liver biopsy, cholestasis, giant cell reaction, focal necrosis, and persistent erythrohemopoiesis are observed. The features are indistinguishable from other forms of neonatal hepatitis. Diagnosis is substantiated by positive serologic tests for rubella antibody. About 20% of the infants die from the total effects of the syndrome. Surviving patients may show complete healing of the hepatitis. A few cases progress to cirrhosis.

Toxoplasmosis

This is an infrequent disease. Infection by the protozoa *Toxoplasma gondii* in utero is usually harmless, and rarely fatal, but may sometimes produce the congenital disease. Encephalomyelitis, chorioretinitis, and hydrocephalus are common features of the syndrome, and hepatitis is a less common component. Jaundice develops within the first 24 hours, along with hepatosplenomegaly. Hemolysis may contribute toward the jaundice. Liver histology reveals portal tract inflammation and macrophages containing the toxoplasma. Prognosis is poor.

Cytomegalic Virus Disease

Although the infection is common among the general public, congenital cytomegalic virus disease as a result of transplacental transmission from mother to fetus is uncommon. Jaundice and hepatosplenomegaly are invariable features at birth. Other findings include purpura, microcephaly, chorioretinitis, and intracranial calcification. Liver histology is indistinguishable from other causes of neonatal hepatitis. Intranuclear inclusions may be found in hepatocytes. Diagnosis rests on serological and virological tests. The virus can be isolated from the liver. Prognosis is generally poor, although mild or subclinical infections have a better outlook.

Herpes Simplex Infection

Primary infection by herpes virus hominis type 1 (simplex) is usually subclinical in early childhood. However, in newborns without protective maternal antibodies, a disseminated form occurs. The source of infection may be the mother, a relative, or a hospital attendant. The condition presents with jaundice, hepatosplenomegaly, and fever. The infant becomes weak and rapidly succumbs. Visible skin and mucous membrane lesions are generally absent. Diagnosis is made at autopsy when typical inclusion bodies are found in the liver and other visceral organs.

Syphilis

This septicemic condition is contracted by the fetus from an infected mother. The severity of the illness is quite variable. Some infants die in a few days, others show symptoms and signs months to years later. The early manifestations involve the liver, spleen, bone marrow, and central nervous system. Jaundice, hepatomegaly, anemia, and albuminuria stand out in the clinical presentation. In the liver teeming spirochetes are found. The lesions may eventually cause hepatic scarring and deformity. Treatment with penicillin prevents progression of late sequelae.

Liver Diseases of Older Infants: Heritable Hyperbilirubinemias

Gilbert's disease, Crigler-Najjar syndrome, Dubin-Johnson syndrome, Rotor syndrome, and recurrent intrahepatic cholestasis are all discussed in Chapter 5.

Reye's Syndrome[14,15]

Although Reye's syndrome (fatty liver with encephalopathy) may affect persons up to 15 years old, it is most common between ages 1 and 3. Typically, the child appears to be recovering from a prodromal illness of upper respiratory infection, when vomiting suddenly occurs. It is followed within 24 hours by central nervous system symptoms: irritability, restlessness, lethargy, convulsions, and coma. The course is rapid, with a high fatality rate. There are no focal neurologic signs, nor meningismus. Papilledema is unusual during the early phase. Hyperpnea is common. Mild to moderate hepatomegaly is detected in about half of the cases. Jaundice is often absent, or mild.

Biochemically, in contrast to other causes of fulminant hepatic failure, the serum bilirubin is normal or slightly elevated. Aminotransferase activity is elevated, prothrombin time prolonged, and blood ammonia levels increased. Hypoglycemia is common in patients under two years of age. A spinal tap yields a clear fluid with normal dynamics, normal cell count, sterile culture, normal protein content, and a low glucose concentration in the hypoglycemic child. Liver histology reveals diffuse small lipid deposits in all hepatocytes. Periportal necrosis, hemorrhage, and cholestasis are also commonly seen. Ultrastructural changes in the liver are not specific. In addition to the fat droplets, the endoplasmic reticulum appears hypertrophied. Microbodies increase in numbers. Mitochondria are distorted by swelling and pleomorphism. At autopsy fat is also found in the kidney, heart, and pancreas. The brain becomes grossly edematous. There is patchy, nonspecific, cortical necrosis.

Differential diagnosis includes the general heading of infections, meningitis, and encephalitis, and other causes of fulminant hepatic failure. Liver function tests should be done in all patients with encephalopathy under the age of 15. Reye's syndrome should be suspected when the patients show high aminotransferase activity with little or no jaundice.[16] A liver biopsy is essential for confirmatory histology. Early diagnosis and medical care have reduced the fatality rate from 50% to 20%.[16]

Treatment includes therapy for hepatic failure, supportive care of the comatose state, and correction of electrolyte imbalance (usually a metabolic acidosis). A prime objective in management is the control of the cerebral edema. Reduction of the increased intracranial pressure by the usage of glycerol and mannitol improves the chances of survival. Therapeutic lowering of the blood ammonia level does not immediately alter the neurologic status. This is different from the response obtained in comatose patients with fulminant hepatic necrosis.

Speculations about etiology abound. The many hypotheses may be grouped under three headings: (1) Viral infections. Herpes, influenza, varicella, coxsackie, echo, and adenovirus groups may all be identified in some but not all cases. The association between influenza and Reye's syndrome has been documented in an epidemic. (2) Toxins. These include aflatoxin, hypoglycin in ackee fruit (cause of Jamaica vomiting sickness), insecticides, pesticides, and salicylates. Epidemiologic evidence linking aflatoxin to encephalopathy in Thailand appears impressive. None of these agents has found wide acceptance as a causative agent. (3) Inborn errors of metabolism. Disturbance of the urea-cycle pathways has some features in common with Reye's syndrome, particularly ornithine transcarbamylase deficiency. The finding in some cases with high serum concentrations of glutamate, alanine, and lysine, low concentrations of arginine, and absence or very low levels of citrulline suggests a deficiency of mitochondrial ornithine transcarbamylase. Citrulline supplements provided to patients result in a decrease of plasma ammonia. About half of the patients with Reye's syndrome show reduced activity of the two mitochondrial enzymes, ornithine transcarbamylase and carbamyl phosphate synthetase, but the three other cytoplasmic enzymes of the urea cycle are normal.[17] The decreased enzyme activities explain the low plasma citrulline, the product of ornithine transcarbamylase, and the elevated blood ammonia, the substrate of carbamyl phosphate synthetase, seen in the disease. Other conditions including the inherited deficiencies of the urea cycle, aspirin poisoning, and alcoholic liver injury do not show this pattern of low mitochondrial but normal cytoplasmic urea-cycle enzymes. The mitochondrial enzymes are reduced during the early stage of Reye's syndrome, and return to normal during the subsequent course. Viral illness in patients with transiently acquired or partial congenital deficiencies of the urea-cycle enzymes may precipitate Reye's syndrome.[18]

It is clear that Reye's syndrome in the United States is not a homogeneous entity but includes at least two subgroups: those with a viral association, and those with an underlying metabolic defect.

Cirrhosis in Newborns

Galactosemia (Chapter 9), Wilson's disease (Chapter 13), congenital hepatic fibrosis (Chapters 9 and 17), polycystic disease (Chapter 17), alpha-1-antitrypsin deficiency (Chapter 9), and cystic fibrosis (Chapter 9) are fully discussed in their respective chapters.

Indian childhood cirrhosis.[19] Also known as infantile (biliary) cirrhosis, the disease appears widespread in India. It affects infants from the first to the third year of life, involving both sexes equally, but sparing the very poor or malnourished. Most studies point to a familial occurrence of the disease. The cause is unknown. Nutritional deficiency, toxins, genetic factors, and viral hepatitis have been variously incriminated. Clinically, the illness may begin like a hepatitis but more often it is insidious with lassitude, low fever, gastrointestinal upset, and abdominal distention.

The liver and spleen become enlarged, and jaundice is present. Liver function tests are abnormal, showing hypoalbuminemia and hypergammaglobulinemia. The alpha-fetoprotein test may be positive.[20] The presence of HB_sAg and smooth muscle antibodies in some cases suggests viral hepatitis as an antecedent cause. Liver histology reveals a hepatitis-like picture in the early stages with patchy necrosis and diffuse mononuclear cell inflammation. Steatosis is not a feature. In progressive cases, fibrosis leads to the development of micronodular cirrhosis. Cholestasis and Mallory body hyalin in hepatocytes are variably present. Death is usual within a year or two of diagnosis.

Tumors.   Tumors and cysts are discussed fully in Chapter 17.

REFERENCES

1. Gellis SS: Jaundice and liver disease in infancy and childhood, in Gen Ref No. 5, pp 47–54.
2. Silverman A, Roy CC, Cozzetto FJ: Pediatric clinical gastroenterology. St. Louis, C V Mosby Co, 1975, pp 400–443.
3. Brough AJ, Bernstein J: Conjugated hyperbilirubinemia in early infancy. *Human Path* 5:507–516, 1974.
4. Calder AA, et al: Increased bilirubin levels in neonates after induction of labour by intravenous prostaglandin E_2 or oxytocin. *Lancet* 2:1339–1342, 1974.
5. Johnson JD: Neonatal nonhemolytic jaundice. *New Eng J Med* 292:194–197, 1975.
6. Editorial: Alpha-1-antitrypsin deficiency and liver disease in childhood. *Brit Med J* 1:758, 1973.
7. Brough AJ, Bernstein J: Liver biopsy in the diagnosis of infantile obstructive jaundice. *Pediatrics* 43:519–526, 1969.
8. Javitt NB, et al: Cholestatic syndromes in infancy: Diagnostic value of serum bile acid pattern and cholestryamine administration. *Ped Res* 7:119–125, 1973.
9. Stiehl A, Thaler MM, Admirand WH: The effects of phenobarbital on bile salts and bilirubin in patients with intrahepatic and extrahepatic cholestasis. *New Eng J Med* 286:858–861, 1972.
10. Landing BH: Protracted obstructive jaundice in infancy with emphasis on neonatal hepatitis, biliary atresia and choledochal cyst, in Gen Ref No. 1, Part B, pp 821–849.
11. Jenner RE, Howard ER: Unsaturated monohydroxy bile acids as a cause of idiopathic obstructive cholangiopathy. *Lancet* 2:1073–1075, 1975.
12. Murphy GM, Signer E: Bile acid metabolism in infants and children. *Gut* 15:151–163, 1974.
13. Lilly JR, Altman RP: Hepatic portoenterostomy (the Kasai operation) for biliary atresia. *Surgery* 78:76–86, 1975.

14. Editorial: Encephalopathy and fatty degeneration of viscera. *Lancet* 2:445–446, 1974.
15. Thaler MM: Reye's syndrome. *Viewpoints Dig Dis* 6:3, 1974.
16. Partin JC: Reye's syndrome (encephalopathy and fatty liver): Diagnosis and treatment. *Gastroenterology* 69:511–518, 1975.
17. Snodgrass PJ, DeLong GR: Urea-cycle enzyme deficiencies and an increased nitrogen load producing hyperammonemia in Reye's syndrome. *New Eng J Med* 294:855–860, 1976.
18. Thaler MM, Hoogenraad NJ, Boswell M: Reye's syndrome due to a novel protein-tolerant variant of ornithine-transcarbamylase deficiency. *Lancet* 2:438–440, 1974.
19. Nayak NC, Ramalingaswami V: Indian childhood cirrhosis. *Clin Gastroenterology* 4:333–349, 1975.
20. Chandra RK: Immunological picture in Indian childhood cirrhosis. *Lancet* 1:537–540, 1970.
21. Zeltzer PM, et al: Differentiation between neonatal hepatitis and biliary atresia by measuring serum-alpha-fetoprotein. *Lancet* 1:373–375, 1974.

HEPATIC GRANULOMAS AND INFECTIONS

16

HEPATIC GRANULOMAS

Infectious diseases of the liver are often diagnosed by means of a liver biopsy. Many of the lesions fall into the category of hepatic granuloma (Table 16.1). Not all diseases associated with hepatic granuloma are, however, infectious. Hepatic granuloma is not an uncommon entity, accounting for 5% of all liver biopsy lesions.[1,2] Four diseases—sarcoidosis, tuberculosis, schistosomiasis and primary biliary cirrhosis—account for 70–80% of all cases with granulomatous hepatitis (the term is used interchangeably with hepatic granuloma) in the United States and Europe.[3] Ordinarily, diagnosis is established by clinical examination, positive culture, chest film, and lymph node and liver histology. In 10–20% of the patients, the cause cannot be determined after an extensive and thorough workup.[4] These patients deserve a trial of antituberculosis drugs to eradicate possible latent infectious foci. A few patients in the group fail to respond to drugs. The cases not infrequently present with a fever of unknown origin.[5] Diagnosis is apparently never established for these rare conditions. If evidence of inflammatory liver disease persists, a trial with corticosteroids may be effective in suppressing both the symptoms and hepatic abnormalities.

Liver biopsy findings are similar for the various types of hepatic granulomas, although subtle changes may indicate some of the causes (Table 16.2; Fig. 16.1). An etiologic diagnosis often requires that the infectious organism be identified. A fragment of fresh and uncontaminated liver should be cultured in all cases of suspected granulomatous disease. Serial sections of the liver specimen should be prepared for examination, especially for locating granulomas which are scarce. Caseation necrosis is not limited to tuberculosis (present in 20–30% of cases); it can also be observed in tularemia, brucellosis, most mycoses, syphilis, and Wegener's granulomatosis. The acid-fast bacilli (AFB) of tuberculosis are demonstrable by staining or by culture isolation in about 15% of cases. AFB are not seen in the liver when the number of organisms is less than 10,000 per gram of tissue. Biochemically, hepatic granulomas,

Table 16.1. Causes of granulomatous hepatitis. [1,2]

---

1. Infection
   a. Bacterial:
      Tularemia, brucellosis, granuloma inguinale, melioidosis, mycobacterial
      diseases (typical and atypical tuberculosis, leprosy)
   b. Fungal:
      Histoplasmosis, coccidiomycosis, North and South American
      blastomycosis, aspergillosis, actinomycosis, nocardiosis, cryptococcosis,
      candidiasis
   c. Parasitic:
      Ascariasis, toxocariasis, schistosomiasis, ancylostomiasis, amebiasis
   d. Rickettsial:
      Q fever
   e. Spirochetal:
      Congenital, secondary, and tertiary syphilis
   f. Viral:
      Cytomegalovirus, lymphopathia venereum, infectious mononucleosis
2. Hypersensitivity
   a. Berylliosis
   b. Drugs: BCG immunotherapy;[21] sulfonamides, phenylbutazone, penicillin,
      diazepam, diphenylhydantoin, halothane, allopurinol, quinidine,
      methyldopa
3. Foreign body:
   Talc granulomas in drug addict hepatitis; silicone fragments in liver, following
   prosthetic heart valve surgery (ball valve variance disease);[22] copper
   sulfate-induced granulomas associated with vineyard sprayer's lung.[23]
4. Unknown:
   Primary biliary cirrhosis; sarcoidosis, Hodgkin's disease and other
   lymphomas, Wegener's granulomatosis, allergic granulomatosis, rheumatoid
   arthritis, chronic granulomatous disease of childhood

---

like other infiltrative diseases of the liver, often display striking elevation
of serum alkaline phosphatase out of proportion to the aminotransferase
increase. The obstructive profile is found especially with sarcoidosis,
syphilis, and infectious mononucleosis.

Sarcoidosis

Sarcoidosis is defined as a multisystemic, apparently noninfectious
granulomatous disease of unknown etiology. Epithelioid granulomas are
commonly found in hilar lymph nodes, lung, liver, spleen, skin, and
phalangeal bones. The Kveim skin test, using an antigen derived from a
sarcoid spleen, is frequently positive, while tuberculin sensitivity and
other indicators of cellular immunity are notably depressed. Hypergam-

Table 16.2. Pathological features of hepatic granulomata.

Disease	Features
Tuberculosis[24,25]	Paucity of granulomata compared to sarcoidosis; scantiness of giant cells and mild surrounding round cell infiltrate; absence of reticulum; caseation necrosis or AFB absent in 50% of cases
Sarcoidosis	More numerous than in tuberculosis; contains many giant cells; well-demarcated surrounding round cell inflammation; presence of paraamyloid
Leprosy	Monocellular granulomas composed of foam cells or foamy Kupffer cells in lepromatous form
Q fever	Rod-shaped fragments in periphery of granuloma, best seen with Lendrun's stain for fibrin
Schistosomiasis	Reactions around ova or chitinous material
Drug-addict hepatitis	Talc granulomas (birefringent material)
Ball valve variance disease	Silicone crystalline fragments

maglobulinemia and hypercalcuria are other important laboratory findings.

Diagnosis is based not only on positive clinical and laboratory features but also on the exclusion of other diseases. The finding of hepatic granuloma, present in 75% of patients, affords a valuable means of confirmation, especially if skin or lymph node lesions are not available. Twenty percent of cases have hepatic manifestations: mild jaundice, pruritus, and hepatomegaly. Serum alkaline phosphatase is strikingly elevated. Sarcoidosis of the liver can proceed to chronic liver disease with marked hepatic dysfunction.[6] Severe hepatic destruction and fibrosis are found on liver biopsy. In the late stages, separation from PBC may be difficult. In Europe, the syndrome of hepatic granuloma and positive Kveim test is considered an early manifestation of sarcoidosis and is treated with corticosteroids.

Tuberculosis[7]

The liver is commonly involved in the different forms of tuberculosis. In acute primary tuberculosis, hepatic granulomas are found in about 55% of cases, usually with little or no evidence of liver dysfunction. AFB are identified in the liver sections by staining or by culture in 10% of the

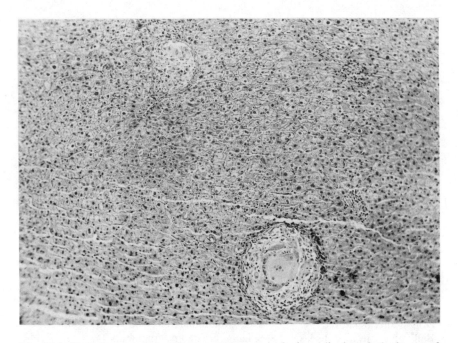

Fig. 16.1. Hepatic granuloma. Two granulomatous foci are displayed, the larger of which contains a central multinucleated giant cell, peripheral epithelioid cells, and lymphocytes. H and E, X100.

patients. The incidence of hepatic lesions is higher in acute miliary tuberculosis, with almost 100% of the biopsies showing granulomas and with demonstrable AFB in 60% of the specimens. Hepatic granulomas are observed in 80% of patients with extrapulmonary tuberculosis and without evidence of pulmonary disease. In chronic pulmonary tuberculosis, the incidence of hepatic granulomas falls to about 25%. Nonspecific histologic features such as Kupffer cell hyperplasia, fatty change, focal hepatocellular necrosis, and inflammation are much more common. AFB are rarely found in the liver. Evidence of hepatic dysfunction is frequent, including delayed BSP excretion and slight hypergammaglobulinemia. However, indexes of parenchymal damage such as serum bilirubin and aminotransferase remain normal. Primary hepatic tuberculosis, much discussed in the past, does not exist as an entity separate from liver involvement in acute miliary tuberculosis.

Syphilis

Syphilis of the liver is rare today. It was once thought that syphilis was a common cause of cirrhosis, but this hypothesis is no longer held. Many of the cases described as cirrhosis following syphilis were probably due to concurrent viral hepatitis or chronic alcoholism.[8] *Treponema pallidum,* the infectious spirochete, may involve the liver in all three stages of syphilis.

Congenital syphilis.   Transplacental crossing of the spirochetes leads to hepatic invasion in teeming numbers, with subsequent liver cell destruction. Should the infant survive, hepatic fibrosis may supervene. Mild jaundice and hepatomegaly are apparent but overshadowed by other manifestations of congenital syphilis.

Secondary syphilis.   Bacteremia in the early stage of syphilis produces liver lesions in about 10% of patients.[9] Clinical features consist of jaundice and an enlarged and tender liver, which subsides after penicillin therapy. The biochemical pattern is characterized by an abnormally high serum alkaline phosphatase (10 × normal) disproportionate to the increase of serum bilirubin and aminotransferase activity.[10] Serum IgG and IgM elevations resemble those found in acute viral hepatitis. Liver histology reveals a moderate inflammation with both polymorphonuclear cells and lymphocytes, hepatocellular disarray, and occasional necrotic areas. Cholestasis is usually absent. In half the cases, spirochetes could be seen in the biopsy specimen.[9]

Tertiary syphilis.   Hepar lobatum is the characteristic gross hepatic deformity. Microscopically, gummas, consisting of caseation necrosis surrounded by fibrous capsules, are deposited in the liver. The resultant cycle of healing and fibrosis yields deep scars and irregular lobulations. The basic lobular pattern of the liver is not disturbed and hence the lesion is not a true cirrhosis.

Infectious Mononucleosis[11]

This acute infection, caused by the Epstein-Barr virus (EBV), is characterized clinically by fever, pharyngitis, and lymphadenopathy, and by laboratory findings of leukocytosis with an absolute lymphocytosis, positive heterophil antibody (antisheep red cells), and EBV antibody response. Confusion with viral hepatitis is possible because in 10% of the patients tender hepatomegaly is present, 5% develop mild and transient jaundice, and 90% have abnormal liver function tests. The abnormalities include mild serum aminotransferase elevation, BSP retention, and raised alkaline phosphatase. Differentiation from viral hepatitis is usually not difficult for the average case, but may be impossible if the hepatic man-

Table 16.3. Comparison between infectious mononucleosis and viral hepatitis.[11]

	Infectious mononucleosis	Viral hepatitis
Etiology	EBV	Hepatitis A or B virus
Fever	Present	Present
Pharyngitis	Present	Absent
Lymphadenopathy	Conspicuous	Inconspicuous
Hepatomegaly	Present in 10%	Present
Splenomegaly	Present in 50%	Mild or absent
Jaundice	5% incidence; mild, transient	Striking and persistent
White cell count	Increased; absolute lymphocytosis with atypical forms	Decreased; relative lymphocytosis
Heterophile antibody	Not absorbed by guinea pig kidney cells	May be present; absorbed by guinea pig kidney cells
Test for HAAb or HB_SAg	Absent	Positive
Liver biopsy	Mononuclear cell infiltration with atypical forms, spotty necrosis	Mononuclear cell inflammation, centrolobular necrosis

ifestations of infectious mononucleosis are severe or prolonged (Table 16.3). Morphologically, the liver shows dense mononuclear cell accumulations in portal tracts and parenchyma. Atypical lymphocytes are included, mimicking the infiltrating cells of chronic lymphocytic leukemia. Small focal hepatocellular necrosis and acidophilic bodies are seen, but lack the centrolobular distribution and diffuseness encountered in viral hepatitis. Cholestasis is usually absent or mild. In other respects, hepatic changes in both viral diseases are exceedingly similar. There is no specific treatment for infectious mononucleosis.

Other viral diseases:

Virus	Clinical features	Liver pathology
Yellow fever: B arbovirus transmitted by mosquitoes	Jaundice mild, hemorrhages due to DIC rather than hepatic failure	Characteristic midzonal necrosis, Councilman bodies, intranuclear viral inclusions present

Other viral diseases (*continued*):

Virus	Clinical features	Liver pathology
Cytomegalo-virus[12]	1. In adults, latent infection	Hepatitis or cirrhosis; intra-nuclear in-clusions seen
	2. Congenital infection usually severe, jaundice and hepatosplenomegaly	Neonatal hepatitis
	3. In compromised host, disseminated course; DIC related to hepatic failure	Hepatitis
	4. May cause per-fusion syndrome	Hepatitis
Rubella	Cataracts, micro-cephaly, con-genital heart disease, hepato-splenomegaly	Giant cell hepa-titis, ? biliary atresia, cirrhosis
"Marburg virus" hepatitis, transmitted by monkeys[13]	Hemorrhages prom-inent due to DIC, high fatality rate	Focal necrosis, steatosis, few cytoplasmic in-clusions, portal inflammation
Herpes simplex[14]	1. In newborn, dis-seminated ful-minant disease with fever, jaundice and hepatosplenomegaly	
	2. In compromised adult host, diffuse infection	Hepatitis, dif-fuse necrosis and inflamma-tion, intra-nuclear inclu-sions common

BACTERIAL INFECTIONS

Leptospirosis

Over 20 serotypes of *Leptospira* are responsible for this disease. Clini-cally, two phases are recognized. The first phase consists of leptospiral dissemination in blood and cerebrospinal fluid, characterized by fever, headaches, and myalgia. The second, or immune phase, appearing after the first week, correlates with the appearance of circulating IgM antibodies. The symptoms are variable but include ocular and central nervous manifestations. A specific variant, Weil's syndrome or disease, is defined as severe leptospirosis, usually due to *L. icterohemorrhagiae*. It is characterized by jaundice, azotemia, hemorrhage, and high fever. Either the hepatic or renal disturbance may predominate. The hepatic manifestations consist of jaundice, right-upper-quadrant tenderness, hepatomegaly, and laboratory findings of mild serum bilirubin increase, moderate elevation of aminotransferase activity, and mild increase of alkaline phosphatase. Liver histology does not parallel clinical severity. There is variable but mild hepatic cell necrosis, slight portal inflammation, and prominent cholestasis. Renal manifestations consist of hematuria, proteinuria, and azotemia. Serious damage to the kidneys takes form as an acute tubular necrosis. The hemorrhagic phenomenon occurs in various organs, attributed to capillary injury.

Diagnosis rests on the culture of organisms from blood or CSF during the first phase of illness, from urine during the second stage, or on serologic testing. Prognosis correlates with the degree of jaundice, varying 15–40%. Drug therapy with penicillin or tetracycline is effective, but must be given early.

Other infectious diseases:

Disease	Clinical features	Liver pathology
Malaria	During acute attacks, mild tender hepatomegaly with variable mild jaundice; abnormal liver tests may be due to toxic effect of plasmodium and not liver damage	Centrolobular necrosis in acute infection of *P. falciparum*; in chronic infection, Kupffer cell increase, round cell infiltration, heavy iron-positive malaria pigment present
Kala-azar, protozoa transmitted by sandflies	Hepatomegaly	Kupffer cell hyperplasia with intracellular Leishman-Donovan bodies
Brucellosis (undulant fever)	Mild tender hepatomegaly sometimes	Granulomas with gram-negative rods; rarely caseation necrosis; may be calcified in chronic cases
Salmonellosis	Jaundice and hepatomegaly during bacteremic phase, in ⅓ of patients	Nonspecific triaditis and liver cell injury

Other infectious diseases (*continued*):

Disease	*Clinical features*	*Liver pathology*
Leprosy	Hepatic signs and symptoms absent	Granulomas with rare or no AFB seen in tuberculoid leprosy; foam cells stuffed with AFB present in lepromatous leprosy

PARASITIC DISEASES

Schistosomiasis[15,16]

Of the three blood trematodes, *Schistosoma mansoni* and *S. japonicum* are more likely to affect the liver than the third member, *S. haematobium*. *S. mansoni* is most common in the western hemisphere; *S. japonicum* predominates in Asia and Southeast Asia; and *S. haematobium* is prevalent in the Middle East and Africa. The adult worm matures in the portal venous system of the liver, where mating also occurs. After copulation, the male and female worms migrate to the small mesenteric veins or, in the case of *S. haematobium*, to the capillaries of the urinary bladder and other pelvic organs. The deposited eggs secrete proteolytic enzymes which destroy the intestinal mucosa before the eggs are excreted into the feces. After reaching fresh water, the eggs hatch liberating ciliated miracidia. The embryos with a life span of 6–8 hours must enter the appropriate snail intermediary host, where asexual reproduction transforms the miracidia into infective cercariae. The cercariae are released into fresh water, and must penetrate human skin within two days or die. In humans, the final hosts, they become schistosmula, gain entrance into the peripheral venules, traverse the right heart and lungs, then enter the systemic circulation to reach the portal veins, where the cycle is repeated.

The chronic, asymptomatic carrier state is much more common than the symptomatic stage. Host susceptibility and high worm burden are determinant factors. Clinically, three stages of infection are recognized. The first stage of cutaneous cercarial penetration is indicated by itching. The second stage of ova dissemination may be manifested by rash, fever, and eosinophilia. The third stage reflects the chronic tissue effects of ova deposition in the intestine, urinary bladder, liver, lungs, and central nervous system. The tissue damage is caused by the ova and its secretions. A soluble egg antigen has been identified which induces a granulomatous hypersensitivity. The intense inflammation, tissue destruction, and granuloma formation occur on the basis of host cell-mediated immune reactions. Intravascular obstruction and fibrosis are the other important pathological changes. Living adult worms by themselves elicit little tissue reaction, except when they die.

Acute schistosomiasis is usually due to *S. japonicum* because the female worm lays the greatest number of eggs compared to the other species. The clinical presentation (Katayama disease) resembles serum sickness. The chronic form becomes manifested as either urinary obstruction or portal hypertension. The liver is involved as part of the hepatosplenic fibrosis. Initially, there is hepatosplenomegaly, but with the passage of years the liver becomes small while the splenomegaly persists. Signs of portal hypertension appear. Pathologically, the early hepatic lesions consist of portal granulomas surrounding the ova. *S. mansoni* eggs are oval with a lateral spine; *S. japonicum* eggs are smaller, with a minute lateral hook; those of *S. haematobium* have a terminal spine.

The late fibrotic stage is characterized by scarring of the finer and intermediate portal venous radicals with distortion of the triads. The classical pattern of pipestem portal fibrosis is recognized by the lobulated capsular surface and the dense portal scarring. This produces a typical presinusoidal type of portal hypertension. As little or no necrosis occurs, hepatocellular function is good. Biochemically, there is little evidence of hepatic dysfunction except for raised serum alkaline phosphatase or mild BSP retention. Hepatosplenic schistosomiasis may be complicated by chronic glomerulonephritis occurring on an immunologic basis, or by protracted *Salmonella* bacteremia. Serological tests include the cercarial slide flocculation procedure. Rectal and liver biopsies are helpful in diagnosis. Ninety percent of patients with rectal eggs have hepatic granulomas. Hepatosplenic schistosomiasis differs from most types of cirrhosis in several important respects.[16] First, the mortality rate of bleeding varices is much lower than in cirrhosis. The liver does not decompensate before or after the variceal hemorrhage. Hepatic function is maintained in the presence of a decrease in portal blood flow because of compensatory increase in hepatic arterial flow. Second, unlike cirrhosis, ascites is uncommon since the portal hypertension is presinusoidal in type. Third, there is an increased incidence of hepatitis B antigenemia in the decompensated stage of hepatosplenic schistosomiasis. The clinical and histologic features of the lesions are indistinguishable from chronic active hepatitis due to other causes. Fourth, hepatosplenic schistosomiasis causes a preferential hypertrophy of the left lobe. The reason is not known.

Treatment is based on drugs such as the trivalent antimony compounds and niridazole. Not all infections require drug therapy, nor is complete eradication of the worms a necessary procedure. Filtration by extracorporeal perfusion for eggs remains an experimental procedure.

Echinococcosis

Also known as hydatid cyst disease, echinococcosis is common in sheep-raising countries where dogs, the definitive hosts, have access to sheep carcasses. Humans, sheep, and cattle are intermediate hosts for the larval (cyst) stage of *Echinococcus granulosus*. A sylvatic focus exists in Alaska and Canada, where wolves act as the definitive hosts. The adult tapeworm resides in the small intestines of canines and excretes eggs from the terminal segments, or proglottids, into the feces. After ingestion by the intermediate hosts, the embryos escape from the eggs, penetrate the intestinal mucosa, enter the portal circulation and are carried to the liver, where they develop into adult cysts. The liver entraps about 70% of eventual hydatid cysts, the lungs 20%, and the remaining 10% passes to bone, spleen, and brain.

Most cysts are unilocular, composed of an external laminated layer and an inner nucleated germinal layer. A third, outermost coat is formed by granulation tissue and fibrosis derived from the host. The peripheral layer frequently becomes calcified. Fluid fills the cyst lumen. The germinal layer gives rise to brood capsules from which scolices develop. The capsules may burst releasing the scolices, forming "hydatid sand." The cycle becomes complete when the dog eats the hydatid cyst of sheep liver. The scolices are released in the canine intestine and develop into adult worms. A second species, *E. multilocularis,* has a similar life cycle, except that small rodents serve as intermediate hosts. *E. multilocularis* is more invasive and destructive than *E. granulosus.* The hydatid cyst in this case is always multilocular.

Hepatic lesions are usually asymptomatic. After years, hepatomegaly and abdominal pains may appear. The enlarging cyst may compress ducts to produce jaundice. An uncomplicated cyst is often silent and presents as an incidental finding at autopsy. Complications include rupture into the peritoneal cavity, biliary ducts, and lungs; secondary infection with bacteria; and anaphylactoid reaction due to release of cyst fluid. Serological tests, especially the indirect hemagglutination test, appear sensitive and specific. The skin (Casoni) test has limited usefulness because of false positives. Occasionally, hepatic calcification can be visualized on a flat plate of the abdomen. Isotopic scanning of the liver should be done for detection purposes. Liver biopsy is best avoided in order to prevent leakage. There is no medical treatment. Surgical excision or drainage affords the only hope of cure. Prognosis is good unless there is a rupture or other complications.

Other parasitic diseases:

Agent or disease	Epidemiology	Clinical features	Liver pathology
Clonorchis sinensis	Endemic in China and Southeast Asia; cyst in poorly cooked fish	Cholangitis, duct stones, liver abscess	Duct inflammation and fibrosis; 15% incidence of cholangiocarcinoma and hepatoma among Chinese in Hong Kong
Fasciola hepatica	Prevalent in sheep- and cattle-raising lands; larvae on contaminated edible aquatic plants, eg, watercress	Like C. sinensis, inhabits biliary tract	Similar to above; not associated with liver malignancy
Ascariasis	Common in Far East; large worm, may get into gall bladder or bile ducts	May be seen on x-ray; cholangitis	Granuloma around ova or worm
Toxocara canis, or T. cati (visceral larva migrans)	Urban disease; usually seen in children, 1 to 4 years old	Hepatomegaly, eosinophilia, fever	Chronic reaction against ova

LIVER ABSCESSES

Pyogenic Abscess[17,18]

Pyogenic abscess of the liver is found in about 0.6% of autopsy material. The abscess complicates in descending order of frequency: biliary traction infection, direct extension from contiguous sites of infection, trauma, bacteremia, pylephlebitis, and cryptogenic causes. The etiology varies with the age of the patients. Infants and young children usually have hepatic abscess secondary to generalized infection. In older children and young adults, trauma and amebic infection represent the major causes. In older and elderly adults, hepatic abscess is usually secondary to biliary tract infection (resulting from obstruction by a stone or by carcinoma) and contiguous infection. The incidence of pylephlebitis as a cause has steadily decreased since the introduction of antibiotics. E. coli accounts for about 50% of infectious organisms, followed by Staphyloccus aureus, Klebsiella-Aerobacter, and anaerobic bacteria. Mixed infections occur commonly. Sterile cultures are obtained in 15% of the cases. Blood cultures are positive in over 50% of the anaerobic type of abscess.[19]

The onset of symptoms is usually acute and superimposed upon the underlying disease. Sudden fever, chills, weakness, prostration, jaundice, and shock point to this condition. Hepatomegaly is common. Sometimes a fluctuant mass may be felt. Leukocytosis, severe anemia, raised serum bilirubin and alkaline phosphatase, and hypergammaglobulinemia are found on laboratory examination. Hepatic scintiscan with ^{99m}Tc sulfur colloid localizes the focal hepatic suppuration in 80–95% of the patients. The use of ^{67}Ga citrate, which concentrates in areas of tumor or inflammation, may increase diagnostic accuracy. Angiography provides another method of confirmation with a diagnostic efficacy comparable to the liver scan.

Pathologically, multiple yellow abscesses or a single cavity lined with a fibrous capsule are noted. A liver biopsy yields pus with a foul odor. Differentiation from amebic abscess can be difficult (Table 16.4). Surgical drainage with antibiotic therapy is the mode of management. Prognosis may be poor, mainly due to late recognition of the condition and the seriousness of the underlying cause. Mortality varies 20–30%.

Hepatic Amebiasis[20]

This disease represents the most frequent extraintestinal complication of intestinal amebiasis. *Entamoeba histolytica,* the causative protozoan

Table 16.4. Comparison between pyogenic and amebic abscess.

Finding	Abscess	
	Pyogenic	Amebic
M > F	0	+ + +
Age over 50 years	+ + +	+
Chest findings	+ +	+ + +
Pleuritic pain	+	+ + +
RUQ pain	+	+ + +
Bloody diarrhea	0	+ + +
Jaundice	+ +	+ +
Abscess cavity	Multiple	Single
Right lobe localization	+	+ + +
Serologic tests	0	+ + +
Foul odor	+ + +	+
Mortality	20–30%	10–20%

From G. L. Barbour and K. Juniper, Jr, *Amer J Med* 53:323–334, 1972.

parasite, locates on the wall of the large intestine. Amebiasis in the United States occurs in about 1-5% of the population. Symptomatic intestinal attacks are characterized by fever, bloody diarrhea, and severe abdominal pains. Mild hepatomegaly is frequent, although there is no evidence that amebas invade the liver at this stage. Whether or not amebic hepatitis precedes abscess development is open to debate. Most observers in India believe there is a precursor stage, consisting of right-upper-quadrant tenderness, hepatomegaly, fever, and leukocytosis in the absence of symptomatic amebic colitis, which responds to chloroquine therapy.

Amebic hepatitis is not considered a specific disorder in the United States or Europe. A liver abscess complicates asymptomatic intestinal infection more commonly than the symptomatic form. The incidence rate is about 5% in all patients with amebiasis. The trophozoites lodge in the intrahepatic portal radicles and produce hepatic necrosis by release of proteolytic enzymes. A hepatic abscess develops insidiously, usually in the posterior portion of the right lobe. This lobe receives most of the portal blood derived from the right colon through the streaming effect of blood flow. Symptoms may occur insidiously or abruptly with chills, high fever, nausea, vomiting, severe upper abdominal pains, and leukocytosis. Confusion with acute cholecystitis, perforated peptic ulcer, and acute pancreatitis is not uncommon. Differentiation from pyogenic abscess can be difficult (Table 16.4). On physical examination, there is tender hepatomegaly. Point tenderness in the posterolateral area of the right lower intercostal spaces is a characteristic finding. The abscess may enlarge upward, elevating the diaphragm and producing basilar atelectasis, costophrenic blunting, and referred right shoulder pain. Jaundice is infrequent.

Liver function tests are normal, except for an occasional rise in serum alkaline phosphatases. Radiologically, the intact amebic abscess lacks a fluid level, calcification, or other density. Isotopic scanning is useful for location of the abscess and for evaluation of therapy. The indirect hemagglutination test is positive in almost 100% of cases, and is valuable for confirmation. Persistent titers in endemic countries renders the serological test more useful for excluding the diagnosis. A liver biopsy yields a characteristic "chocolate or anchovy sauce." The exudate contains no leukocytes, unless secondarily infected with bacteria, and usually no amebas. Trophozoites may be found in the abscess wall on biopsy in 20-50% of cases. In 10% of cases, the abscess ruptures into the right pleural cavity or lung.

Treatment consists of drug therapy, using chloroquine or emetine, both of which are concentrated by the liver. Metronidazol (Flagyl) may also be prescribed. Drainage of the amebic abscess is not required in all instances. Combined with chemotherapy, aspiration hastens resolution. Mortality is listed as 10-20%.

REFERENCES

1. Guckian JC, Perry JE: Granulomatous hepatitis: An analysis of 63 cases and review of the literature. *Ann Intern Med* 65:1081–1100, 1966.
2. Guckian JC, Perry JE: Granulomatous hepatitis of unknown etiology: An etiologic and functional evaluation. *Amer J Med* 44:207–215, 1968.
3. Editorial: Granulomas of the liver. *Lancet* 2:1079–1080, 1975.
4. Fitzgerald MX, Fitzgerald O, Towers RP: Granulomatous hepatitis of obscure aetiology: Diagnostic contribution of Kveim testing and anti-tuberculosis therapy. *Quart J Med* 40:371–383, 1971.
5. Simon HB, Wolff SM: Granulomatous hepatitis and prolonged fever of unknown origin: A study of 13 patients. *Medicine* 52:1–21, 1973.
6. Maddrey WC, et al: Sarcoidosis and chronic hepatic disease: A clinical and pathologic study of 20 patients. *Medicine* 49:375–395, 1970.
7. Bowry S, et al: Hepatic involvement in pulmonary tuberculosis: Histologic and functional characteristics. *Amer Rev Respir Dis* 101:941–948, 1970.
8. Editorial: Syphilis and hepatic cirrhosis. *Lancet* 1:28–29, 1970.
9. Feher J, et al: Early syphilitic hepatitis. *Lancet* 2:896–899, 1975.
10. Sherlock S: The liver in secondary (early) syphilis. *New Eng J Med* 284:1437–1438, 1971.
11. Sherlock S: Infectious mononucleosis, in Gen Ref No. 15, pp 635–637.
12. Reller LB: Granulomatous hepatitis associated with acute cytomegalovirus infection. *Lancet* 1:19–22, 1973.
13. Bechelsheimer H, Korb G, Gedigk P: The morphology and pathogenesis of "Marburg virus" hepatitis. *Human Path* 3:255–264, 1972.
14. Lee JC, Fortuny IE: Adult herpes simplex hepatitis. *Human Path* 3:277–281, 1972.
15. Warren KS: Regulation of the prevalence and intensity of schistosomiasis in man: Immunology or ecology? *J Infect Dis* 127:595–609, 1973.
16. Reboucas G: Clinical aspects of hepatosplenic schistosomiasis: A contrast with cirrhosis. *Yale J Biol Med* 48:369–376, 1975.
17. Rubin H, Swartz MN, Malt R: Hepatic abscess: Changes in clinical, bacteriologic and therapeutic aspects. *Amer J Med* 57:601–610, 1974.
18. De la Maza LM, Naern F, Berman LD: The changing etiology of liver abscess: Further observations. *JAMA* 227:161–163, 1974.
19. Sabbaj J, Sutter VL, Finegold SM: Anaerobic pyogenic liver abscess. *Ann Intern Med* 77:629–638, 1972.
20. Barbour GL, Juniper K Jr: A clinical comparison of amebic and pyogenic abscess of the liver in sixty-six patients. *Amer J Med* 53:323–334, 1972.
21. Hunt JS, et al: Granulomatous hepatitis: A complication of B.C.G. immunotherapy. *Lancet* 2:820–821, 1973.
22. Ridolpi RL, Hutchins GM: Detection of ball variance in prosthetic heart valves by liver biopsy. *Johns Hopkins Med J* 134:131–140, 1974.
23. Pimentel JC, Menezes AP: Liver granulomas containing copper in vineyard sprayer's lung: A new etiology of hepatic granulomatosis. *Amer Rev Respir Dis* 111:189–195, 1975.

24. Hughes M, Fox H: A histological analysis of granulomatous hepatitis. *J Clin Path* 25:817–820, 1972.
25. Alexander JF, Galambos JT: Granulomatous hepatitis: The usefulness of liver biopsy in the diagnosis of tuberculosis and sarcoidosis. *Amer J Gastroenterology* 59:23–30, 1973.

TUMORS OF THE LIVER

17

Metastatic tumors of the liver outnumber primary hepatic cancers by a ratio of 20 or 30 to 1. In nearly one-third of all autopsies metastatic tumors are found in the liver, the common primary sites being the lung, gastrointestinal tract, and breast. Gross umbilication due to central necrosis or fibrosis usually indicates metastases rather than primary tumor. Although secondary tumors are often multiple, 10% show a solitary nodule. Tumors invade the cirrhotic and noncirrhotic livers with equal avidity. The cirrhotic process does not protect the liver from metastases. Patients with hepatic metastases usually do not survive more than a year after diagnosis, except when the metastases are derived from a carcinoid tumor or neuroblastoma of the adrenal gland. Both secondary tumors are associated with prolonged life expectancy.

Primary tumors are derived from normal components of liver structure (Table 17.1).

BENIGN TUMORS

Hemangioma

Cavernous hemangioma is probably the most common of all primary liver tumors. The lesions are small (usually found incidentally at autopsy) but may enlarge during pregnancy and become symptomatic. In children, large hemangiomas present as hepatomegaly, with or without other congenital angiomas elsewhere.

Liver Cell Adenoma

Often misdiagnosed either as a cirrhotic nodule or as a hepatoma, the lesion consists of uniform hepatocytes somewhat larger than normal, often separated from surrounding normal parenchyma by a capsule. The liver-cell-cord pattern is usually disturbed and no triads or bile ducts are

Table 17.1. Classification of primary liver tumors.

Type	Site of origin	Age and sex preference	Gross feature
Benign variants:			
Liver cell adenoma	Hepatocyte	Childbearing women	Single or multiple, usually in right lobe
Bile duct adenoma	Bile duct	Adult men	Single, small, subcapsular
Bile duct cystadenoma	Bile duct	Middle-aged males	Large, multilocular
Hemangioma	Blood vessel	Any age	Single or multiple, small
Hemangioendothelioma	Blood vessel	Infant girls	Well encapsulated, potentially malignant
Malignant variants:			
Hepatocellular carcinoma (hepatoma)	Hepatocyte	Young and middle-aged males	Single or multiple, cirrhotic background
Cholangiocarcinoma	Bile duct	Adults	May be massive and diffuse
Cystadenocarcinoma	Bile duct	Adults	Well-delineated lesion
Malignant hemangio-endothelioma (angiosarcoma)	Blood vessel	Adults	Multiple, hemorrhagic nodules
Hepatoblastoma	Mixed epithelial and mesenchymal cells	Young boys	Usually a solitary mass in right lobe

observed (Fig. 17.1).[1,2] Increased vascularity is a common feature, which predisposes toward hemoperitoneum. This adenoma is more frequently found in females, because of its association with the use of oral contraceptives.[3,4] Malignant conversion does not occur. Differentiation from hepatocellular carcinoma may be difficult (Table 17.2). Liver biopsy is inadvisable because of the increased risk of hemorrhage from the vascular parts. The tumor should be resected surgically both for diagnosis and for a cure.

MALIGNANT TUMORS

Hepatocellular carcinoma (75–85%) and cholangiocarcinoma (5–10%) are the most common types of malignant tumors.

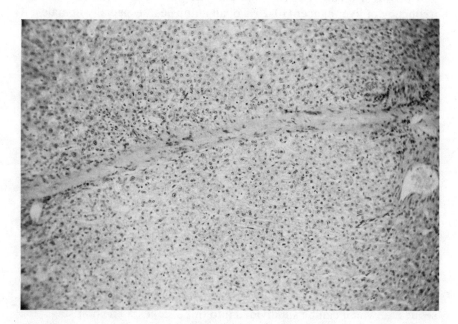

Fig. 17.1. Hepatic adenoma. The capsule demarcates the adenoma (upper field) from normal parenchyma (below). H and E, X100.

Table 17.2. Contrast between hepatic adenoma and hepatocellular carcinoma.

	Hepatic adenoma	Hepatocellular carcinoma
Age, sex	Young female	Older male
Association	Oral contraceptives	Cirrhosis
Clinical presentation	Asymptomatic, hemoperitoneum	Hepatic dysfunction, hepatomegaly
Laboratory test	? ?	↑ AFP ↑ Prolyl hydroxylase
Liver histology	Bland liver cells, deformed vasculature, missing triads, pushing borders, cirrhosis absent	Atypical liver cells, less prominent vascularity, missing triads, infiltrating borders, cirrhosis present
Course	Benign	Fatal

Hepatocellular Carcinoma[5,6]

The frequency of hepatocellular carcinoma (hepatoma) varies strikingly by geographic location (Table 17.3).[7] The reasons for the variation are not known. Most areas of Africa and parts of Southeast Asia show a high frequency of liver cancer (10–20% of all autopsies), especially in males; it is uncommon in North America (less than 0.7% of all autopsies in the United States) and Western Europe; and rare in Central and South America. The highest incidence is in the Bantu males in Mozambique, where in the younger age group the rate is about 500 times that of a comparable group in the United States. Among adults, males are affected more frequently than females by a ratio 4:1. The peak age incidence is 40–60 years, with a smaller peak before age 20. In Africa, the average age is a decade earlier, about 30 years of age.

Etiologic associations.   Seventy-five percent of hepatomas arise from a background of macronodular cirrhosis. The association between hepatoma and cirrhosis is lower in Africa, about 50%. The proportion of cirrhosis of all types that develops into hepatoma is about 2% in the United States, in contrast with over 20% in Uganda. The frequency of carcinoma complicating the cirrhosis of hemochromatosis is high, reaching 15% in Australia. It is believed that cirrhosis in itself is not precancerous, but that the hyperplastic nodule plays a primary role. Liver carcinogenesis in humans and experimental animals proceeds in a stepwise sequence, which can be subdivided into three stages.[8] The first stage, the initiation process, consists of interaction between highly reactive chemi-

Table 17.3.   Incidence rates of liver cancer in human males.

Area	Incidence of liver cancer (per 100,000)
Mozambique	98.2
Johannesburg	14.2
Singapore	5.5
United Kingdom	3.0
Yugoslavia	1.9
New York	1.8

From T. A. Connors, *Biochem Soc Trans* 1:912–917, 1973.

cal carcinogens, ionizing radiation, or virus and target cell macromolecules, primarily DNA. The event may be either short- or long-term. Permanent damage to DNA involves relatively few cells, since very few combinations of reactive molecular sites and metabolic effects can occur to initiate the carcinogenic process. Biologically, a new focal population of hepatocytes is induced, differing from the original normal population in being resistant to the cytotoxic effects of the carcinogen. The new hepatocytes proliferate in response to the demand for cell regeneration produced by the cytotoxic environment. The normal hepatocytes remain suppressed by the cytotoxic damage.

The selective growth of the new focal population produces the hyperplastic nodule, characteristic of the second stage of carcinoma evolution. Hepatocytes in hyperplastic nodules are arranged in two or more cell-thick plates and show tubularization. Biochemically, these cells lack glucose-6-phosphatase and adenosine triphosphatase and lose their ability to accumulate iron and break down glycogen. Other markers such as alpha-fetoprotein and a newly described antigen, preneoplastic antigen, may appear during this stage.

The transition of the premalignant change to carcinoma comprises the third and final stage. During the interval other influences on the liver such as drugs and various metabolic conditions may affect the development of the autonomous hepatocellular population.

Hepatocarcinogenesis

There are innumerable chemicals which can induce liver cancer in animals, but only a few are implicated in human hepatocarcinogenesis. Among the candidates, aflatoxin, synthetic sex hormones, ethanol, hepatitis B virus, and nitrosamines are implicated in the development of hepatocellular carcinoma (Table 17.4). Vinyl chloride and thorotrast are associated with angiosarcomas.[9,10]

Aflatoxin.[11,12] This mycotoxin, isolated from the fungus *Aspergillus flavus*, contaminated the groundnuts of poultry feed, which caused an epidemic of acute hepatic necrosis and death among turkeys in 1960. Since then, it has been extensively studied as a potential human carcinogen. Aflatoxin is separable into 12 structurally related compounds, pentacyclic chemicals with one or two six-membered lactone rings. Aflatoxins B_1 and G_1 are the main components of the toxic extracts, which show marked carcinogenic activity in rats, rainbow trout, and ducks. As little as 0.1 part per billion of aflatoxin fed continuously over 20 months results in 10% tumor induction in the rainbow trout. Although species variations exist, aflatoxin elicits a predictable sequence of hepatic changes, namely, periportal or centrolobular necrosis, followed by marked duct proliferation in triads and eventual carcinoma. Cirrhosis is neither a prerequisite nor a concomitant event in the process.

Table 17.4. Clinical antecedents of liver tumors.

Agent or drug	Association
Hepatitis B virus	Less convincing carcinogen in the United States than in Africa and Asia
Alcohol, hemochromatosis	Variable carcinogens; up to 15% develop hepatomas
Oral contraceptives	Benign tumors or vascular lesions; may bleed, and cause intraabdominal crisis
Synthetic androgens	Long-term usage in high doses required; few cases reported; ? reversible lesions
Vinyl chloride	Potent occupational hepatotoxin
Thorotrast	Latent periods of 10–20 years; no longer in use
Arsenic	Also causes cirrhosis
Clonorchis sinensis	Accounts for 15% of all liver carcinomas in Hong Kong
Aflatoxin, other mycotoxins	Interesting, but no definitive evidence as human hepatocarcinogens
Adult cirrhotics with alpha-1-antitrypsin deficiency[42]	Up to 30% complicated by neoplastic change

The mycotoxin inhibits both RNA and DNA polymerase activity. The effect is similar in some respects to actinomycin D. The toxins of *A. flavus* are widely distributed in many foodstuffs, notably peanuts, in areas where liver cancer is common. The causative link between aflatoxin and human hepatoma is not entirely proved. There are some discordant findings. Aflatoxin given over a three-year period has not produced liver carcinoma in subhuman primates. Although this does not exclude its oncogenic potential, aflatoxin is probably not a strong carcinogen in primates. Most epidemiologic studies report an association between the high level of aflatoxin in local diets in Thailand and Africa and the increased incidence of hepatoma in these areas. However, other studies do not note such a correlation in some locales of Thailand and India. However, it is conceivable that aflatoxin may act synergistically with HB_SAg or other carcinogens to produce liver cancer. Preexisting liver injury, whether produced by virus or toxins, potentiates the carcinogenicity of aflatoxin.[13] Other mycotoxins such as steriogmatocystin, leuteoskyrin, islanditoxin, sporidesmin, rubratoxin, and ochratoxin also have hepatotoxic and possibly hepatocarcinogenic properties. Their relevancy to human disease is obscure at the moment.

Ethanol.   Pure ethanol does not produce hepatoma in animals. Although an experimental model is lacking, there is epidemiological data which links alcohol consumption to the development of hepatoma. The appearance of the tumor in alcoholic patients with cirrhosis is on the increase.[14] It is not known whether alcohol itself or some constituent in it is the responsible agent. In some areas of the world alcohol is contaminated. Local beverages produced in Zambia are shown to contain dimethylnitrosamine, a well-known experimental carcinogen.

Hepatitis virus.   An increased incidence of HB_SAg is found in some areas where liver carcinoma occurs frequently. For example, there is 40% antigen positivity in patients with hepatoma in Greece,[15] 70% in Uganda,[16] and 80% in Taiwan.[17] Negative association is also recorded. In Singapore only 3% of 114 Chinese patients with hepatoma gave a positive HB_SAg reaction compared to a 4% rate in blood donors.[18] The association between the hepatitis virus antibody and hepatoma is even more significant than that with the viral antigen. The prevalence of HB_CAb (anti-HB_C) is higher than the reported prevalence of HB_SAg or HB_SAb among patients with hepatoma.[19] In the United States, West Africa, and Hong Kong, HB_CAb is found 2–6 times more often in cases of hepatoma than in comparable normal groups. Furthermore, the titers of HB_CAb detected are higher than the low concentrations of HB_SAg found in hepatoma patients. The timing of the exposure is another important factor. Infection with the hepatitis B virus in utero and in early infancy is more likely to lead to the eventual development of hepatoma than exposure during other periods of life. An association has been reported in Japanese families between HB$_S$Ag being transmitted from mother to child, and the later occurrence of cirrhosis and hepatoma.[19] The epidemiological data suggest that hepatitis virus is an antecedent factor in the development of hepatoma. Liver cell dysplasia, in which cellular enlargement, nuclear pleomorphism, and multinucleated cells are seen in cirrhotic nodules, may represent a precursor stage in the transition of viral hepatitis to liver cancer.[20] The oncogenic potential of the virus has not been demonstrated in animals.

Nitrosamines.   The chemical identification of this potent group of carcinogens is a difficult and complex task which has prevented thorough epidemiological study of the compounds in foodstuffs. The carcinogens do occur in spoiled food and certain plant extracts. Some evidence points to their role in the pathogenesis of esophageal carcinoma in countries where the incidence is high. A recent report has identified a nitrosamine substance in salt-dried fish which forms the staple diet of the Cantonese in Hong Kong.[21] The finding could account for the increased frequency of hepatoma in the area.

Sex hormones.   To date at least five cases of idiopathic aplastic anemia (Fanconi's syndrome) which were treated with synthetic androgens for 10–15 months have developed hepatoma.[22] The association appears significant. Some of the hormonal-related tumors have also regressed after withdrawal of the drug. Both epidemiological and animal studies support the thesis that an "androgenic environment" predisposes toward the development of hepatocellular carcinoma.

Human and spontaneous hepatoma in certain strains of mice are 3–6 times more common in males. Chemical induction of hepatomas is facilitated by concomitant administration of testosterone. It appears that prolonged use of androgens may cause liver cell hyperplasia and subsequent carcinomatous transformation. The association between oral contraceptive usage and development of liver cell tumor is well documented.[3,4] The duration of use, particularly after 60 months, and the type of synthetic estrogen in the pill are important determinants of risk.[2] Mestranol-containing compounds are more often associated with liver cell adenomas than are other types of estrogens.

Histologically, the pattern ranges from an adenoma to a hamartomatous-appearing lesion, with fibrosis and proliferated bile ducts or dilated blood cysts.[23] Because of the increased vascularity, the tumors may bleed and produce life-threatening hemorrhage in about one-third of the patients. For this reason, and for the purpose of diagnosis, elective resection is recommended.

Clinical Presentation

The clinical manifestations are those of the underlying cirrhosis. Hepatomegaly appears in 70% of the patients, abdominal pain in 60%, and abdominal mass in 40%.[24] Jaundice is present in 15% of the patients, and fever in 10%. Three common modes of presentation are described: (1) right-upper-quadrant pain and a mass, with weight loss or ascites in 70% of patients; (2) hepatic deterioration without a palpable mass in 10% of patients; (3) right-upper-quadrant pain, jaundice, and presumed cholecystitis in 10% of the cases. Occasionally, the ascites may become bloody. In some instances, an acute abdominal crisis may result from hemoperitoneum.

Hepatoma should be suspected in cirrhotic patients who suddenly develop an enlarged liver, ascites, worsening hepatic status and tests, an arterial murmur heard over the liver, or unusual hormonal signs (Table 17.5).[25] The finding of an elevated alpha-fetoprotein level or increased prolyl hydroxylase activity in patients with longstanding liver disease[26] should also raise the diagnosis.

Hepatic Tests

The abnormalities reflect the cirrhotic background. Serum alkaline phosphatase is usually disproportionately higher than is the increase of aminotransferase. The serum alpha-fetoprotein frequently exceeds 500 ng/ml and appears in close to 95% of Caucasian and non-Caucasian patients. The quantitative level of AFP varies widely, and carries no prognostic or clinical significance (see Chapter 2). There is no correlation between the duration of the symptoms, the size and type of tumor, and patient survival. The test is not specific for hepatomas, although the levels in other diseases are generally not as high. AFP can be detected in viral hepatitis, teratocarcinomas of the testis, and metastatic gastric carcinoma of the liver.[27]

A second diagnostic enzyme change for hepatoma is the extremely high levels of serum prolyl hydroxylase. The liver contains a large amount of this enzyme which hydroxylates proline to form hydroxyproline during collagen synthesis. Liver injury in such conditions as viral hepatitis, cirrhosis, and extrahepatic cholestasis, and in methoxyflurane anesthesia releases prolyl hydroxylase into the general circulation. The concen-

Table 17.5. Humoral and other unusual manifestations of liver cancer.[25]

Effect	Mechanism	Comment
Polycythemia	↑ erythropoietin or ↑ erythropoiesis-stimulating factor	Occurs in 50% of Chinese patients
Hypoglycemia	↑ rate of glucose utilization or ↓ rate of glucose production	Occurs in 30% of Chinese patients
Hypercalcemia	↑ circulating parathyroid hormone-like material	Levels may reach 20 mg/dl without bony metastases
Carcinoid syndrome[43]	↑ serotonin	
Hyperlipemia, hypercholesterolemia	? ↓ negative-feedback synthesis of hepatic cholesterol; ? intrahepatic cholestasis	Found in 33% of Ugandan patients
Precocious puberty	? ↑ gonadotropin hormone	More likely to occur with hepatoblastoma
Dysfibrinogenemia	?	
Cystathioninuria	?	
Porphyria cutanea tarda	?	
Variant alkaline phosphatase	?	
Very high levels of serum vitamin B_{12} content and B_{12} binding protein[44]	?	

trations are not at the levels seen in hepatoma. Tumor occurrence may be localized by radioisotopic scanning and a celiac arteriogram.

A liver biopsy affords another useful means of diagnosis. About 70–80% of patients with either primary or secondary liver cancers can be detected on needle biopsy. Grossly, the tumor may appear nodular, massive, or diffuse (Fig. 17.2). The histological appearance is sometimes difficult to distinguish from liver cell adenoma or cirrhotic nodule. The presence of the cirrhotic background contrasts with the subtle morphologic change of the hepatoma. Cellular atypism may be inconspicuous. Altered hepatocytes, slightly different from normal, form irregular cords which mimic the usual plate pattern (Fig. 17.3). The sinusoids and the reticulum framework are distorted. Triads disappear completely or are

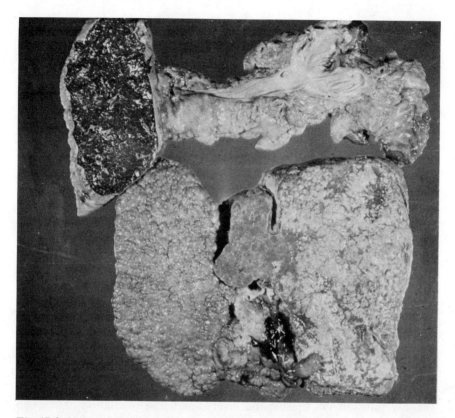

Fig. 17.2. Hepatocellular carcinoma. The massive tumor replaces most of the right lobe (upper L). Note the cirrhotic background. The splenomegaly (lower right) and dilated splenic vein reflect portal hypertension secondary to the cirrhosis.

diminished in numbers. The invasion of veins and encroachment of neighboring nodules may be observed. Distinctive growth patterns have been described: trabecular, acinar, solid, scirrhous, atypical, and clear cell. They carry no prognostic significance. Bile production is a characteristic feature. In the neoplastic cells, the glycogen content is usually low. Mallory bodies are rarely found.

Management

Therapy in adults is directed toward palliation. In children, major resection is considered essential, if feasible. The operation carries a high mortality rate. In adults, the resection rate is low because of rapid growth and late diagnosis. Lobectomy, wedge resection, radiation, chemo-

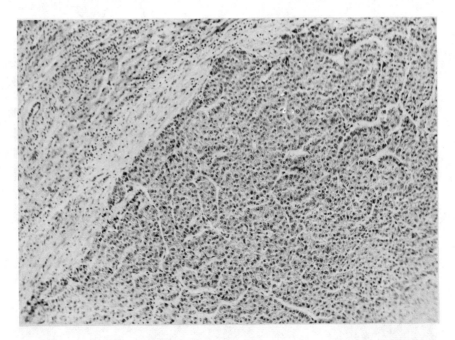

Fig. 17.3. Hepatocellular carcinoma. The tumor cells are in rosette formation (left) and resemble normal hepatocytes in the cirrhotic nodule (right lower corner). H and E, X100.

therapy infusion via the hepatic artery, and transplantation have been employed with varying, but generally poor, salvage rates. Survival beyond a year after diagnosis is rare.

Cholangiocarcinoma

Cholangiocarcinomas do not show the sex distribution, association with cirrhosis, and AFP production found in hepatocellular carcinomas.[6] Cholangiocarcinomas arise from bile duct epithelium, forming acinous or papillary structures lined by mucus-secreting cells. Fibrosis is an abundant component, occasionally providing a sclerotic pattern which simulates a metastatic adenocarcinoma. Carcinomas of the main hepatic ducts, especially at the bifurcation, produce a relentless cholestasis that is frequently misdiagnosed unless an adequate cholangiogram is performed. Cholangiocarcinomas sometimes arise in patients who have had thorotrast exposure, *Clonorchis sinensis* infestation, hemochromatosis, polycystic disease, and rarely chronic ulcerative colitis. About 15% of all primary carcinomas of the liver in Hong Kong are cholangiocarcinomas related to infection with *C. sinensis*.[28] Ductal inflammation, stenosis, fibrosis, and hyperplasia elicited by the Chinese liver fluke precedes the actual appearance of the bile duct carcinoma by about 10 years. Eradication of the fluke should reduce the incidence of cholangiocarcinoma in the area. The results of treatment are as dismal as those for hepatoma.

Malignant Hemangioendothelioma[9,29,30]

Injection of thorotrast, once used as a radiographic contrast medium, produces after a latent period of about 20 years malignant hemangioendothelioma (angiosarcoma), hepatoma, cholangiocarcinoma, mesothelioma, and meningioma.[31] The vascular tumor is often grossly bulky and hemorrhagic. Dense, ionizing, thorotrast deposits are observed in the tumor masses. The second cause of human angiosarcoma represents an occupational hazard among process workers making polyvinyl chloride (P.V.C.) from vinyl chloride (V.C.). There is no indication that P.V.C. is dangerous in itself or that it depolymerizes to V.C. Unreacted, free V.C. monomer may be present in newly made P.V.C. and could be released on storage. In rats exposure to V.C. at concentrations of 50 ppm causes liver angiosarcoma. A long exposure period of 10–20 years is apparent in workers who develop the tumor. V.C. may also produce multisystemic disease with scleroderma-like features, Raynaud's circulatory phenomenon, acroosteolysis, thrombocytopenia, splenomegaly, and liver injury. The latter may proceed to portal fibrosis with portal hypertension.

Other uncommon associations of the malignant vascular tumor are chronic arsenic intoxication, prolonged exposure to gamma rays, and primary hemochromatosis. Microangiopathic hemolytic anemia may be an uncommon complication. Histologically, angiosarcoma consists of pleomorphic tumor cells with large hyperchromatic nuclei, giant forms, but infrequent mitoses, which line irregular vascular channels (Fig. 17.4). In some tumor areas the cells appear elongated and spindle-shaped. Cirrhosis is present in 20–40% of the cases.

Hepatoblastoma[32,33]

Hepatoblastoma, hepatocellular carcinoma, and rhabdomyoblastoma form the most common primary malignant tumors of the liver in infants and children. Hepatoblastoma occurs more frequently than the other two tumors. It is almost always seen prior to age two. Hepatocellular carcinoma and rhabdomyoblastoma are found in older children.

Histologically, hepatoblastoma consists of epithelial, mesenchymal, or mixed epithelial-mesenchymal components. The epithelial parts feature both fetal and embryonal-type hepatocytes. The mesenchymal components include primitive spindle cells, osteoid tissue, cartilaginous foci,

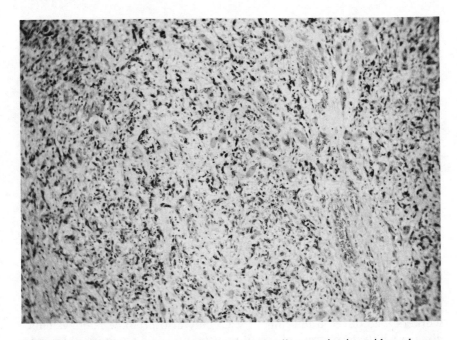

Fig. 17.4. Angiosarcoma. Dark, spindle-shaped cells grow in sinusoids and compress the liver cords. H and E, X100.

and muscle cell elements. Mitoses are infrequently observed. The morphological pattern in rhabdomyoblastoma is composed of bizarre giant and spindle cells, some of which reveal cross striations, indicating derivation from muscle cells.

Hemangioendothelioma[34]

The female/male ratio for this tumor is 2:1; it usually appears before the age of six months. It may be associated with hemangiomas elsewhere, or with other congenital anomalies. Although considered benign, the tumor does have a malignant potential. Jaundice and hepatomegaly are common findings. Other cases present with abdominal distension, vomiting, and diarrhea. Congestive heart failure is often the outstanding feature due to arteriovenous shunts that form the tumor. A rare complication is microangiopathic hemolytic anemia, which results as erythrocytes are damaged during their passage through the tumor bed. Histologically, there is an orderly proliferation of small blood vessels or an aggressive pattern with darker and pleomorphic endothelial cells. Partial hepatectomy, hepatic artery ligation, steroids, and radiation therapy have all been tried in order to control the tumor.

CYSTS OF THE LIVER[35,36]

Single or multiple cysts of the liver are not common (Table 17.6). The most frequent cystic lesion is the solitary unilocular cyst, lined by a cuboidal epithelium and presumably derived from bile ducts. Found in 17 of 100,000 abdominal operations, they are detected in the fifth to sixth decade of life, affecting females more often than males. Solitary cysts are not accompanied by other congenital anomalies. Rare malignant degeneration is recorded.

Congenital Cysts (Polycystic Disease of the Liver)[37]

In this disorder the liver alone or both the liver and kidneys are involved. The several varieties encountered are summarized in Table 17.7. The cyst fluid which accumulates appears to be in equilibrium with the plasma fluid in terms of similar osmolarity and electrolyte concentrations. This suggests that the cyst lining is freely permeable to inorganic ions.[38] In addition, albumin and immunoglobulins are present and may have a role in cyst growth by acting as osmotically active expanders.

Table 17.6. Cysts of the liver.[35,36]

I. Congenital
  1. Solitary cyst
  2. Polycystic disease
     a. With or without polycystic kidney
  3. Congenital dilation of common bile duct
     (choledochus cyst)
  4. Focal dilation of intrahepatic bile ducts
     (Caroli's disease)
     a. Combined with congenital hepatic fibrosis
     b. Combined with medullary sponge kidney
  5. Proliferative cysts (cystadenomas)
  6. Lymphocytic, endothelial, dermoid cysts
II. Infection
  1. Hydatid cyst, amebic cyst, pyogenic abscess
III. Traumatic
  1. Blood and degenerative cysts
IV. Inflammatory
  1. Retention cyst due to biliary obstruction
V. Unknown etiology
  1. Peliosis hepatis, associated with androgenic therapy
     and advanced tuberculosis

Table 17.7. Polycystic diseases of the liver and kidney.

| | | | | Pathology | | | |
| | | | | Kidney | | Liver | |
Type	Inheritance	Mode of presentation	Typical progress	Gross	Dilated renal tubules	Dilated bile ducts	Periportal fibrosis
Perinatal	Autosomal recessive	Bilateral renal masses	Rapid uremia and death	Bilateral symmetrical uniform cysts	> 90% involved	All affected	Minimal
Neonatal	Autosomal recessive	Bilateral large kidneys	Progressive renal failure	Bilateral symmetrical uniform cysts	60%	All affected	Mild
Infantile	Autosomal recessive	Bilateral large kidneys; hepatosplenomegaly	Chronic renal failure; systemic and portal hypertension	Bilateral symmetrical uniform cysts	25%	All affected	Moderate
Juvenile (congenital hepatic fibrosis)	Autosomal recessive	Hepatomegaly	Portal hypertension	Few cysts	< 10%	All affected	Cirrhosis
Adult	Autosomal dominant	Renal masses	Uremia; systemic hypertension	May be unilateral; irregular cysts	Variable but usually > 80%	A few	Absent or minimal

From H. Blyth and P. G. Ockenden, *J Med Genet* 8:257–284, 1971.

Focal Dilation of Intrahepatic Bile Ducts[39]

In the pure form of this condition, also known as Caroli's disease, the whole liver is transformed by ectasia of the intrahepatic bile ducts with cavity formation. The symptoms are the result of biliary stasis, cholangitis, and lithiasis. The liver is dark and enlarged. Sectioning discloses dilated ducts filled with pus or stones. On microscopic examination, scar tissue surrounds the triads containing the ectatic and inflamed ducts. Cirrhosis does not occur. The recurrent infection is rarely complicated by amyloidosis. Prognosis in general is poor.

Choledochus Cyst

Choledochus cyst, or cystic dilation of the common bile duct, affects girls primarily, and before the age of 10 in 80% of the cases. It is not caused by mechanical obstruction or by other neighborhood lesions. The condition is apparently congenital and idiopathic. It may be a variant of neonatal obstructive cholangiopathy. The clinical manifestations consist of pain, jaundice, and an abdominal mass. The cyst usually grows to large dimensions, causing outlet obstruction. As a result, the liver becomes enlarged and cirrhotic with ascending cholangitis. Laboratory findings confirm an obstructive process, with a marked rise in serum alkaline phosphatase. Radiographic visualization with an oral or intravenous cholangiogram is diagnostic. Results of surgical treatment are usually good.

Peliosis Hepatis[40,41]

Morphologically, two varieties are described: parenchymal, in which blood-filled spaces are not lined by endothelium, and multifocal necrosis is prominent; and angiomatoid, in which the hemorrhagic spaces possess an endothelial coat. The lesions are rare; they have been reported after the use of androgenic or estrogenic steroids. Peliosis hepatis also is noted in advanced tuberculosis at autopsy. The initiating factor is probably hepatocellular necrosis with secondary formation of blood-filled spaces. Intraperitoneal hemorrhage, hepatic failure, and hepatorenal syndrome may complicate peliotic lesions.

REFERENCES

1. Phillips MJ, et al: Benign liver cell tumors: Classification and ultrastructural pathology. *Cancer* 32:663–670, 1973.
2. Edmondson HA, Henderson B, Benton B: Liver-cell adenomas associated with use of oral contraceptives. *New Eng J Med* 294:470–472, 1976.

3. Editorial: Liver tumors and steroid hormones. *Lancet* 2:1481, 1973.

4. Editorial: Liver tumors and the pill. *Brit Med J* 3:3–4, 1974.

5. El-Domeiri AA, et al: Primary malignant tumors of the liver. *Cancer* 27:7–11, 1971.

6. MacSween RNM: A clinicopathological review of 100 cases of primary malignant tumors of the liver. *J Clin Path* 27:669–682, 1974.

7. Connors TA: Liver cancer: Induction and treatment. *Biochem Soc Trans* 1:912–917, 1973.

8. Farber E: Pathogenesis of liver cancer. *Arch Path* 98:145–148, 1974.

9. Editorial: Vinyl chloride, P.V.C. and cancer. *Lancet* 1:1323–1324, 1974.

10. Visfeldt J, Poulsen H: On the histopathology of liver and liver tumors in thorium dioxide patients. *Acta Path Microbiol Scand* 80A:97–108, 1972.

11. Newberne PM, Butler WH: Acute and chronic effects of aflatoxin on the liver of domestic and laboratory animals: A review. *Cancer Res* 29:236–250, 1969.

12. Wogan GN: Mycotoxins and liver injury, in Gen Ref No. 6, pp 161–181.

13. Editorial: More on the aflatoxin-hepatoma story. *Brit J Med* 2:647–648, 1975.

14. Brunt PW: Alcohol and the liver. *Gut* 12:222–229, 1971.

15. Hadziyannis S, et al: Hepatitis-associated antigen and alpha fetoprotein in primary liver-cell carcinoma in Greece. *Gut* 12:764, 1971.

16. Vogel CL, et al: Serum alpha-fetoprotein in 184 Ugandan patients with hepatocellular carcinoma: Clinical, laboratory and histopathologic correlations. *Cancer* 33:959–964, 1974.

17. Tong MJ, et al: Hepatitis-associated antigen and hepatocellular carcinoma in Taiwan. *Ann Intern Med* 75:687–691, 1971.

18. Simons MJ, et al: Australia antigen in Singapore Chinese patients with hepatocellular carcinoma. *Lancet* 1:1149–1151, 1971.

19. Maupas P, et al: Antibody to hepatitis-B core antigen in patients with primary hepatic carcinoma. *Lancet* 2:9–11, 1975.

20. Anthony PP, Vogel CL, Barker LF: Liver cell dysplasia: A premalignant condition, *J Clin Path* 26:217–223, 1973.

21. Fong YY, Walsh E O'F: Carcinogenic nitrosamines in Cantonese salt-dried fish. *Lancet* 2:1032, 1971.

22. Johnson FL, et al: Association of androgenic anabolic steroid therapy with development of hepatocellular carcinoma. *Lancet* 2:1273–1276, 1972.

23. O'Sullivan JP, Wildring RP: Liver hamartomas in patients on oral contraceptives. *Brit Med J* 3:7–10, 1974.

24. Ihde DC, et al: Clinical manifestations of hepatoma. *Amer J Med* 56:83–91, 1974.

25. Margolis S, Homcy C: Systemic manifestations of hepatoma. *Medicine* 51:381–391, 1972.

26. Keiser HR, Vogel CL, Sadikali F: Protocollagen proline hydroxylase in sera of Ugandans with hepatocellular carcinoma. *J Nat Cancer Inst* 49:1251–1255, 1972.

27. Kelleher J, et al: Alpha-fetoprotein in metastatic gastric carcinoma. *Gut* 15:401–403, 1974.

28. Belamaric J: Intrahepatic bile duct carcinoma and C. sinensis infection in Hong Kong. *Cancer* 31:468–473, 1973.

29. Makk L, et al: Clinical and morphologic features of hepatic angiosarcoma in vinyl chloride workers. *Cancer* 37:149–163, 1976.
30. Thomas LB, et al: Vinyl-chloride-induced liver disease: Banti's syndrome and angiosarcomas. *New Eng J Med* 292:17–22, 1975.
31. Selinger M, Koff RS: Thorotrast and the liver: A reminder. *Gastroenterology* 68:799–803, 1975.
32. Keeling JW: Liver tumors in infancy and childhood. *J Path* 103:69–85, 1971.
33. Dehner LP, Ishak KG: Vascular tumors of the liver in infants and children: A study of 30 cases and review of the literature. *Arch Path* 92:101–111, 1971.
34. Pollard SM, Millard-Sadler GH: Malignant haemangioendothelioma involving the liver. *J Clin Path* 27:214–221, 1974.
35. Ameriks J, Appleman H, Frey C: Malignant nonparasitic cyst of the liver. *Ann Surg* 176:173–177, 1972.
36. Sanfelippo PM, Baehrs OH, Weiland LH: Cystic disease of the liver. *Ann Surg* 179:922–925, 1974.
37. Blyth H, Ockenden BG: Polycystic disease of kidneys and liver presenting in childhood. *J Med Genet* 8:257–284, 1971.
38. Fisher J, et al: Polycystic liver disease: Studies on the mechanisms of cyst fluid formation. *Gastroenterology* 66:423–428, 1974.
39. Fevery J, et al: Congenital dilation of the intrahepatic bile ducts associated with the development of amyloidosis. *Gut* 13:604–609, 1972.
40. Naeim F, Cooper PH, Semion AA: Peliosis hepatis: Possible etiologic role of anabolic steroids. *Arch Path* 95:284–285, 1973.
41. Bagheri SA, Boyer JL: Peliosis hepatis associated with androgenic-anabolic steroid therapy: A severe form of hepatic injury. *Ann Intern Med* 81:610–618, 1974.
42. Eriksson S, Hägerstrand I: Cirrhosis and malignant hepatoma in α_1-antitrypsin deficiency. *Acta Med Scand* 195:451–458, 1974.
43. Primack A, et al: Hepatocellular carcinoma with the carcinoid syndrome. *Cancer* 27:1182–1189, 1971.
44. Waxman S, Gilbert HS: A tumor related vitamin B_{12} binding protein in adolescent hepatoma. *New Eng J Med* 289:1053–1056, 1973.

MISCELLANEOUS TOPICS

18

Toxemia of Pregnancy

Hepatic lesions are common, though inconstant, in the eclamptic state, and bear no relationship to the clinical severity of the disease. Patients with the severest hepatic changes may survive. Clinical manifestations are dominated by convulsions, coma, fever, and pulmonary edema. There is little symptomatic evidence of liver involvement. The characteristic hepatic lesion is periportal hemorrhagic necrosis, with thrombosis of the small periportal vascular channels. The lesion may extend to involve the center of the hepatic lobule. In rare cases, extensive subcapsular hemorrhage may develop and rupture into the peritoneal cavity with fatal consequences. The cause of the hepatic alterations is ascribed to vasospasm and disseminated intravascular coagulation.

The Liver in Ulcerative Colitis

The frequency of abnormal liver histology and function tests varies widely with different reports. The discrepancies arise because of the differences in the severity and disease stage of the colitis that is under study.[1,2] Liver abnormalities are apparently not related to age at onset of colitis; complications involving the eyes, skin, or joints; hepatotoxic drugs; or previous jaundice. Chronic liver disease is associated with the extent of colitis, especially when the entire colon is inflamed, and colitis of long duration. Only 10–20% of the patients becomes symptomatic with jaundice and hepatomegaly. Liver histology and biochemical tests correlate poorly, especially if either one shows only minor abnormalities.

Liver histology. The most frequent alteration is fatty change, followed by pericholangitis (Table 18.1). The term pericholangitis is incorrect, as it implies that the site of inflammation is the bile duct. Portal triaditis appears to be a more accurate description and will be used in this text. Fibrosis, bile duct proliferation, amyloid deposition, and bile duct carcinomatous transformation occur rarely. Cirrhosis and chronic active hepatitis also are uncommon sequelae.

Table 18.1.   Histological changes in the liver of ulcerative colitis. [1,2]

Histological change	Frequency, %
Fatty change	5–50
Portal triaditis	5–45
Bile duct proliferation	1–15
Fibrosis	1–15
Hepatocellular necrosis	0–10
Cholestasis	5
Amyloidosis	1
Granuloma	0–5
Cirrhosis	2–4
Chronic active hepatitis	1
Cholangiocarcinoma	1

Biochemical tests.   Among the various tests alkaline phosphatase, aminotransferase, BSP retention, and serum bilirubin are useful in detecting hepatic dysfunction, which occurs more frequently than histological abnormalities. Other biochemical procedures contribute little to the information derived from these hepatic tests. Serum albumin and globulin are often altered in ulcerative colitis, but these changes do not necessarily reflect the hepatic status. Except in severe or chronic liver disease, histology and biochemical dysfunction do not parallel each other.

Etiology.   Several theories have been proposed but none of them is completely satisfactory. First, there is portal bacteremia which is popularly held as the etiologic cause. This is, however, poorly substantiated. Cultures for both bacteria and their L forms of 45 liver biopsies proved uniformly sterile except for four contaminated cases.[2] Second, an autoimmune mechanism is postulated. Evidence for the assumption is lacking. In one report, immunoglobulin levels, thyroglobulin antibodies, antinuclear factor, and immunofluorescent tests for human colon antibodies were similar in those with or without hepatic dysfunction.[2] Third, the hepatic lesions in ulcerative colitis may reflect previous viral hepatitis. There is no proof for this view. The incidence of $HB_S Ag$ is no higher in those with liver disease than in those without liver involvement.

Treatment.   There is no effective therapy available for the liver complications of ulcerative colitis. Antibiotics and corticosteroids have been used without demonstrable benefit. A total colectomy is said to result in the arrest or regression of liver disease by some clinicians, but is denied by others.[3]

The Liver in Regional Enteritis

Hepatic dysfunction is detected in about 30% of the patients with regional enteritis. Biochemically, there is a rise in serum alkaline phosphatase or increased BSP retention.[4] Clinical symptoms of liver involvement are usually absent. Hepatic lesions resemble those seen in ulcerative colitis and include triaditis, fatty change, portal fibrosis, and granuloma. Unlike ulcerative colitis, gallstones are found frequently (34% in one series) in patients with regional enteritis.[5]

Liver Transplantation

Orthotopic liver homotransplantation, which involves the removal of the host liver and its replacement with a homograft, is a more common operation than axillary grafting, in which an extra liver is inserted. Liver transplantation has been performed for biliary atresia; primary and secondary liver malignancies; biliary, alcoholic, and cryptogenic cirrhosis; fulminant hepatic failure; Wilson's disease; hepatorenal syndrome; glycogen storage disease; and other metabolic disorders.[6] The operation is technically difficult, and most patients are in poor physical condition. The immediate postoperative mortality is about 30%. Long-term results are poor. Only 2 of the 27 patients from the Cambridge/King's College Hospital series are alive after 3½ years; in the Denver series by T. E. Starzl, 18 out of 83 patients with orthotopic liver grafts survived a year; 9, more than 2 years; and 2 are approaching 5-year survival.[7,8] Homograft rejection is not the primary obstacle to success. The immunogenic property of the liver does not appear to be as severe as that of the skin, kidney, or heart. Availability of donors, better preservation of the donor graft, the construction of a normal biliary drainage, and the prevention of new tumor growth are among the major problems waiting resolution. The survival of liver grafts has been hampered by several major postoperative complications; these are discussed below.

Biliary fistula from anastomotic leaks or biliary obstruction. This occurs in one-third of the patients. The role of ischemia, bacterial or viral infection, rejection phenomenon, and mechanical obstruction is uncertain, but each may contribute to the pathogenesis.

Acute graft rejection. This complication usually occurs within a week after transplantation. Clinically, the jaundice is accompanied by a sharp rise in serum aminotransferase activity and an elevation in alkaline phosphatase. Liver histology shows features consistent with acute rejection: portal inflammation with plasma cells and immunoblasts, focal parenchymal necrosis and inflammation, and centrolobular cholestasis. MIF production, the hepatic scan, and cholangiogram are also abnormal. The acute rejection phenomenon is usually reversible with immunosuppressive therapy.

Chronic rejection. Immunologic destruction of the transplant develops despite immunosuppression two months or later after surgery in 10–20% of cases. The onset of the rejection may be gradual or sudden; biochemically, it resembles complete or nearly complete biliary obstruction. Severe hyperbilirubinemia and marked elevations of both serum alkaline phosphatase and aminotransferase are present. Bile disappears from the stool but appears in the urine. Progressive deterioration is the general rule, although the interesting complication of cirrhosis has been recorded. Liver morphology displays sparse cellular infiltration, intense cholestasis, and marked subintimal thickening of the hepatic arteries. The vascular changes mimic those of the kidney graft suffering from chronic rejection. Chronic rejection is thought to involve humoral antibody-mediated tissue destruction rather than altered cellular immunity.

Septic infarction. This syndrome is characterized by the following triad: gram-negative septicemia, sudden and marked elevation of serum aminotransferase, and a persistently absent area of isotope labeling in the homograft. The underlying factor is related to acute rejection or to hepatic arterial thrombosis. Treatment consists of surgical drainage or resection, and increase of immunosuppressive drugs.

Recurrence of disease. The complication may be encountered with primary liver carcinoma and HB_SAg-associated liver disease. Tumor recurrence is described in transplanted livers for patients with porta hepatis ductal adenocarcinoma. This is probably due to incomplete removal of the growth at the initial hepatectomy. Inspection of homograft at the site of the resected liver with hepatoma has confirmed the explosive appearance of secondary deposits. For this reason, T. E. Starzl does not treat primary liver carcinoma by liver transplantation. One patient with HB_SAg-positive, chronic active hepatitis developed the same progressive lesion in the graft. Liver transplantation does not ablate the serum autoantibodies associated with the liver disease in graft recipients.

Increased risk of new primary malignancies. Development of new tumors, particularly lymphomas, is documented for liver transplant patients as with other groups treated with prolonged immunosuppressive therapy.

Liver Disease in Renal Transplant Recipients

Hepatic abnormalities are found in 10–40% of patients following 1–3 months of renal transplantation.[9,10] Onset of liver disease may exceed a year in posttransplant patients with chronic liver disease. High-spiking fevers or signs of acute renal rejection often precede liver dysfunction. Bilirubinemia generally ranges 2–5 mg/dl; aminotransferase rarely exceeds 500 IU/l; and alkaline phosphatase fluctuates at levels of 10–30 K.A. (King-Armstrong) units. There are three types of clinical presentation. In the first type, patients may experience an acute, anicteric, and self-limited hepatic disorder. The illness is often associated with seroconversion to cytomegalovirus, or with culture of the virus from the liver or urine. HB_SAg may be identified in some of the cases. In the second type, a few patients develop acute fulminant hepatic failure. In the third and most common type, the patients develop chronic liver disease. Infection with cytomegalovirus, herpesvirus, and hepatitis B virus is common in this group. The incidence of viral infections is similar to that found in patients who do not develop liver injury. However, in most cases the etiology of the chronic liver disease is not apparent. Twenty percent of these patients show one or another circulating autoantibodies (SMA or M antibody).[9] Progression to cirrhosis occurs in about 25% of the cases with chronic liver disease. Azathioprine and other drug-induced hepatotoxicity is not a common cause of liver dysfunction in the postrenal transplant patients. Azathioprine may produce a cholestatic type of liver damage which is dose-related and reversible. If azathioprine-induced injury is implicated, the drug should be discontinued in favor of cyclophosphamide.

Hepatitis B antigenemia in recipients does not alter the outcome of kidney transplants.[11] There is no correlation between hepatic dysfunction or graft survival with antigenemia acquired before transplantation or in the posttransplant period.

Hyperalimentation

Hyperalimentation involves the parenteral administration of solutions containing 15–20% glucose, 4–7 g amino nitrogen in a protein hydrolysate, vitamins and salts per liter.[12] Approximately three liters of the hypertonic solution (4 × isotonic) is given daily to seriously ill and debilitated postoperative or otherwise cachetic patients. The benefits derived in terms of nitrogen balance, weight gain, and improved appearance are impressive.

Serious complications are not infrequent, and are related either to infections or metabolic problems.[13,14] Both the parenteral solution and the indwelling catheter are common sources of contamination. Infections, particularly fungal, are reported in about 10% of the cases. Metabolic complications are related to the glucose, which may produce a solute diuresis and occasionally a hyperosmolar nonketotic coma; to the amino acids, which may give rise to hyperammonemia, azotemia, and hyperchloremic acid; and to the calcium-phosphorus content, which may result in a hypercalcemia and hypophosphatemia. Liver abnormalities are common. Clinically, jaundice (particularly in infants) and hepatomegaly may occur.

Hepatic tests reveal elevations of alkaline phosphatase and aminotransferase activity. Enzyme induction secondary to accelerated glucose metabolism or hepatotoxicity resulting from amino acid imbalance may account for the biochemical changes. The burden of excess ammonia affects patients with marginal hepatic reserves by precipitating coma. Liver biopsies may show either fatty infiltration or cholestasis with eosinophiles in periportal fields. Ultrastructurally, disorganization of the endoplasmic reticulum with loss of ribosomes, mitochondrial swelling, and fat deposition are observed.[15] The cause of the fatty liver is not known. Mechanisms which might account for the effect include increased lipid synthesis in the liver, decreased hepatic oxidation of fatty acids, increased peripheral mobilization of fatty acids, and choline deficiency. The role of the excess glucose may be important. Hypertonic glucose administered to rats produces a fatty liver. The addition of amino acids does not prevent the fat deposition in the liver.

CRST Syndrome

The syndrome of calcinosis cutis, Raynaud's phenomenon, sclerodactyly, and telangiectasia (CRST) is considered a benign variant of scleroderma. CRST is associated with primary biliary cirrhosis,[16,17] and rarely partial nodular transformation of the liver.[18] Scleroderma does not cause liver disease, although hepatomegaly, disturbed liver function tests, and cirrhosis have been reported. Recent experience discounts liver involvement in scleroderma. The telangiectasia of CRST is identical to that encountered in Rendu-Osler-Weber (ROW) syndrome. Bleeding is infrequent and family history is absent in CRST, both of which occur in ROW disease. The difference between the two syndromes appears relative and a matter of degree. ROW disease can be associated with hepatic lesion. The multiple telangiectasias in the liver act as hepatic artery-hepatic vein shunts which can bleed and cause fibrosis. The deformed liver becomes cirrhotic in the end stage.

Malignant Lymphomas Involving the Liver: Hodgkin's Disease

At autopsy 65% of cases with Hodgkin's disease show hepatic involvement.[19] Diagnosis of hepatic lesions during life depends on the stage of the disease and the method of diagnosis. Clinical symptoms (fever, sweating, marked weight loss), hepatomegaly, liver function tests including BSP retention and alkaline phosphatase, and hepatic scans are of no value in predicting liver involvement but rather indicate Hodgkin's disease elsewhere in the patient. Alkaline phosphatase is high in advanced Hodgkin's disease, whether the liver is affected or not. Patients in the third stage of the disease with clinical involvement of the abdominal lymph nodes and spleen have a 20% incidence of liver lesions detected by liver biopsy.[20,21] The percentage is somewhat higher when peritoneoscopy is also used. The incidence rate of positive histology by liver biopsy falls to near zero in the absence of splenomegaly. It is obvious that liver biopsy alone cannot perform the function of staging in Hodgkin's disease. About 70–90% of patients in every clinical stage will fail to show hepatic involvement on a single liver biopsy attempt. Positive histology must include the atypical reticulum cells of the Reed-Sternberg variety, which may be found only after multiple sectioning of the liver specimens. About 10% of the livers may reveal isolated, noncaseating granulomas without Reed-Sternberg cells,[22] in the presence of clinical Hodgkin's disease. This is not considered evidence for liver involvement.

Non-Hodgkin's Lymphoma

In lymphocytic lymphoma, the liver biopsy is positive in about 40% of cases.[23] Clinically, this correlates well with hepatomegaly. Peritoneoscopy increases the percentage but also has a 50% rate of false negatives. With the categories of mixed lymphocytic-histiocytic and histiocytic lymphomas, a positive liver biopsy is obtained in 10% of the patients. Peritoneoscopy discloses additional cases by a factor of 2 or 3. Hepatomegaly does not indicate liver involvement for the latter two types of lymphoma. For all three forms of lymphoma, liver function tests correlate poorly with hepatic deposits of tumor.

The Liver in Multiple Myeloma

About 40% of the patients with multiple myeloma have hepatomegaly due to massive plasma cell infiltration of the liver.[24] Jaundice, splenomegaly, and an exudative ascites (protein > 2.5 g/dl) occur less frequently. The ascites is not caused by secondary peritoneal disease. The fluid accumulation represents an outpouring of protein-rich hepatic lymph seen in postsinusoidal portal hypertension. Increased BSP retention, raised serum alkaline phosphatase, mildly elevated aminotransferase (<150 IU/l), and hypoalbuminemia correlate with the histologic abnormalities. The morphologic pattern consists of either tumor mass formation or diffuse sinusoidal infiltration by plasma cells. The latter finding resembles the liver of patients with chronic myelogenous leukemia. Other nonspecific histologic alterations include fatty change, hemosiderosis, mild necrosis, and a few granulomas. Extramedullary hematopoiesis and amyloidosis are observed infrequently. Chemotherapy for multiple myeloma does not appreciably diminish the frequency of abnormal hepatic function tests. Drug treatment does not reduce the incidence of myeloma in the liver.

Sickle Cell Disease

Hepatic dysfunction is frequent, and is more severe in the homozygous than in the heterozygous condition. This can be ascribed to hepatocellular anoxia secondary to sinusoidal aggregation of sickled red cells, fibrin platelets, and to the occasional presence of increased collagen and basement-membrane thickening in the spaces of Disse. The pathological changes may cause transient and reversible portal hypertension. Infarct may develop and may heal by fibrosis or cirrhosis. Anabolic steroids and surgical procedures may induce jaundice in patients with the sickling diathesis.

Hemobilia

Hemobilia refers to hemorrhage into the intrahepatic or extrahepatic bile ducts. The condition is rare. Less than 400 cases have been reported in the literature.[25] The causes are traumatic in over half of the cases. The traumatic category includes nonsurgical, blunt hepatic trauma producing intrahepatic hematoma or arteriobiliary fistula, and surgical trauma, particularly with surgery at the porta hepatis. Among the nontraumatic causes, aneurysms of the hepatic artery, erosion into the cystic artery by gallstones, hepatic neoplasms, and hepatic abscess due to biliary ascariasis (tropical hemobilia) are included. The cardinal clinical triad consists of paroxysmal right-upper-abdominal pain, jaundice, and gastrointestinal hemorrhage. Serum bilirubin elevation and raised alkaline phosphatase reflect the biliary occlusion due to clot formation. A rare diagnostic sign is the presence of a filiform blood clot, formed in the biliary tree, in the vomitus or stool. The only definitive diagnostic procedure is selective celiac arteriography. Hepatic scintiscan and splenoportogram are not adequate methods since they usually do not reveal the arterial lesions. Treatment is surgical and directed toward stopping the arterial bleeding. Mortality is high, about 25%.

Vitamin Imbalance:
Hypervitaminosis A

The liver stores vitamin A primarily as biologically inactive palmitate ester in fat-storage (Ito) cells. It is released into the general circulation when acted on by retinol esterase, as retinol bound to retinol-binding protein (RBP) and prealbumin. Palmitate ester itself is not toxic to the liver. In animals large doses of vitamin A induce lysosomal and mitochondrial damage. Vitamin A toxicity probably occurs when the capacity of RBP to transport the vitamin is exceeded.[26] The excess vitamin A appears in serum as retinyl esters associated with lipoproteins. The unusual vitamin-lipoprotein complex exposes cell membranes to the detergent activity of vitamin A, resulting in membrane instability. In addition to its carrier functions, RBP prevents cell damage by vitamin A. In humans, the smallest dose leading to intoxication is 41,000 IU taken daily over an eight-year period.[27] Chronic hypervitaminosis A in children and adults produces hepatomegaly, abnormal liver function tests, occasional cirrhosis, and ascites. The liver dysfunction generally consists of mild elevations of serum alkaline phosphatase, BSP retention, and prothrombin test. Other manifestations of vitamin A intoxication include dry skin, hair loss, fatigue, bone pain, and signs of increased intracranial pressure.

Pathologically, vitamin A accumulates preferentially in the centrolobular areas of the liver (increased to about 10 times normal), detectable by its fluorescent property. The vitamin in fat storage cells may induce a central fibrocongestive lesion, with perisinusoidal fibrosis and congestion.[28] The picture mimics the central hyaline sclerosis of alcoholic hepatitis, early Budd-Chiari syndrome, and myedema involving the liver. Obstruction of the hepatic vein outflow leads to cirrhosis and portal hypertension. In mild and early cases, the hepatic lesions are reversible upon withdrawal of the vitamin.

Hypovitaminosis A

Decreased levels of vitamin A and RBP are recorded in patients with acute viral hepatitis, chronic active hepatitis, and cirrhosis. Both vitamin A and RBP levels are correlated with serum zinc concentration. With improvement in viral hepatitis, all three parameters return to normal range. The hyposmia, and indirectly anorexia, of acute viral hepatitis are associated directly with hypovitaminosis A and depressed circulating RBP, and vary inversely with the plasma bilirubin level.[29] Zinc containing retinene reductase catalyzes the conversion of retinol (vitamin A alcohol) to retinal (the aldehyde form), a reaction necessary for normal vision. Either vitamin A or zinc deficiency may result in night blindness, which occurs not infrequently in chronic liver disease. Zinc is also a constituent of liver alcoholic dehydrogenase which can catalyze the retinol to the retinal step. The identity of alcohol dehydrogenase and retinene reductase is probable. Ethanol is said to inhibit competitively testicular formation of retinal. This secondarily leads to aspermatogenesis, decreased testosterone production, and other feminizing features.

Hypervitaminosis B$_3$

Nicotinic acid, the dietary precursor of nicotinamide, is converted to the amide derivative, nicotinamide, which functions metabolically as nicotinamide adenine dinucleotide (NAD). Large doses of nicotinic acid are used therapeutically to treat hypercholesterolemia (up to 9–10 g/day) and schizophrenia. Occasional reports of hepatic injury have followed. Histologic abnormalities of parenchymal cell damage, cholestasis, and portal fibrosis are observed on biopsy material.[30] Discontinuing the medication results in improvement of abnormal liver function tests.

Vitamin D$_3$ Vitamin D$_3$ (cholecalciferol) is first hydroxylated in the liver at the C25 site in the side chain to give 25-cholecalciferol (25-HCC). The intermediate compound is transported on a carrier protein to the kidney where hydroxylation at the C1 position in the A ring yields the highly active 1,25-dihydrocholecalciferol (1,25-DHCC); 1,25-DHCC represents the biologically active metabolite of vitamin D$_3$ which stimulates intestinal transport of calcium, among other biochemical responses.[31] The feedback control regulating the renal synthesis of 1,25-DHCC depends on the changes in the serum-calcium concentration associated with variations in dietary calcium intake, or with mediation by parathyroid hormone. The occurrence of osteomalacia in epileptics is correlated with prolonged, anticonvulsant drug therapy.[32] Phenobarbital and diphenylhydantoin both induce the hydroxylation enzyme in the liver and accelerate the metabolism of cholecalciferol. This action depletes the hepatic stores of the vitamin and lowers the serum level of 1,25-DHCC. The biochemical indexes of osteomalacia (low serum calcium, elevated phosphorus and alkaline phosphatase) are indirectly the result of drug induction of the liver enzyme responsible for vitamin D activation.

REFERENCES

1. Eade MN: Liver disease in ulcerative colitis: I: Analysis of operative liver biopsy in 138 consecutive patients having colectomy. *Ann Intern Med* 72:745–787, 1970
2. Perrett AD, et al: The liver in ulcerative colitis. *Quart J Med* 40:211–238, 1971.
3. Eade MN, Cooke WT, Brooke BN: Liver disease in ulcerative colitis: II: The long-term effect of colectomy. *Ann Intern Med* 72:489–497, 1970.
4. Perrett AD, et al: The liver in Crohn's disease. *Quart J Med* 40:187–209, 1971.
5. Cohen S, et al: Liver disease and gallstones in regional enteritis. *Gastroenterology* 60:237–245, 1971.
6. Editorial: Liver transplant. *Lancet* 2:29–30, 1974.

7. William R, Smith MGM: Liver transplantation: A clinical and immunological appraisal, in Gen Ref No. 9, pp 433–466.
8. Williams R, et al: Liver transplantation in man: The frequency of rejection, biliary tract complications, and recurrence of malignancy based on an analysis of 26 cases. *Gastroenterology* 64:1026–1048, 1973.
9. Ware AJ, et al: Spectrum of liver disease in renal transplant recipients. *Gastroenterology* 68:755–764, 1975.
10. Berne TV, et al: Hepatic dysfunction in recipients of renal allografts. *Surg Gynecol Obstet* 14:171–175, 1975.
11. Chatterjee SN, et al: Successful renal transplantation in patients positive for hepatitis B antigen. *New Eng J Med* 291:62–65, 1974.
12. Moore FD, Brennan MF: Intravenous feeding. *New Eng J Med* 287:862–864, 1972.
13. Dudrick SJ, et al: Parenteral hyperalimentation: Metabolic problems and solutions. *Ann Surg* 176:259–264, 1972.
14. Fleming CR, et al: Total parenteral nutrition. *Mayo Clin Proc* 51:187–199, 1976.
15. Jacobson S, Ericsson JLE, Obel A-L: Histopathological and ultrastructural changes in the human liver during complete intravenous nutrition for seven months. *Acta Chir Scand* 137:335–349, 1971.
16. Lyon-Murray IM, et al: Scleroderma and primary biliary cirrhosis. *Brit Med J* 3:258–259, 1970.
17. Reynolds TB, et al: Primary biliary cirrhosis with scleroderma, Raynaud's phenomenon and telangiectasia: New syndrome. *Amer J Med* 50:302–312, 1971.
18. Lurie B, et al: CRST syndrome and nodular transformation of the liver: A case report. *Gastroenterology* 64:457–461, 1973.
19. Givler RL, et al: Problems of interpretation of liver biopsy in Hodgkin's disease. *Cancer* 28:1335–1342, 1971.
20. Bagley CM Jr, et al: Liver biopsy in Hodgkin's disease: Clinicopathologic correlations in 127 patients. *Ann Intern Med* 76:219–225, 1972.
21. Belliveau RE, Wiernik PH, Abt AB: Liver enzymes and pathology in Hodgkin's disease. *Cancer* 34:300–305, 1974.
22. Kadin ME, Donaldson SS, Dorfman RF: Isolated granulomas in Hodgkin's disease. *New Eng J Med* 283:859–861, 1970.
23. Bagley CM Jr, et al: Diagnosis of liver involvement by lymphoma: Results in 96 consecutive peritoneoscopies. *Cancer* 31:840–847, 1973.
24. Thomas FB, Clausen KF, Greenberger NJ: Liver disease in multiple myeloma. *Arch Intern Med* 132:195–202, 1973.
25. Bismuth H: Hemobilia, *New Eng J Med* 288:617–619, 1973.
26. Smith FR, Goodman DS: Vitamin A transport in human vitamin A toxicity. *New Eng J Med* 294:805–808, 1976.
27. Muenter MD, Perry HO, Ludwig J: Chronic vitamin A intoxication in adults: Hepatic, neurologic and dermatologic complications. *Amer J Med* 50:129–136, 1971.
28. Russell RM, et al: Hepatic injury from chronic hypervitaminosis A resulting in portal hypertension and ascites. *New Eng J Med* 291:435–440, 1974.

29. Henkin RI, Smith FF: Hyposmia in acute viral hepatitis. *Lancet* 1:823–826, 1971.

30. Winter SL, Boyer JL: Hepatic toxicity from large doses of vitamin B_3 (nicotinamide). *New Eng J Med* 289:1180–1182, 1973.

31. Kodicek E: The story of vitamin D from vitamin to hormone. *Lancet* 2:325–329, 1974.

32. Editorial: Anticonvulsant osteomalacia. *Lancet* 2:805–806, 1972.

AFB	acid-fast bacilli
AFP	alpha-1-fetoprotein
ALA	delta-aminolevulinic acid
AlAT	L-alanine aminotransferase, formerly (S)GPT
AMP	cyclic 3′, 5′-adenosine monophosphate
AsAT	aspartate aminotransferase, formerly (S)GOT
ATP	adenosinetriphosphate
BSP	bromsulphalein
BUN	blood urea nitrogen
CAH	chronic active hepatitis
CEA	carcinoembryonic antigen
CF	complement fixation
CPH	chronic persistent hepatitis
CSF	cerebrospinal fluid
DIC	disseminated intravascular coagulation
DNA	deoxyribonucleic acid
DNCB	dinitrochlorobenzene
EBV	Epstein-Barr virus
EEG	electroencephalogram
GI	gastrointestinal
HAAg	hepatitis A antigen
HAAb	hepatitis A antibody
HAV	hepatitis A virus
HB_cAb	hepatitis B core antibody
HB_sAb	hepatitis B surface antibody
HB_sAg	hepatitis B surface antigen
HBV	hepatitis B virus

LCAT	lecithin-cholesterol acyltransferase
LP-X	lipoprotein-X
LT	lymphocyte transformation
MIF	macrophage migration inhibition factor
MW	molecular weight
N	normal
NAD(H)	nicotinamide adenine dinucleotide (reduced)
NADP(H)	nicotinamide adenine dinucleotide phosphate (reduced)
PAS	periodic acid Schiff (stain)
PBC	primary biliary cirrhosis
PBG	porphobilinogen
PHA	phytohemagglutinin
PPD	purified protein derivative, tuberculin
PS(S)	portal-systemic (shunt)
PTH	posttransfusion hepatitis
RE(S)	reticuloendothelial (system)
(S)ER	(smooth) endoplasmic reticulum
UDP	uridine diphosphate
UTP	uridine triphosphate
V.C.	vinyl chloride
VH	viral hepatitis

GENERAL REFERENCES

1. Becker FF (ed.): *The Liver: Normal and Abnormal Functions,* parts A and B. New York, Marcel Dekker, 1975.
2. Bucher NLR, Malt RA: *Regeneration of Liver and Kidney.* Boston, Little Brown and Co, 1971.
3. Davidson CS: *Liver Pathophysiology: Its Relevance to Human Disease.* Boston, Little Brown and Co, 1970.
4. Elias H, Sherrick JC: *Morphology of the Liver.* New York, Academic Press, 1969.
5. Foulk WT (ed.): *Diseases of the Liver.* New York, McGraw-Hill, 1968.
6. Gall EA, Mostofi EK (eds.): *The Liver by 34 Authors.* Baltimore, Williams and Wilkins, 1973.
7. Leevy CM: *Evaluation of Liver Function in Clinical Practice.* Indianapolis, Lilly Research Laboratories, 1974.
8. McDermott WV Jr: *Surgery of the Liver and Portal Circulation.* Philadelphia, Lea and Febiger, 1974.
9. Popper H, Schaffner F (eds.): *Progress in Liver Diseases,* vol 4. New York, Grune and Stratton, 1972.
10. Popper H, et al (eds.): Nomenclature, diagnostic criteria and diagnostic methodology for diseases of the liver and biliary tract. Fogarty Intern. Proc. No. 22, US Government Printing Press, 1974 (book edition in press).
11. Popper H (ed.): Cirrhosis. *Clin Gastroent* 4:225–463, 1975.
12. Schaffner F, Sherlock S, Leevy CM (eds.): *The Liver and Its Diseases.* New York, Intercontinental Medical Book, 1974.
13. Scheuer PJ: *Liver Biopsy Interpretation,* ed 2. Baltimore, Williams and Wilkins, 1973.
14. Schiff L (ed.): *Diseases of the Liver,* ed 4. Philadelphia, Lippincott, 1975.
15. Sherlock S: *Diseases of the Liver and Biliary System,* ed 5. Oxford, Blackwell Scientific Publications, 1975.
16. Tygstrup N (ed.): Viral hepatitis. *Clin Gastroent* 3:239–474, 1974.